Janet Pleshette has written on alternative medicine for *Over 21, She, Weightwatchers, Womancraft, Here's Health, Prevention, Healthy Living* and various Australian and American publications. She is a member of the Medical Journalists' Association and a co-founder, with Dr James Lambert Mount, of the Natural Health Foundation. This is her first book.

'Once upon a time there were three little sisters,' the Dormouse began in a great hurry; 'and their names were Elsie, Lacie and Tillie; and they lived at the bottom of a well—'

'What did they live on?' said Alice, who always took a great interest in questions of eating and drinking.

'They lived on treacle,' said the Dormouse, after thinking a minute or two.

'They couldn't have done that, you know,' Alice gently remarked; 'they'd have been ill.'

'So they were,' said the Dormouse; '*very* ill.'

FROM *Alice in Wonderland* by Lewis Carroll

HEALTH
ON YOUR PLATE

JANET PLESHETTE

Hamlyn Paperbacks

HEALTH ON YOUR PLATE
ISBN 0 600 20377 8

A Hamlyn Paperback
Published by Arrow Books Limited
17–21 Conway Street, London W1P 6JD

A division of the Hutchinson Publishing Group

London Melbourne Sydney Auckland
Johannesburg and agencies throughout
the world

First published in Great Britain by
Hamlyn Paperbacks 1983
Reprinted 1983 and 1984

Copyright © 1983 by Janet Pleshette

Printed and bound in Great Britain by
Hazell Watson & Viney Limited,
Member of the BPCC Group,
Aylesbury, Bucks

The author and publishers would like to thank
all the copyright holders who have kindly granted
us permission to quote or reproduce their work
in this book.

Contents

Author's Note   6
Foreword   7
Introduction   9

Part One: All about Foods   19
  Carbohydrates · Fats · Fibre · The Modern Food
  Industry · Protein · Salt · Sugar · Tea and Coffee ·
  Vitamins and Minerals · Vitamins · Minerals · Trace
  Minerals · Orthomolecular Therapy or Megavitamins ·
  Whole Foods · Bonus Foods and Supplements ·
  Biochemic Tissue Salts · Brewer's Yeast · Cider
  Vinegar · Evening Primrose Oil · Garlic · Ginseng ·
  Honey · Kelp · Lecithin · Liver · Molasses · Muesli ·
  Pollen · Propolis · Raw Juices · Royal Jelly · Spirulina ·
  Sprouting Seeds and Grains · Wheat Germ · Yogurt

Part Two: Eating for Specific Purposes   139
  Breast-feeding · Children and Food · Compatible
  Eating · The Eyes and Food · Fasting · Hair and Food ·
  Macrobiotics · The Menopause · Nails and Food ·
  Older People and Food · The Pill · Pregnancy,
  Lactation and Food · Skin and Food · Teeth and Food ·
  Vegetarian and Vegan Eating

Part Three: Illnesses – The Nutritional Approach   217
  Allergies to Food · Arthritis and Rheumatism · Asthma
  and Hay Fever · Bronchitis and Emphysema · Cancer ·
  Constipation · Cystitis · Diabetes · Fatigue · Heart and
  Artery Disease · High Blood Pressure · Hyper-active
  Children · Low Blood Sugar · Migraine · Multiple
  Sclerosis · Obesity · Pre-menstrual Tension · Stress ·
  Varicose Veins and Piles

Part Four: Nature Cure and Food Therapy   309
  Nature Cure · Food Therapy: The Diet

Acknowledgments   403
Appendix   405
References   408
Index   421

Author's Note

This book is written for people who eat.

It is written on the assumption that its readers, already familiar with the delights of food, would like to know more about the relationship between what they put into their stomachs and the quality of their lives.

It draws a distinction between foods that enhance good health and foods that can damage it.

If you are well, you will find out how to eat so you can stay that way.

If you are ill, you will find detailed descriptions of successful, medically-backed nutritional treatments for many illnesses. Before beginning any treatment, it is best to see a qualified medical practitioner who can advise on your general fitness to embark on such a treatment.

This book could not have been written without the comments and support of many eminent doctors and naturopaths whose names are listed separately. I hope that I can get their work – and their nutritional philosophy – over to you.

Dedicated to my son, with all the numbers

Foreword

I recommend this book to the general public and to all professional therapists, both orthodox medical and alternative practitioners, who will find it contains a mine of information that is often hard to come by.

The book is written from a point of view that understands that orthodox scientific medicine and the traditional vitalistic therapies are both parts of a greater whole. The author demonstrates that the scientific method proves naturopathic ideas are correct whenever it is applied to them. Nor does the book fail to mention the importance of the mind in the production of disease, but being about food it does not emphasize that aspect – to do that could have doubled its length.

I congratulate Janet Pleshette on having written this book. It should sell as well as those of Adelle Davis, which means I think it's a winner. I wish it the success it undoubtedly deserves.

Dr Alec Forbes, M.A., D.M., F.R.C.P.
Bristol 1983

Introduction

'How do I feel today? I feel as unfit as a fiddle.'
OGDEN NASH

Too many of us are sick now. Too many people are forced to carry the burden of chronic degenerative illness, with its harsh effect on the quality of life. Away from Third World famines, we in the West have our health problems, too.

We can go to the moon – but we can't *cure* asthma, rheumatism or diabetes. We can build a computer which will beat us at chess – but we can't control the rising tide of Western illness.

One in five people in the West will die of cancer. One in four will die of heart disease. The incidence of these two diseases has doubled over the past 25 years, but survival rates for the commonest types of cancer have remained virtually unchanged for the same period of time.[1] Only one person in 50 will escape arthritic or rheumatic degeneration by the age of 70. There are about 600 000 known diabetics in the UK and probably another 600 000 who have mild diabetes without knowing it. About half the people in the UK are too fat, and one of the pharmaceutical industry's best sellers is the laxative.

A health league has been drawn up by computing infant, maternal and middle-aged deaths. Sweden is the healthiest nation, followed by the Netherlands, Norway, Switzerland, Denmark and Japan. England and Wales come a depressing seventh. The USA comes twenty-first.[2]

There are two classes of diseases – infections, and the chronic degenerative illnesses. It is often stated that now we have conquered the infections with the miracle drugs, the chronic degenerative diseases are next on the list. It is true that these diseases need to be dealt with. But it is not true that we have overcome infections entirely with drugs.

A comparison of death rates from scarlet fever, diphtheria, whooping cough and measles shows that nearly 90% of the total decline in mortality between 1850 and 1965 occurred *before* the introduction of widespread immunization and

[1]For references SEE page 409

antibiotics.[1] Immunization has almost wiped out polio, and vaccines have helped to bring down the incidence of whooping cough and measles. We must look elsewhere, however, for an explanation of the lowered incidence of most other infections.

Behind the decrease in both infant mortality rates and infectious disease is the enormous improvement in public health measures. Our food and water are clean. We use disinfectants to kill germs, we have better sanitation, cleaner air, better housing with less overcrowding; our families are smaller and we enjoy a generally higher standard of living. The Welfare State holds a net under us and we don't starve. These public health measures have done a lot to reduce infections such as TB, cholera, typhoid fever and smallpox. Of course, medicine has played a part in this; but not the main role.

Against all this improvement must be set the rising incidence of chronic degenerative disease. In this area, orthodox medicine is largely powerless.

'I will give no poisonous drug, even if asked to.'
HIPPOCRATIC OATH

Doctors now are surrounded by avalanches of drugs which they are both trained and encouraged to prescribe.

What is a drug? A very wide definition is 'medicinal substance' (*Concise Oxford Dictionary*). Another definition is 'any substance which can alter the structure or function of the living organism' (*Medicines: A Guide for Everybody* by Peter Parish). This includes vitamins and other nutrients.

But we could perhaps define a drug as something foreign to the body. This discriminates between nutrients, which are familiar to and needed by the body, and substances unfamiliar to it *in that exact quantity or form.*

Let us take an example: Insulin is desperately needed by the body. Without insulin injections a diabetic may die. But insulin for injection comes from cattle and not from the actual individual receiving it, who is biochemically unique in all his body processes and products. It is not administered, either, in the same amounts and at the same frequency as would happen naturally. So we would define injected insulin as a drug.

To sharpen the distinction between substances your body naturally needs and foreign chemicals introduced into it – do you really believe that your headache is caused by a deficiency of aspirin?

There are no drugs without undesirable side-effects. When a drug is taken, its adverse side-effects are balanced against the dangers of the illness. The risk in this balancing act is not taken by the doctor. It's taken by the patient.

The Vice-Dean of the British College of Naturopathy and Osteopathy, Dr I.P. Drysdale, believes that 85% of drugs now prescribed should not be used at all. He suggests that the remaining 15% should be prescribed in a more intelligent, discriminating way.

What do drugs do? They attack, not the cause of the illness, but its *symptoms*.

Drugs do not cure chronic degenerative illnesses. They suppress symptoms and ignore causes. Drugs for high blood pressure, for instance, must be continued by the patient indefinitely. The high blood pressure has not been corrected permanently. It has only been lowered for the duration of the drug's effects. This condition, like any degenerative illness, may have many causes, and it is the causes that matter and not the symptom of high blood pressure itself.

In the case of an infection, an antibiotic is a Magic Bullet to kill the bacteria. The body has a germ skulking around inside it, so you take aim, fire your pill and Hey Presto – the germ is flat on its back and the person is well again. Unfortunately, the drug is very often not a bullet, but a mallet. In hitting the germ it takes a swipe at the unfortunate patient as well. A healthy person has an immune system which wipes out infections with a deadly and sophisticated accuracy unmatched by any drug.

However valuable they may be in some instances, drugs always introduce toxins into the body which it then has to cope with as well as the illness. Recovery often takes place not because of the drug treatment, but in spite of it.

We are all worried about the side-effects of drugs. But we also hear about the extensive and expensive testing of new drugs which can take years of work. This may make us feel safe. It is somewhat disconcerting, therefore, to discover that many of the common drugs have never been subjected to the rigorous trials now in operation. These drugs date from before the Medicines Act of 1971, which tightened up the regulations.

Antibiotics encourage the development of resistant strains

of bacteria in us and have even been blamed for causing a new VD strain.[3] There have been several deaths due to sensitivity to penicillin. Reserpine for high blood pressure can cause suicidal depression and it was alleged in the House of Commons early in 1979 that tricyclic anti-depressants could do the same. Quinine is still being used to treat night cramps; one of the side-effects after repeated average doses is blindness.[4] Clofibrate, for reducing high blood fat levels, was associated with a 25% increase in deaths in the people on whom it was tested.[5] In spite of the boom in cancer drugs, and constant talk of the miracle which is always just around the corner, the majority of these drugs damage normal cells, causing dreadful side-effects and sometimes precipitating cancer themselves.

Drugs destroy nutrients in the body. Antibiotics and sulpha drugs destroy the intestinal bacteria which make B vitamins in the gut. Aspirin destroys folic acid and vitamins C and K. Barbiturates destroy vitamins C, folic acid and other B vitamins. Corticosteroids destroy vitamin C and zinc.

There is a new class of illness with us – iatrogenic. This means an illness caused by the adverse side-effects of a prescribed drug or drugs. It is estimated – conservatively – that about 10% of sick people are made worse or given another illness by orthodox medical treatment.[6] This figure does not of course include those who are ill without realizing that the illness is due to their prescription. Drug-induced side-effects and illnesses have been called diseases of medical progress. Perhaps we should ask in which direction we are progressing . . .

In 1971 the Committee on Safety of Medicines was formed. It sifts drug reports sent in from chemists, doctors, dentists and medical literature. In 1980 the Committee received over 100 000. It is not obligatory to report a drug's adverse effects and a doctor may shrink from doing so, not wishing to admit that his prescription made Aunt Maisie have a fit. These reports are therefore only the tip of the iceberg.

About a quarter of GPs complete their prescription forms inadequately.[7] Nearly one quarter of these GPs actually make a mistake when writing out a prescription. Not much fun for the chemist and even less for the patient.

Putting a chemical into a person is as dangerous as putting a knife into him. It's even more dangerous when it's the wrong chemical.

*'The desire to take medicine is perhaps the greatest feature
which distinguishes man from animals.'*   SIR WILLIAM OSLER

In England, every tenth night of sleep is drug-induced. 19% of
British women and 9% of men take a tranquillizer during any
one year.[1] We in Britain take more than 10 000 million tablets
of aspirin, phenacetin or paracetamol each year. Every day,
250 000 people are taking five or more painkillers.[8]

Like any other business, a drug company is there to make
money. In common with the breweries and the tobacco
companies, they answer our demand for chemicals. They
foster the idea of the Magic Bullet.

The healthy profits of the drug industry influence the
absurd cost of the National Health Service. The total UK
profits of the drug industry for 1977 were £78.9 million before
tax.[9] The estimate for the cost of the NHS for 1981/82 is £11.1
billion.[10]

British drug firms spend over £15 million a year advertising
their products to the medical profession. Open the newspaper
called the *General Practitioner*. There will be a beautifully-
produced full-page colour advertisement for a drug, with the
side-effects and contra-indications in extremely small print.
This contrasts with the frequent reports on damage from drugs
on the neighbouring pages. Without their advertisers, medical
journals would go out of business.

Please heal me, doctor, but don't ask me to change

We in the West lean on our doctors. We get the medical care
which we demand. We cannot entirely blame 'them' – the drug
companies, the orthodox medical profession – for the attitudes
and therapy which we, the public, ask from them.

A GP said recently, 'If my patient expects a remedy for a
cold I will give him an antibiotic. He will be better in seven
days, but he may still be suffering from the side-effects of the
drug. If I give him no drug he will still be better in about the
same time. But he may feel that I have neglected him.' A
Health Education Council leaflet appearing in doctors'
waiting rooms is headed 'Be prepared to leave this surgery
empty-handed. The doctor may not give you a prescription.
His advice may be all that you need.' How many of us are
satisfied with this?

Many doctors try very hard not to be walking prescription

pads. They try to stop their patients stuffing themselves with too much food or poisoning themselves with alcohol or tobacco. The blame for their failure cannot be laid upon them; it is the responsibility of the patient. The doctor who spares time for someone when he has a waiting room full of sniffling anxious people has done his best in difficult circumstances. The patient who does not implement his doctor's advice, demanding pills instead, is passive and immature.

The idea of personal responsibility for health is less than alluring. It takes change and effort – now. We prefer to wait for an illness to happen, then we take it to the doctor and expect to be given a cure.

Ian Kennedy, in his 1980 Reith Lectures, criticized attitudes to health, putting part of the blame on to us, the patients, and adding, 'you can only make the right choices as to food or lifestyle if you have the proper information'. This book will give you part of that information.

'Medicina curat, natura sanat'

This old Latin tag is taken now to mean 'medicine cures, nature heals'. But that is not the original meaning. It used to mean 'medicine cares, nature heals'. The doctor can only point you in the right direction.

It's the body that does the work of healing and the practitioner and his patient who encourage an environment where healing can take place. It's the clotting factors, acting quickly to congeal your blood, which stop that cut from bleeding you to death. It's the white blood cells that overwhelm and destroy an infection which has broached your first line of defence, the skin. The body will try to throw off any illness, any imbalance, if it is given the chance; its capacity to do so is strengthened, or hampered, by the choices you make about the way you live.

'Organism; organized body with connected inter-dependent parts sharing common life.' CONCISE OXFORD DICTIONARY

There is a medical philosophy older than the Magic Bullet. This interprets ill-health as disharmony; a state of 'dis-ease' existing within the whole body and affecting the whole person.

A human being is a miraculously complex arrangement of parts which are all influenced by, and influence, each other.

He or she is not a collection of bits which can profitably be examined separately. Your depression might be partly due to what you eat or it might be the result of a long period of worry and chronic tension. A superlative diet and relaxation classes would help. Your constipation is probably due mainly to what you eat, and a bag of bran is better for you than a laxative.

Nature cure, or naturopathy, treats the whole person. It is a mainstay of alternative medicine.

'For far too long, traditional systems of medicine and modern medicine have gone their separate ways in mutual antipathy. Yet are their goals not identical?' DR HALFDAN MAHLER, Director-General of the World Health Organization.

Alternative (or traditional) medicine is a modern growth industry. The undoubted successes of acupuncturists, herbalists, naturopaths and osteopaths highlight the failures of orthodox therapy.

This field used to be the last resort of the old, the desperate and the very sick. They would visit an alternative practitioner not because they believed in him but because he was their only hope. Now his waiting room is full of younger people, aware of the beginnings of illness and willing to do something about it.

The natural therapists, however, are up against not only many orthodox doctors, but the charlatans on their own fringe, those unqualified practitioners who make such good ammunition for alternative medicine's detractors. Ideas are muddy and confused from some of the extremists in the field. We cannot go 'back to nature' – whatever that may mean. The days when we could bask in the sun catching fruit (unsprayed) as it fell from the tree are over – if they ever existed. We have exchanged the horrid risks of natural living for the just as horrid risks of unnatural living.

We must learn to go forward *with* nature, instead of enthusiastically setting out to destroy her. The modern food industry in particular must change to meet our growing knowledge. Research is providing more and more incontrovertible links between our food and our illnesses and this proof can no longer be belittled or ignored.

In November 1964, the prestigious researcher John Yudkin was invited to speak at a conference in Paris organised by La

Fondation pour le Progrès de l'Alimentation, a scientific body allegedly entirely independent, but whose work is supported by the French food industry. After the conference the proceedings were being put together in the form of a book. Yudkin had described in his paper the growing evidence that sugar could play a part in some of our Western diseases and he stated that people ate too much sugar because they liked the taste of it. He was asked to delete this passage from the book and refused. His paper was not included in the final published version. Here is an example of a leading nutritionist being denied expression by an organization which purports to be unbiased.

'Striving after health until he makes himself sick.' From *Try Being Healthy* by DR ALEC FORBES, pub. Langdon 1976.

Let us now whisper the dreaded word 'crank'. We've all seen them – although of course it's never you or me. People whose concern for their own health is so obsessive that it overrides everything else. People who spend their evenings counting the vitamins in their soup or rubbing carrot juice on their kneecaps or being miserable and uncomfortable and anxious in a host of other ingenious ways. They are easily recognizable; the thing worshipped has to be perfect, it has to work all the time, and it has to be the *only way*.

Alternative medicine is not perfect, it will not work all the time, and it is not the only way. In his book *Good Health Through Natural Therapy* Dr E.K. Ledermann writes, 'No school of medicine can claim to be all-sufficient. While it is correct to trust the self-healing power of nature, it is not correct to trust this power absolutely. If a patient fails to respond to natural treatment, or if his condition is such that no response to natural treatment can be expected, then the resources of scientific modern medicine must be made available.' Both orthodox and alternative medicine have a common goal – that of healing the sick. Why can't they work together?

'La destinée des nations dépend de la manière dont elles se nourrissent.'   BRILLAT-SAVARIN

Good food is an important part of getting well and staying well. A hundred years ago, our food might have been pest-ridden. Now, it is clean. But pests will not eat some of it.

Not only is there widespread ignorance among the general public about nutrition, there is pretty much the same situation in the orthodox medical profession as well. Unbelievably, there is *only one* department of nutrition in an undergraduate medical school in this country – Southampton. At the Middlesex Hospital, Dr Gaston Pawan gives part-time lectures in nutrition to some of the students. This appalling gap in medical education is the reason why many doctors have taken the trouble to educate themselves on the subject – thereby vastly enhancing their skills as healers. I have never met a doctor who has regretted for one moment this extra study and profound change of attitude.

This book is written to describe the relationship between our health and what we eat and it gives detailed nutritional therapy for many of our modern chronic degenerative diseases.

If we could stop ourselves from getting ill in the first place, how much better that would be. The nutrition explained and recommended here will go a long way towards keeping you fit and free from illness.

If a person is going to use dietary means to get well, he will need an explanation both of his illness and of the dietary treatment. It is wrong to treat people like children or blithering idiots who cannot understand and accept the truth. This can be a life-saving distinction – for instance, in a serious disease like multiple sclerosis, early diagnosis is imperative if the nutritional treatment is to stand a chance of success.

There are some things I have had to leave out. I have only been able to touch briefly on the relationship between mind and body (SEE *Cancer and the Mind*, page 269). It could be argued that almost all illness is psychosomatic but it was quite impossible to include this vast area.

I have also given only brief leads for those who are interested in following up the other alternative therapies available. To have left these out would have been very unfair, but to have gone into them fully would have made the book too long.

This book is in four sections. The first part describes the constituents of food, discussing both whole foods and the modern food industry, together with supplements and foods of special nutritional value.

The second section sets out the connection between diet and the various stages of life – for example, childhood, pregnancy and lactation, old age – and describes the best way to eat for good eyesight, healthy skin and hair, and so on. It discusses special ways of eating (vegetarianism, veganism, macrobiotics) and the benefits of fasting.

The third section deals with our long-term degenerative diseases, giving nutritional therapy. This section is linked to the *Food Therapy Plan* – a professionally devised dietary which will help you to recover. The rationale behind this approach is set out in the *Nature Cure* section.

I wish you well.

Books mentioned in this section
Medicines: A Guide for Everybody by Peter Parish (Penguin 1980)
Good Health Through Natural Therapy by E.K. Ledermann (Pan 1978).

PART ONE

All About Foods

Carbohydrates

There are three main groups of carbohydrates – sugars, starches and fibre.

Sugar (sucrose and glucose) and refined starches are the most concentrated sources. Flour, cakes, bread, biscuits, breakfast cereals, pastry, honey, potatoes and preserves are good sources. Fruits, vegetables and their juices, nuts, alcoholic drinks and milk all contain a little. Even meat has a little starch, and part of the fat you eat is turned into glucose.

The first two groups of carbohydrates, sugars and starches, are used for producing energy. The last group, fibre, has a different role to play. In moderation, carbohydrates are indispensable. In excess, they are stored as fat.

When discussing food and health, it is essential to distinguish between unrefined and refined carbohydrates.

Unrefined carbohydrates

These are the best. They contain their original vitamins and minerals plus their fibre, intact. They are found in whole-grains, including wholemeal flour and brown rice, and in bran (the best source of fibre), legumes and pulses (including peas, beans and lentils), nuts and dried fruits, root vegetables, fruits and leafy vegetables and fruit and vegetable juices.

Refined carbohydrates

White flour and white sugar are refined carbohydrates. White flour has had most of its nutrients milled out – including the fibre – after which a few of them are put back. White sugar has been entirely stripped of all its nutrients and left that way (SEE *Sugar*, pages 61–5).

Fibre

Fibre is not a nutrient. But it is an essential part of our food and there is no substitute for it. It is not digested, but acts to propel food wastes along the gut so that they are quickly and efficiently expelled (SEE *Fibre* pages 35–42).

Carbohydrates deprived of their fibre – refined – are a major cause of many of our Western diseases. It is now accepted that the absence of fibre can contribute to obesity since refined foods do not fill you up. It is easy to see, too, that constipation, varicose veins and piles can be caused or aggravated by the slow, difficult passage of bowel contents. Fibre definitely reduces the absorption of cholesterol and a high-fibre diet tends to be a low-fat diet and vice versa; it is thought therefore that fibre has a role to play in the prevention of heart and artery disease by helping to cope with harmful fats. Over-eating of refined carbohydrates upsets the equilibrium of the bowel micro-organisms, and this is thought to contribute to inflammation of the appendix, gall bladder and kidneys. All these conditions are rare in communities where refined carbohydrates are not eaten.

We should remember, however, that refined foods have been robbed of their vitamins and minerals as well as their fibre. This must also play a part in the causation of illness.

Refined vs Unrefined
Even if we leave out the question of the vitamins, minerals and fibre found in unrefined carbohydrates and lacking in the refined varieties, there is still a big difference between the two. Refined carbohydrates are not just lacking in certain essentials; they can be actively harmful.

Refined sugar (sucrose) is easily digested. It quickly floods the system, and demands insulin from the pancreas in order to be metabolized as well as using up B vitamins. The rapid rise of blood sugar levels caused by the entry of sucrose, therefore, is followed by an output of insulin from the pancreas which lowers the blood sugar again. (As a result of the over-reaction of the pancreas, low blood sugar (SEE *Low Blood Sugar*, pages 340–5) can follow the ingestion of a lot of sucrose.) Later, there is a rise in blood triglycerides (a kind of fat) levels too, and even some hormones are affected. It is thought that adult-onset diabetes, as well as being partly inherited, is most likely among people who eat refined, low-fibre carbohydrates, because diabetes can be encouraged by over-working the pancreas, forcing it to deal with sudden floods of white sugar.

This quick rise in blood sugar levels caused by the immediate absorption of sucrose lays stress on the body's coping mechanisms.

The less refined the carbohydrate, in general, the longer it takes to be used by the body. Unrefined, high-fibre carbohydrates release a slow, constant stream of glucose into the bloodstream at about two calories a minute. This is just what the body needs. With a steady, consistent supply of glucose provided in this way, there is always something good cooking inside you and keeping a steady blood sugar level. You rarely have a low blood sugar problem, and the need for insulin to deal with the glucose is reduced.

The US Senate Select Committee on Nutrition and Human Needs of 1977 recommended that we should double our intake of unrefined carbohydrates, eating starchy foods rich in fibre which contain their original nutrients. With this increase in the right kind of carbohydrates, fat intake would be substantially reduced as well.

Fats

This is a complex area and I have gone into it in considerable detail. Readers who don't want to plough through the whole section might prefer to read the summary at the end.

'Fats' is a word I feel I should whisper.

We hear so much about the harm that fats can do to our hearts now that we take a quick furtive look round the room before that extra helping of cream. So let's elucidate.

Some fat is absolutely essential. It's needed for the development of brain, nerves and certain body processes and is found in every cell. It carries the fat-soluble vitamins A, D, E and K round the body and is thought to help in the use of the B vitamins. Fat or sugar cells help to make some proteins and hormones and to grow friendly intestinal bacteria. Fat helps to support the internal organs and a thin layer under the skin protects the muscles and nerves and helps to maintain body temperature; fat reserves are used during fasting. And – very importantly – fats produce energy. In fact fats may rival carbohydrates as an energy source. A gram of fat gives more energy than a gram of carbohydrate plus a gram of protein (it also gives nine calories, though – quite a lot).

Fats are widely used in our eating because they make the

food taste better and they sustain us, taking a long time to digest. A cook would be completely lost without fats. We eat, however, much more fat than we actually need.

Types of fat

A particular food will have about 15 different fatty acids in differing amounts. We can group these into saturated, poly-unsaturated and monounsaturated fats. Each food has a characteristic mixture of these and one will predominate.

In general, saturated fats are solid at room temperature and foods containing mostly saturated fats are meat, milk, eggs, butter and cream.

Polyunsaturated fats are soft or liquid at room temperature and are found in green leaves, seeds, nuts, beans and fish as well as in the oils extracted from these foods (but palm and coconut oils are rich in *saturated* fats).

Monounsaturated fats (olive oil is monounsaturated) are neutral and need not concern us here.

Saturated fats have, so to speak, their hands full – of hydrogen atoms. Polyunsaturated fats have spare links in their structure waiting for hydrogen atoms. Unsaturated fats, included with them here, have rather fewer spare links.

Saturated fats are used for energy. They can be made by the body from sugar, starch or protein and any surplus is stored in large bulges, which is perhaps why they are called 'visible' fats.

The polyunsaturated fats are structural, used for building, and are found everywhere in the body. These fats include the essential fatty acids, of which more below.

Concerning the ratio of fats in our food, it should be noted that the free-range animal reared for meat has more poly-unsaturated fats in its carcase and fewer saturated fats than the fatstock animal. Additionally, Dr Michael Crawford of the Nuffield Laboratory of Comparative Medicine has shown that the modern intensively-reared cow may have about 30% fat and 55% lean, while a cow free to select its own food and range over the land has a carcase fat of about 4% and a lean tissue mass of about 80%. This is a huge difference; it does not apply however to all kinds of meat.

Essential fatty acids (EFAs)

These, sometimes still called vitamin F, are found in poly-unsaturated fats. The most important are linoleic acid, linolenic acid and arachidonic acid. It is now evident that if linoleic acid is supplied in the diet, the body can make the other two, provided several other nutrients are present. Linoleic acid is found in seeds, nuts and beans (and their oils), linolenic acid in green leaves, arachidonic acid in some vegetables and animal tissue.

These fatty acids are concerned in many tasks including brain and nerve construction and hormone formation. Human breast milk is rich in them, and they are vital for the growing baby. EFA deficiencies can produce eczema, dry and scaly skin, dry hair and will damage growth and reproduction in laboratory animals. When they are lacking the body may change sugar to fat very quickly as though it is trying to produce the missing nutrients. This quick change makes the blood sugar plummet and you will get as hungry as a wolf. EFA shortages accompany a deficiency of their end-product, the prostaglandins. Prostaglandins are found in almost every cell in the body. They are involved in the immune system's reaction to disease and have far-reaching effects on the circulation. Research is uncovering more and more information about them (SEE *Evening Primrose Oil*, page 111).

Some nutritionists believe that EFA deficiencies are common. Swedish scientists have estimated that our intake of one of them, linolenic acid, has halved since the beginning of the century. The EFAs in oils, nuts, seeds and green leaves are unstable and likely to go rancid and they are often destroyed when the food is processed. According to Dr Michael Crawford this destruction by hydrogenation of the EFAs is the most serious problem in food processing today (SEE *A couple of villains*, page 33).

Fish oils contain a class of fatty acids known as EPA (eicosapentaenoic acid) and DHA (docosahexaenoic acid), which can lower elevated blood cholesterol levels (*Journal* of the American Medical Association, 12 February 1982), and reduce the over-stickiness of blood clotting factors while raising the amount of substances called high-density lipo-proteins (Dr Tom Sanders, Queen Elizabeth College, London). Work on these fatty acids began fairly recently.

Cholesterol
This is another word I feel I should whisper. American

biochemist Richard Passwater has pointed to the existence of a new neurosis – cholesterophobia. . . .

Cholesterol is a benign, essential substance found everywhere in the body, but principally in the brain and nerve sheaths. It is used for making bile salts (its name means 'bile solid'), vitamin D and hormones and in the absorption of fat-soluble vitamins and fatty acids. It is yellowish-white, fatty and rather like porridge.

Cholesterol is found only in animal fats – eggs, milk, cheese, butter, meat, cream and pastries, and, of course, in food fried in animal fats. Vegetable fats contain no cholesterol. This is only part of the story, however. Cholesterol is manufactured by almost all the tissues in the body but chiefly by the liver, and usually the amount of cholesterol in the blood seems to be determined largely by the amount made by the liver. Some workers, therefore, believe that the amount of cholesterol we actually take in is a secondary consideration, since our bodies make it for us, especially when we eat more food than we need.

So if cholesterol is necessary and natural, what has happened to turn it into the artery-clogging White Menace?

Cholesterol circulating freely in the blood is taken to the liver and muscles where it is used or stored. But it is the cholesterol which does not make the journey and which attaches itself to the linings of arteries, blood vessels and capillaries that causes the trouble. This is a main ingredient of arterial plaques which stick to the arteries, narrowing them and increasing the possibility of heart trouble by impeding the circulation of the blood. So some researchers say that it is not the level of colesterol circulating in the blood that matters. It's the *undissolved* cholesterol, lining and therefore narrowing the blood vessels, which does the damage. Others believe that the level of cholesterol in the blood is vitally important. So let's play safe, and assume that the latter is the case.

The level of cholesterol in the blood is affected both by the amount we eat and the amount we make. We can cut down on the amount we eat simply by cutting our intake of saturated fats. Concerning the cholesterol we make, it has been found that large, infrequent meals stimulate the liver to pour out more cholesterol. It is not difficult to cut down on too many eating binges; they're not good for you in many other ways, either.

When researchers look at the way cholesterol behaves in the

bloodstream things get more complicated. It is not used by the body in isolation any more than any other substance. There are many nutrients which help to control the cholesterol and use it in the right way, so that it passes along the bloodstream without forming into lumps and sticking to the walls.

For insrance, cholesterol and lecithin (SEE *Lecithin* page 121) are needed together. When the liver is healthy, it will turn out both these substances in exactly the right balance. Laboratory animals when fed a lot of cholesterol-containing foods plus lecithin *do not* develop artery damage, and lecithin has repeatedly been found to play a major role in dissolving fats and keeping the bloodstream healthy. Another experiment echoes this conclusion: human volunteers who were fed large amounts of egg yolk powder (the equivalent of about fifteen eggs a day) submitted to a blood test at the end of the experiment. Of the thirteen volunteers, only two showed a high blood cholesterol level.[1] Eggs contain both cholesterol and lecithin.

Easy rider   Cholesterol does not swim through the blood – it rides. It usually attaches itself to high-density lipoproteins (HDLs) and low-density lipoproteins (LDLs). The HDLs hang on to their cholesterol and help it on its way. The LDLs, on the other hand, release their load very easily so that it can stay, undissolved, in the circulatory system and cause trouble. These two substances, therefore, have a major effect on how much cholesterol is dropped by the wayside.

It has been found that there is a hereditary factor in the ratio of the protective HDLs to the less protective LDLs; encouragingly, however, we have quite a lot of influence over the other, environmental, factors. The valuable HDLs are highest in non-smokers, underweight people, moderate drinkers, people taking vigorous exercise and those eating vegetable-rich[2] low-fat diets with plenty of natural fibre (SEE *Fibre* page 35).

Cholesterol and the B vitamins   Other nutrients exerting influence on the level and solubility of blood cholesterol are the B vitamins choline, inositol and pyridoxine (B6). If these essential vitamins are lacking the cholesterol level rises and it tends to form lumps. American nutritionist Adelle Davis cites research showing that choline will protect laboratory animals from the heart and artery damage which other animals sustain on the same high-cholesterol diet without choline.

Current research suggests that it is vitamin *B6*, or pyridoxine, that is most involved in artery health. Laboratory animals on a high-cholesterol diet were protected from artery damage by supplements of this vitamin, and work with human patients confirms this, establishing that a B6 deficiency can encourage a high blood cholesterol level.[3] The protective effect of B6 involves a sufficient intake of protein together with the mineral magnesium.

The B vitamins, therefore, play a vital part in the maintenance of a healthy bloodstream and arteries. Since the contraceptive pill destroys B6, can this drug be accused of contributing to our rising figures for artery damage and heart disease?

Cholesterol and the essential fatty acids The fact that the essential fatty acids in some oils can lower blood cholesterol is the reason for the current swing in favour of polyunsaturated fats. Experiments reinforce the view that animals given EFAs fare well, even on a high-cholesterol diet, and support the theory that a deficiency of these acids, or something wrong in the way they are used, is an important factor in artery disease. It is now agreed that essential fatty acids are vital in the utilization of both cholesterol and other saturated fats. They also help the liver to manufacture lecithin which, as we have seen, helps to dissolve these fats.

But we cannot assume that, because a fat or oil appears to be polyunsaturated, it will contain its natural quotient of essential fatty acids. I will discuss this point in detail under *Oils* pages 29–30.

The continuing story of cholesterol Fresh and rancid cholesterol are very different.

When the cholesterol in foods is allowed to go rancid, the chemicals formed in the process do more damage to the circulatory system than the original fresh cholesterol.[4]

The cholesterol or its derivatives in powdered eggs, powdered whole milk, custard, pancake mixes and similar foods can oxidize, or go rancid, very easily, and when this happens contaminants are formed. It is probable, too, that foods such as smoked fish, meat and sausages may have their cholesterol content changed in the smoking process. Afterwards, they are usually stored at room temperature, allowing the oxidation and consequent cholesterol deterioration to

continue. This also applies to some cheeses and is yet another
argument for eating fresh foods.

There is no doubt that, *when mishandled by the body*,
cholesterol is a menace. Its tendency to silt up the arteries and
reduce the blood supply can affect hearing and sight, cause leg
cramps and interfere with the oxygen supply to the brain, as
well as add to the risk of heart disease. There is also a possible
link between cholesterol deposits and the ageing process – not
surprising when you consider what these unnatural deposits do
to the circulation and therefore to the transport of nutrients
and wastes. Some researchers in fact accuse it of being
responsible for most of the symptoms of ageing, saying also
that cholesterol plaque waterproofs the capillary walls,
preventing water from passing from the blood into the cells
and tending to dehydrate them. The body of a young man is
70% water – and the body of an old man may be only 60%.

The complete picture   There are many primitive peoples of
widely differing ethnic stock – for instance, the Somalis and
the Samburus of east Africa and the early Eskimos – who have
always eaten a great deal of animal fat but who do not suffer
from heart or artery disease to any significant extent. It is
encouraging to read, too, that yet more long-suffering
laboratory animals, on a 'high butter diet' with plenty of
vitamins and mineral supplements and 20% protein, did not
sustain any artery damage. They simply put on weight.[5]

It is clear, therefore, that it is the *total nutrition* available to
the body, including the B vitamins and minerals involved as
well as fats, that matters in arterial health. These substances
can deal with the blood cholesterol in a natural, effective way,
preventing it from causing any damage. Roger Williams
confirms this in his book *Nutrition Against Disease* and says
that the amount of fat or cholesterol consumed is more or less
inconsequential.

The oils
We have seen that fats which are soft, or liquid, at room
temperature are mostly polyunsaturated. Let's look at how the
original seeds are persuaded to give up their polyunsaturated
oils.

There is a marked nutritional difference between refined
and unrefined oils.

Refined oils   In our modern world, happy peasants do not sit around on the baked earth, beating the daylights out of some seeds to get a little dark, fragrant oil. Things are more organized now.

Refined oils go through a process involving about fifteen separate steps. The oil-bearing materials – seeds, nuts or beans – are ground, steamed, then mixed with chemicals which act as solvents. The mixture is then heated to drive off the solvent, but solvent residues are sometimes left in very small quantities. The chemicals used as solvents are petroleum-based, and it was stated at the International Union against Cancer in 1956 that 'since various petroleum constituents, including certain mineral oils and paraffin, have produced cancer in man and experimental animals, the presence of such chemicals in food appears to be objectionable, particularly when such materials are heated to high temperatures.'

The oil is then washed with caustic soda, bleached, filtered and deodorized, which removes the lecithin, minerals and vitamin E. Chemicals are then added to prevent the oil going rancid (its own natural antioxidants having been removed!).

One of the essential fatty acids, linolenic acid, is often processed out of refined oils because it is unstable and goes rancid easily. Many oils are partly hydrogenated too, again to improve their keeping qualities, and this process saturates some of their fats. So we end up with a product which is pale, odourless, long-lasting – and unnatural. In particular, since the ingestion of any polyunsaturated fat puts up the body's need for the vitamin E which naturally accompanies that fat, it is unwise to process out this important vitamin along with the other antioxidants present.

Unrefined oils The two methods of extracting oil to be sold as 'unrefined' are pressure extracted and the expeller method. A simple hydraulic press is used for pressure extraction and this method is now rare. The more usual expeller method uses a screw or press to squeeze out the oil.

In both methods the pressure used will itself generate heat of up to about 120°C. So the term 'cold-pressed' is a misnomer and serves only to distinguish an unrefined oil from a refined variety. Although this temperature is mild indeed compared to those reached in the processes for refining oil, an American manufacturer of unrefined oils commented tersely that he'd like to see the inventor of the term 'cold-pressed' actually bathing in the oil as it emerged from the extraction process.

The difference
We have seen that refining oils destroys most of their
nutrients. About 0.6mg of vitamin E is needed for each gram
of polyunsaturated fatty acid eaten.

Natural oils contain chlorophyll, carotenoids (for forming
vitamin A), the natural preservatives lecithin and vitamin E
(sesame oil also carries the antioxidant sesamol), and the
minerals copper, magnesium, calcium and iron.

There is another important difference between refined and
unrefined oils. The heat used in refining oils can reach about
235°C. The oils are often held at this high level for several
hours, and it is this prolonged high heat which is damaging.

In one study,[6] heated oil was given to laboratory animals
with an average ration of cholesterol, producing artery damage
more pronounced than that sustained by animals on the same
diet but without the oil. Repeated experiments on this subject
point to the strong possibility that refined (i.e. heated) and
unrefined oils behave differently in the body, because oils are
damaged by such high heats. It is apparently the *unrefined* oils
which offer some protection against artery disease. Roger
Williams, who has been through this area with care and
unrivalled expertise, states in *Nutrition Against Disease* that,
'most commercial "polyunsaturated" vegetable oils are
possibly productive of atherosclerosis and should be avoided
by the consumer.'

Science News Letter for 16 June 1951, reported clinical tests
showing that a remedy for high blood cholesterol was found to
be the phospholipids (lecithin) found in unrefined oils. It also
appears that a diet high in polyunsaturates which does not also
include the natural antioxidants (principally vitamin E, but
also selenium and vitamin C), may produce artery damage and
cellular ageing in man.[7] This ageing consists of ceroid pigments
which are found in damaged arteries.

Laboratory animals fed large quantities of polyunsaturated
fats are more susceptible to cancer than those fed saturated
fats. It is postulated that an intake of vitamin E which
balances the intake of polyunsaturated fat (a combination
naturally present in unrefined oils) may keep down the cancer
incidence.

It's time, therefore, that some hard thinking was done on
the crucial difference between refined and relatively unrefined
polyunsaturated oils.

Too many polyunsaturates?

We are not equipped to handle large quantities of *any* kind of fat. After all, oils come mostly from seeds. In order to eat unseparated from its natural source the amount of oil we gaily tip into the frying pan and on to the salad, we would have to chomp our way through small mountains of seeds and nuts – not an appealing prospect.

It is therefore not altogether surprising that recent work shows that too much polyunsaturated fat is not any better for you than too much saturated fat.

We have already seen that laboratory animals are more susceptible to cancer when they are fed a lot of polyunsaturated fats. During human trials to test the effects of polyunsaturated fats, these fats accompanied a high incidence of cancer.

Writing in the *British Medical Journal* for 20 January 1979, Sir John McMichael reports that some vegetable oils (and hardened fats) 'can be more damaging to arteries than butter', saying that 'there are other hazards to heart muscle from vegetable oils'. In further discussing the role of fats in heart disease, he continues 'thus the polyunsaturated diet does not prevent coronary heart disease, but might even be suspected of contributing to its development'. Besides stale cholesterol, other harmful substances are produced when polyunsaturated fats are allowed to go rancid, and these 'free radicals' damage tissue and can encourage cancer.

It is clear, therefore, that there are dangers in polyunsaturates if they are eaten to excess. Could those who eat a lot of poly-unsaturated fat, thinking that it will protect them against heart and artery disease, be actually adding to the risk?

To cap all this, adding polyunsaturates to the diet without reducing the other fats taken will cause an increase in weight.[8]

Too many saturates?

It is now widely accepted that the cholesterol-bearing saturated fats are harmful in excess. Three of the saturated fatty acids (lauric, palmitic, myristic – the last found in butter) have been found to raise the blood cholesterol level. Animal fat is acid-forming, too, and can cause digestive problems, and there is some evidence that a diet heavy in animal fats as well as in polyunsaturates may put up the incidence of cancer. Fibre, or roughage, comes into the picture too. People either eat lots of fat with little fibre, or lots of fibre with little fat, and in his book *Taking the Rough with the Smooth* Dr Andrew Stanway comments that the way the body handles fat seems to vary according to the amount of fibre in the diet.

A couple of villains

A *hydrogenated fat* is an unnatural substance. It is a vegetable fat or oil which has been changed by man so that it has become saturated and in this process the essential fatty acids are destroyed. What remains is a solid fat or a liquid, partly hydrogenated, oil, which is very long-lasting. Hydrogenated fats are found in margarines, refined salted oils, many snack foods, and in fast and fried foods.

Trans-fatty acids are produced when fats are hydrogenated. When these artificial fats finally go rancid, they form carcinogenous substances. Researchers believe that trans-fatty acids can alter cell membranes, too, allowing cancer-forming substances to pass through more easily. They raise blood cholesterol levels and put up the body's need for one of the EFAs. In a paper written for the Clinical Research Institute, Montreal, David F. Horrobin writes, '30% to 40% of the LA (cislinoleic acid, an EFA in its natural form) in margarine and foods prepared from hydrogenated oils may be in the trans form.'

How much fat?

In the UK, 42% of our calories are eaten in the form of fat. *This is far too much*, and the Royal College of Physicians and the British Cardiac Society warned in a 1976 report that it should be reduced to at least 35%. Many naturopaths advise a greater drop, sometimes to as low as 5%, in accordance with the naturopathic principle of drastically reducing all fats.

We have a limited amount of an enzyme which the body needs for the metabolism of fatty acids. It also looks after nerve tissue and our immunity against illness, including cancer. If we eat too much fat, so much of this enzyme is used in processing that fat that not enough is left over for other tasks and health will suffer as a result.

It is without doubt a common-sense measure to cut down on our dietary fats as well as to increase the quality of our food so that we can deal with those fats more efficiently. Even a diet of whole grains, beans, seeds and green leaves would supply enough essential fatty acids for health without any extra fat being added at all. We have to realize that, although fats are pleasant and satisfying in our food, the amounts we take in at present are not only unnecessary but actively harmful.

SUMMARY

1 Fats are widely used in the body.

2 There are broadly three types – polyunsaturated (soft at room temperature) and saturated (hard at room temperature), and EPA with DHA. Polyunsaturated fats are found mostly in seeds, nuts, beans, their unrefined oils and green leaves; saturated fats mostly in animal fats. EPA and DHA are found in fish oils.

3 Polyunsaturated fats contain essential fatty acids, one of which is vital to us.

4 Cholesterol is a useful substance, both found in our food and made by the body. We often eat too much cholesterol however and – more importantly – we often handle it inefficiently in our bodies.

5 We can cut down on our cholesterol intake by cutting down on animal fats. In general, this may help to lower blood cholesterol.

6 We can handle cholesterol in our bodies more efficiently by taking in more B vitamins and by making sure we get enough essential fatty acids. We are not likely to be short of the protein which is another necessary factor in this process.

7 Polyunsaturated fats can be just as harmful, in excess, as saturated fats, but in different ways. This is particularly true of refined, highly processed oils.

8 We should therefore:

Eat less of all fats.

Eat plenty of wholegrains including wholemeal bread for the B vitamins and natural fibre.

Eat unrefined, 'cold-pressed' oils (obtainable from a health store – check the label), seeds, nuts, beans, green leaves.

Avoid fried, processed, smoked and 'fast' foods.

Information

Relaxation techniques have been shown to lower high blood fats. Please see *Additional Therapies* section at end of book (page 381) under *Relaxation*. Autogenic Training is effective here.

Books mentioned in this section
Nutrition Against Disease by Roger Williams (Bantam 1978).
Taking the Rough with the Smooth by Andrew Stanway (Pan 1982).

Fibre

'The big mistake in nutrition has been removing the part of food that doesn't provide nutrients, but is enormously valuable as a protection against disease.'   SURGEON DENIS BURKITT

What is fibre?

Dietary fibre is the modern name for roughage. By this we mean the part of a plant that, when it is eaten, is not digested in the small intestine. It consists of the walls of plant cells, and its qualities vary according to its source. There is more fibre on the outside layers of seeds and vegetables and the peel of fruit. Dietary fibre is found only in plants – the term does not refer to the fibrous parts of meat. It is a complex group of substances and research into it continues.

Food sources of fibre are cereals, legumes, root vegetables and some leafy vegetables, nuts and fruits. Dried fruits have more fibre weight for weight because most of the water has been removed, and fresh fruits and vegetables correspondingly less because of their high water content. All the same, a fresh apple owes its shape, solidity and texture to its supporting fibre, without which it is just a few mouthfuls of apple juice.

Fibre is something we have been assiduously removing from our food for many years – in particular we take great care to process out nearly all the fibre – known as bran – from our flour. (We also remove the wheat germ, leaving only the endosperm from which refined white flour is made.) We carefully peel most of our vegetables, throwing the peel away. This makes an enormous difference to our food: as a result of all this refining, we in the West usually eat far too little fibre. Our intake has decreased over the years and we now take about 15 to 25 grams a day. In Third World countries, people eat three to five times this amount; it is only Western man who eats concentrated starches and sugars without fibre and only Western man who commonly suffers from a long list of chronic degenerative diseases including constipation, obesity, appendicitis, diabetes, heart disease, etc.

Fibre has long been considered a useless substance, but in fact it plays a crucial part in health. It is in the news now, having been given the official seal of approval after many years of painstaking work by doctors and researchers. A recent report by the Royal College of Physicians[1] has summarized this work, giving a cautious but definite boost to the fibre enthusiasts. (The naturopaths have been supporting fibre for rather longer.)

What does fibre do?
Its main effect is on the wastes in the bowel. Fibre passing along the gut holds water and encourages gas and bacterial action. This means that stools are bulky, soft, and expelled from the body without effort. When fibre is missing from the diet, too much water is absorbed from the wastes as they travel along the bowel and stools are hard, dry and difficult to expel. Fibre's main function, therefore, is to encourage a natural, easy bowel action and prevent constipation.

It is quite simple to find out if you are constipated. If your stools are hard, small and dark and you have to strain in order to get rid of them, then you are. It is not a question of how regularly you pass them. If your food takes a long time to get through your body – if the 'transit time' is relatively long – then you may indeed produce regular stools, but they will have spent too long inside you. The substance essential to help the wastes on their way and cut the transit time to a shorter, healthier length is fibre (SEE *Constipation* pages 282–6).

In countries where fibre is eaten naturally in the diet, transit time is about 30 hours. For us in the West it can be three days in youngsters, or as long as two weeks in older people. Although fibre almost always accelerates the transit time, if this is very fast the fibre may actually act in the opposite way and slow it down. Colonic pressure – the pressure measured inside the bowel – is lower with plenty of fibre in the diet, and this is healthier too.

Fibre and disease

We have seen the influence that fibre has on bowel action and therefore on one of our Western scourges, constipation. Diverticular disease is a condition where pouches are formed in the gut from internal pressures generated by the muscular strain of pushing along hard, small faeces. Previously, this disease was treated with a bland, smooth diet; but now doctors are seeing the error of their ways and most are treating diverticular disease with a high-fibre diet which softens and increases the wastes so that they are moved along easily and quickly.

Piles (haemorrhoids) are thought to be largely due to the pressures of an overloaded bowel and the need to strain at stool.

These difficulties are relieved by dietary fibre. Because of its link with constipation, a fibre deficiency is thought to contribute to piles and varicose veins too (SEE pages 382–7).

Dietary fibre can help to reduce obesity. A high-fibre diet fills you up more so that you tend to eat less. Fibre has little or no calories, needs a lot of chewing, and can also decrease the absorption of other foods.

Researchers have found that diabetics on a high-fibre diet need less insulin, and the report on this work[2] concludes that certain types of dietary fibre may be useful in treating diabetics.

Unrefined carbohydrates are digested more slowly and sugars are released gradually, giving a steady, consistent supply of energy. This is unlike the fast rise of blood sugar after a meal of refined carbohydrates, which puts a strain on the pancreas, forcing it to respond by pouring out large amounts of insulin. An overworked pancreas can lead to disbetes. The treatment of diabetes with a high-fibre diet is given further encouragement in the Royal College of Physicians' Report which concludes that replacing refined carbohydrates in the diet by whole carbohydrates could reduce the risk of non-insulin-dependent diabetes. The slower absorption of foods eaten with their natural fibre means that fibre is also helpful in the treatment of low blood sugar (SEE *Low Blood Sugar*, pages 340–5).

Links have been traced between heart disease and the eating of refined carbohydrates, but conclusions are hard to pin down. People on high-fibre, low-fat diets (for instance, vegetarians) tend to have low blood cholesterol levels, and on the whole they suffer less from heart disease. 'Fibre', says surgeon Denis Burkitt, 'modifies the metabolism of cholesterol and bile acids, both of which are implicated in the causation of gallstones and coronary heart disease – although there would be many other factors as well.'[3] Burkitt, a leader in dietary fibre research, points out that a high-fat diet is always a low-fibre diet, and a high-fibre diet is always a low-fat diet.

A high-fibre-diet tends to lower the blood pressure of hypertensive patients[4] but this is hard to measure because the drugs used for this condition can cause the blood pressure to fluctuate. High pressure predisposes people to heart disease.

Small, hard, slow-moving stools increase the risk of large bowel cancer. The longer transit time of these stools means that the intestinal bacteria have more time to change the digestive bile acids and food pollutants into potentially cancer-causing compounds, and these compounds have more time to work on the bowel lining too. Dietary fibre, by diluting carcinogens and giving a naturally faster transit time, helps to protect against this.

Fibre needs to be thoroughly chewed and during this process the particles act abrasively on the teeth, helping to keep them clean and massaging the gums and thereby helping to prevent tooth and gum disease. The thick saliva produced by fibrous foods is thought to protect the stomach against over-acidity.

Conrad Latto, former consultant surgeon at the Royal Berkshire Hospital in Reading, insisted before operating that his patients take bran, to reduce the risk of thrombosis. This was continued after surgery. In the eight years that he followed this practice he had only one case of a clot in the lung – the man would not eat his bran! It seems, therefore, that fibre helps to prevent deep vein thrombosis.

Irritable bowel syndrome has been successfully treated with fibre, which is helpful for many other diseases. For instance, hiatus hernia, a common condition where a small pouch of the stomach protrudes through the diaphragm, is thought to be caused by straining at stool. This need to strain can be abolished by adding fibre to the diet.

Although it is generally thought that only the fibre found in cereals is effective, research has also shown that pectin, the fibre found in the skin of fruits, vegetables and sunflower seeds, will lower blood cholesterol levels and increase the amount of cholesterol in the wastes given off by the body.[5] It appears, therefore, that although cereal fibre is thought to be the most important, fruit and vegetable fibre has its uses too and demands further investigation.

In conclusion, the Royal College of Physicians' Report says that, in identifying illnesses directly connected with a lack of fibre, 'the clearest indications come from disorders of the bowel function – constipation and the spastic type of the irritable bowel syndrome. When we pass from what may be regarded as the direct effect of fibre increasing stool bulk, the benefits become less clear cut, but may still be appreciable.'

Fibre and . . .
There is one vitally important point that needs to be made. *Fibre is not a substance in isolation.*

If a person eats plenty of fibre, he is, in addition, getting the nutrients which accompany it. If he takes his fibre in wholemeal bread, he will also be getting all the vitamins, minerals, protein and oil which are wrapped up in the whole grain used to make the bread. If he takes his fibre in fruits and vegetables, he is getting all the benefits associated with these foods. Unless you feed somebody with fibre on its own in a laboratory experiment, you cannot rule out the fact that the benefits of fibre may be partly due to the nutrients included in the whole cereals, fruits and vegetables which contain it.

This argument also applies to bran. Readers will see from Table 1 (page 40) that bran contains several minerals and some vitamins together with a little protein and fat.

To discuss the benefits of fibre fairly, therefore, we must include the benefits that both whole cereals (containing bran, endosperm and germ), and whole fruits and vegetables can give us.

This rather complicates what we all thought was a nice simple issue. . . .

The argument against fibre
Fibre contains phytate, which has been thought to impair the absorption of zinc, iron and calcium.

Researching into the impaired absorption of zinc which occurs with the consumption of wholemeal bread and other fibre-rich foods, Dr John Reinhold of the Pennsylvania Nutrition Research Project carried out studies into the

1: Average analysis of Allinson Natural Broad Bran

Grams per 100 grams

Dietary fibre	*44.00*
Protein	*14.10*
Fat	*5.50*

Milligrams per 100 grams
Minerals

Sodium	*28.00*
Potassium	*1160.00*
Calcium	*110.00*
Magnesium	*520.00*
Iron	*12.90*
Copper	*1.34*
Phosphorus	*1200.00*
Zinc	*16.20*
Sulphur	*65.00*
Chlorine	*150.00*

Vitamins

B1 – thiamine	*0.89*
B2 – riboflavin	*0.36*
B3 – niacin	*29.60*
B5 – Pantothenic acid	*2.40*
B6	*1.38*
Biotin	*14.00* micrograms
Folic acid	*260.00* micrograms
Vitamin E	*1.60*

By kind permission of Allinson.

different kinds of bread eaten in Iranian villages. He established that villagers eating a lot of unleavened wholemeal bread were indeed deficient in zinc. However, in those places where the wholemeal bread was made with yeast from a leavened dough like Western bread, he found no mineral deficiencies, even though in some villages bread makes up 75% of the total diet.[6] Leavening the bread, it appears, destroys the phytate.

Commenting on the alleged malabsorption of calcium caused by phytate, leading fibre expert Denis Burkitt wrote to me; 'it is a complete red herring that phytate in binding

2: Percentage of dietary fibre in food

	%
Wheat bran	44.0
100% unrefined wholemeal flour	9.6
85% extraction flour	7.5
Refined white flour (for comparison only)	3.0
Soya flour	14.3
Wholemeal bread	8.5
Hovis (UK)	4.6
White bread (for comparison only)	2.7
All-Bran	26.7
Puffed Wheat	15.4
Weetabix	12.7
Shredded Wheat	12.3
Grapenuts	7.0
Muesli (Country Store – this figures varies according to brand)	7.4
Ryvita rye crispbread	11.7
Rice, brown, boiled	5.5
Rice, white, boiled (for comparison only)	0.8
Almonds	14.3
Fresh coconut	13.6
Brazil nuts	9.0
Peanuts	8.1
Hazelnuts	6.1
Corn on the cob, boiled	4.7
Spinach, boiled	6.3
Broccoli tops, boiled	2.9
Spring greens, boiled	3.8
Brussel sprouts, boiled	2.9
Cabbage, boiled	1.8
Cauliflower, boiled	1.8
Celery, raw	1.8
Fruit, fresh	0.5 to 4.5*
Fruit, dried	7 to 24*

From The Composition of Foods *by A.A. Paul and D.A.T. Southgate (HMSO). Last two entries* from* Nutrition in General Practice, *1.11.79, by Sheila Bingham.*

calcium can have ill effects. The calcium is actually liberated again further down the bowel.'

Probably adaptation to phytate in the long term is the common-sense view, since we have been eating foods complete with their fibre for thousands of years.

In our enthusiasm for bran, we should perhaps bear in mind that we are in fact adding a substance to our food which has been removed from the germ and starchy endosperm with which it grows. Even bran, therefore, could be called a 'refined' food – because the germ and the endosperm have been refined out of it. Although its addition to our food can be very beneficial, bran on its own is sometimes a little indigestible, particularly for the elderly. It can cause flatulence for a week or two in anyone of any age who is not used to it, and should be started gently (please SEE *Constipation*, page 282, for more advice on taking bran).

Sources of dietary fibre
Eat wholemeal bread, wholegrain pastas, wholewheat flour, (digestive biscuits are made from wholewheat flour), brown rice. Many breakfast cereals now are whole cereals or contain added bran. When possible eat vegetables in their skins – scrub them, do not peel them (potatoes, for instance).

Eat nuts, dried fruits, lentils, peas and beans; these are all good sources of fibre.

The foods in Table 2 (page 41) contain good percentages of fibre.

Recommended reading
Don't Forget Fibre in Your Diet by Denis Burkitt (Martin Dunitz 1979)

The Modern Food Industry

'There is now a battle being waged in every supermarket in the land for space in your stomach and intestines.'   DR RICHARD MACKARNESS

To discuss the part that the modern food industry plays in our lives, we must start with the soil.

Cold Comfort Farm . . .

The topsoil, from which our crops are harvested and on which our animals graze, is teeming with life. It contains bacteria, fungi, worms and other creatures, which enrich the humus and help to produce the nutrients taken up by the plants and later by the animals. Soil fertility depends on its micro-life.

Farmers apply artificial fertilizers direct to their soil in an attempt to produce better crops. When soluble, these chemicals can be toxic to the soil population. With few bacteria in it, and therefore less humus, the soil can easily become poor and eroded by wind and rain. The farmer then applies yet more fertilizer to try to put matters right.

Artificial fertilizers crowd out other minerals naturally present in the soil. So nowadays many soils – and therefore many crops – are deficient in minerals. The application of chemical fertilizers made up of only a few minerals impedes the uptake of the others and unbalances the whole mineral pattern. Many crops lack potassium, for instance. Liming can prevent the release and uptake into the plants of cobalt, nickel, manganese and zinc. Superphosphate can lead to a copper deficiency and prevent the uptake of niobium and vanadium.

Plants become less resistant to disease, and less nourishing for the animals and for us. Nitrate fertilizers increase the total crop yield – but they depress the quality of the protein harvested; in general the protein content of our crops is falling.[1] The vitamin C content of Brussels sprouts is affected by the manganese level in the soil. Nitrogenous fertilizers can affect the vitamin B2 levels in spinach crops.

Plants vary, therefore, in their nutritive value according to the value of the soil in which they grew. A plant cannot change one element into another. If it has iron, copper, zinc, calcium, potassium and phosphorus in its makeup, these elements must have come from the soil in which it grew. If the plants are mineral-deficient, then obviously the cattle eating those plants and grazing on that grass will be too.

The body can adjust if necessary to low intakes of a mineral. But at what cost? This question is largely unanswered.

'Organic' can mean several things. In a sense, plants always grow organically – that is, working together with the life in the soil and dependent on it. But in this context, 'organic' means 'produced without artificial fertilizers or pesticides' (*Concise Oxford Dictionary*).

It has been found that cows fed on organically grown crops give more milk on less feed.[2] Some German research has shown that organic manure, plus nitrogen potash and phosphate fertilizers, gives the highest yields and the best quality crops. Perhaps it is possible to combine the cruder benefits of artificial fertilizers with the natural, more balanced influence of compost and manure.

The demands of the food industry, however, do not mean that only our crops, and as a result our meat, may be nutritionally unbalanced. Besides fertilizers, other chemicals come into the picture. Crops are sprayed to kill off insects and prevent disease. Peaches, apples and cherries are sprayed on the tree and will carry spray residues when sold; one fruit may have several different sprays on it. Once a crop has been treated with an insecticide or solvent mixture, there is often no known way of removing the residue. The sprays become part of the fruit, vegetables and grains thus treated. Fruit is sometimes artificially coloured, and growth-promoting hormones and other chemicals are used by farmers to protect animals and crops from pests and to increase yield.

Synthetic hormones are planted into the flesh of livestock, and antibiotics and tranquillizers are added to feed. Fish and poultry are dipped into antibiotic solutions.

Crops and animals near smelting plants or busy road junctions can carry an accumulation of lead, and fish in water into which factory effluent is discharged can contain mercury and other harmful chemicals. These amounts are only rarely enough to be obviously toxic. But the damage being done may well be subtle, building up over many years. This slight poisoning can clearly be seen in people who are sensitive to the chemicals and who suffer an allergic reaction to them.

Our daily bread
What is in the supermarket wet cardboard? If this is the Staff of Life, is it safe to lean on it?

Once again, let's go back to the crop itself.

Modern strains of wheat have been developed for high gluten and carbohydrate yield, often at the expense of the balance of nutrients found in the previous strains. The oil content of modern wheat, for instance, is lower.

When the wheat has been harvested, the grain is separated out and the bran and wheat germ removed. The remainder of the wheat grain – the starchy endosperm – is used for the white flour from which most of our bread is made. Flour is processed at different percentages of extraction; 70% extraction means that the flour contains 70% of the original germ and bran, and 95% means that it contains correspondingly more. In his book *The Food and Health of Western Man* Dr James Lambert Mount states that *'the reinstitution of flour of extraction rate 95–100 per cent would do more for the health of this country's people than any other single measure in the field of nutrition'* (Mount's italics).

Flour refining is carried out by steel rollers, which finally brought this process to a peak of efficiency when they were introduced round about 1880. Besides removing the germ and the bran – the most nutritious parts – the rollers operate at high speeds and temperatures and therefore the fragile B vitamins, vulnerable to heat, can be destroyed.

In an attempt to put something back, regulations passed in 1963 (and amended in 1972) require white flour to have iron, niacin, thiamine and calcium added to it. This does not stop white flour, however, from being lower in magnesium by 40%,

3: The modern food industry

The refining of flour to 70% extraction rate involves the following losses of nutrients from wholewheat flour:

Fibre	80%
Vitamin E	100%
Pyridoxine	84%
Thimaine	80%
Biotin	77%
Nicotinic acid	77%
Folic acid	68%
Riboflavin	67%
Pantothenic acid	50%
Manganese	85%
Magnesium	75%
Phosphorus	70%
Potassium	50%
Iron	50%

Trace elements: Lithium, Boron, Copper, Cobalt.

From The Food and Health of Western Man *by James Lambert Mount (by kind permission of Precision Press, Publishers).*

chromium by 71.4%, cobalt by 69.4%, copper by 69.8% and zinc by 77.4% than whole, unrefined flour.[3] Other nutrients removed from white flour are vitamin E, some protein, all the bran, most of the B vitamins including riboflavin, pantothenic acid, pyridoxine, folic acid and biotin. Table 3 shows how many nutrients are lost.

It is often argued that in unrefined flour there is more phytic acid, and that this acid prevents the body from taking up zinc, calcium and iron. But most of the phytic acid is broken down by the yeast during baking, so it does not cut down the zinc uptake if the bread is leavened, as it usually is.[4] I am told by fibre expert Denis Burkitt that the calcium is in fact satisfactorily absorbed by the body.

The toxic mineral, cadmium, is found in increased amounts in white bread, because white flour consists of the endosperm part of the grain where cadmium collects. The cadmium/zinc ratio in wholewheat flour is only 1/65, but in refined flour it is 1/26.[5]

Additives used in the making of white bread and other refined flour products include:

BLEACHING AND IMPROVING AGENTS
Chlorine dioxide
Potassium bromate
Ammonium or potassium persulphate
Benzoyl peroxide
Chlorine (cake flours)
Sulphur and dioxide (biscuits)

EMULSIFYING AGENTS
Super glycerinated fats
Stearyl tartrate
Lecithin

PRESERVATIVES
Propionic acid
Calcium or sodium propionate
Acetic acid
Mono calcium phosphate[3]

It is not possible to discuss all these additives. They are not all suspect – lecithin is a valuable nutrient. But calcium propionate, which keeps bread fresh, inhibits the enzyme which enables the body to assimilate calcium (it is however naturally present in cheese). Chlorine dioxide destroys the vitamin E content in white flour – what there is left of it.

It is not surprising that Dr Richard Mackarness, trying stoneground wholemeal flour on some of his patients who were allergic to white bread, found that they could tolerate wholemeal bread quite happily. He concludes that the chemical manipulation and treatment of white flour may make it allergenic.[6]

White flour, by depriving the body of the natural fibre it needs in order to work properly, is one of the factors believed to be responsible for the modern outbreak of colon and related diseases which increasingly plague Western man (SEE *Fibre* pages 35–42).

One experiment which seems to support the nutritional value of white bread is that conducted by McCance and Widdowson and reported in the Medical Research Council report 287. Some German children were given white bread with their food and their fellows were given wholemeal. At the end of the experiment, there were no differences in the health of the two groups.

This work however was only conducted over a year, so caution was expressed by the two scientists in their conclusion. The children in both groups were in fact eating an above-average diet, excellent in many respects, from which it would have been easy for their bodies to make up the deficiencies existing in the white bread. Unfortunately, this is not always the case.

It can take twenty years for people to develop the chronic diseases such as diverticular disease and piles which are thought to result from a lack of fibre in the diet.

Let's not get cranky and be afraid to eat a couple of biscuits because they are made of refined flour and refined sugar. The occasional cake or biscuit will obviously make little difference.

But bread is a staple food and many of us eat it several times a day. The fact that wholemeal bread has more nutrients – including fibre – than white has been established by analysis and we should not expect the other foods in our diet to make up for our refined, denatured bread.

How many refined, processed foods, lacking in essential nutrients, can we eat before we no longer have any 'fail-safe' foods to fall back on?

Convenience foods

'Convenience foods are assumed to be eaten infrequently and are thus subject to more lenient additive regulations'.
SHEILA BINGHAM, *Nutrition*

'It has been predicted that in 1980 no less than 80 per cent of all the housewife's food purchases will be in convenience form.'   ALLAN CAMERON, *Food – Facts and Fallacies*

Convenience foods are lovely. Just open a packet or a can and – hey presto! – everybody can sit down and eat.

Eat what?

Convenience foods have to be tough. They have to withstand storage, handling, transport, freezing, reheating, and still stay acceptable to the public. Since the 1960s, there has been a boom in these foods, and in the development and use of chemical stabilizers, flavours, extenders, colours, preservatives and antioxidants to keep them fresh and help them sell in a cut-throat market. The additive market in the UK is now worth about £150 million a year. Food technology has grown during the last hundred years to cope with the size and complexity of modern society and it is assumed that foods which will stay fresh and delicious indefinitely are both desirable and inevitable. The housewife is encouraged by seductive advertising – particularly on television – to associate convenience foods with easily prepared, delicious meals and the shining faces of her happy family.

Food, however, is supposed to nourish us as well as taste good and fill our stomachs. Two main things happen to the convenience food before it reaches your plate. Firstly, essential nutrients are taken out. Secondly, chemical additives are put in.

Vitamins and minerals Let's look at what happens to the vitamins and minerals in our food while it is being processed, starting with the vulnerable and essential vitamin C.

When stored, spinach can lose half its vitamin C in 24 hours. Vegetables which are blanched before being canned, frozen or dried lose from 10% to 50% of their vitamin C, depending on the method used. Deep frozen vegetables can lose 30% to 55% of their vitamin C – but they may still contain more, when frozen, than their wilting greengrocer counterparts. This vitamin is reduced by about 15% in a canned vegetable, depending on the temperature and length of storage, and up to

20% loss occurs in fruits which are freeze-dried. Air drying may destroy all of it.[7]

The thawing of frozen meat can cause up to 40% loss of the B vitamin thiamine. Heating foods to process them causes loss of vitamins A, C and E, and the B vitamins. Canning, which involves heating the vacuum-sealed food in a salt or sugar syrup for about half an hour, destroys nearly half the B1 content; other losses are C, the other B vitamins, and minerals which leach into the liquid and which may be poured away (canned spinach was found to have lost 81.7% of its manganese, 70.6% of its cobalt and 40% of its zinc). Frozen peas and beans are washed in EDTA which removes essential minerals.[8]

Processing, therefore, depletes the original vitamin and mineral content of the food.

Additives Today's corpse keeps longer. There are more preservatives in it – from today's food. This may be good for the undertaker. But is it good for the corpse?

Food additives are used to improve the appeal and lengthen the shelf-life of convenience foods. Not all additives are suspect. Some have been used for centuries and are relatively harmless – sugar, salt, vinegar. Some are good for you – lecithin and vitamin C. But the number of these additives is increasing every year, and many of them are the subject of debate. These chemicals are tested on laboratory animals before being released and put on the market. But they are only tested for causing cancer and cell damage – and only on animals. Dr B.F. Feingold, who has pioneered additive-free foods as a treatment for hyper-active children, writes, '. . . the time-honoured idea that synthetic additives can be judged simply from routine carcinogenic and mutagenic standards is out of date and dangerous. Advances in medical science would indicate that neurological and behavioural effects may now be added to the examinations. It is folly to assume that a synthetic chemical, declared free, within limits, of acute toxic properties, is also automatically free of damage to various body systems.' It has been found that many people thought to be allergic to certain foods are only allergic to the additives in them. For instance, some people react with respiratory distress to the fungicide impregnating citrus fruit packed in crates.

In any case, a laboratory animal is not a human being. Their physiology differs from ours in many respects. Ulcerative colitis can be produced in the guinea pig by a vegetable gum called carrageen which is quite harmless to us. Why not the other way around? Several additives have passed laboratory tests without having had any effects on the animals, but have afterwards been banned as further information came to light.

There is no single, universally accepted test for measuring the harm which may be done by additives. Most additive tests, as well as being limited to cancer and mutagenic damage, are short-term and do not tell us what happens over the long span of a *human being's* life. The laboratory animals are killed and dissected after they have been eating the additive, but this will only show up evidence of obvious harm, and not any subtle changes that may have taken place.

This way of testing each individual chemical on its own is really more suitable for drugs. Because additives *are not taken alone*. They are eaten, year after year, together with other additives in our food, and should therefore be tested in this way. Dr Michael Crawford in his book *What We Eat Today* comments that the safety standards of new drugs have been rigorously tightened in recent years, and it is time that a similar tightening was applied to food additives. Dr G. Roche Lynch, Home Office pathologist, toxicologist and world authority on forensic medicine, also expresses doubts about the safety of additives and this concern is echoed by an editorial in *The Lancet* of 16 August 1979 – 'the question of the *ultimate effect* (my italics) of food additives on man is still unanswered'.

Nitrates and nitrites are salt-like chemicals added to meats to preserve them and give flavour and colour. Both combine with certain amines to form nitrosamines, which can cause cancer. They are used in preserved meats, sausages, salami, hot dogs, hamburgers and canned meats.

Trans-fatty acids are produced when fats are hydrogenated to make them last longer. It is thought that, when repeatedly heated, trans-fatty acids can change cell membranes in such a way that carcinogenous substances can pass through more easily. This could happen to the oils used in a fish and chip shop. When burnt, frying oils can also contain acrolein, a poison. Rancid foods often contain a harmful chemical, malonaldehyde, which is formed when fatty acids decompose. Stale cholesterol, which has been found to harm the arteries of laboratory animals more effectively than fresh, is often found in powdered whole milk, smoked foods, and some cheeses.

It is true that all food is a collection of chemicals. But over the centuries we have been eating, in general, the right collections of chemicals for us. What is disturbing – and dangerous – is that we are putting other chemicals in our food which do not add to its nutritive value and which are completely new to our bodies. The effects of these chemicals, *in the way in which they are taken by us*, have not been tested.

Books mentioned in this section
The Food and Health of Western Man by James Lambert Mount (Precision Press 1979)
Nutrition by Sheila Bingham (Corgi 1977)
Food-Facts and Fallacies by Allan Cameron (Faber 1973)
What We Eat Today by Michael Angus Crawford and Shelagh Crawford (Spearman 1973)

Protein

The word *proteios* is Greek for 'first, holding first place'. The Dutch chemist Mulder who gave protein its name described it as 'unquestionably the most important of all known substances in the organic kingdom. Without it, no life appears possible on our planet.'

We are about 20% protein. It makes up skin, hair, nails, cartilage, muscles and tendons and the organic framework of our bones. We need protein for metabolism and to maintain our internal environment – for instance to control the water balance in the tissues. Protein is necessary for the formation of antibodies to fight infection.

Of our food, only protein has nitrogen, an element essential for life, and since nitrogen is constantly being excreted from the body, it must be replaced.

Protein can be compared to a house built of bricks. There must be as many different kinds of houses built with bricks as there are architects to design them. But the kinds of *bricks* are limited. The bricks from which the proteins are made are known as amino acids, and there are about 20 of them. It is, of course, the way the bricks are put together that makes one house different from its neighbour. And in the same way it is the many *combinations* of amino acids which make the proteins different from each other.

Of these 20 or so amino acids, eight are vital because they cannot be made by the body (children need nine). These substances are called the essential amino acids or EAAs, and they need to work together. Their names are isoleucine, leucine, lysine, methionine, phenylalanine, threonine, tryptophan, valine and perhaps histidine. We have an internal pool of amino acids from tissue breakdown, digestive secretions and food, and this pool helps to even out any temporary imbalance.

During the digestion of protein it is broken down into its component amino acids which can then be used by the body cells. Each type of cell has a distinctive protein need. Many proteins carry vitamins and minerals along with them, and enzymes (which facilitate chemical processes) are made of protein.

We have seen that it's the building bricks, the amino acids, that matter and not the proteins themselves; the parts and not the whole. But it's the whole we see, of course, when we tackle the steak on our plate, or cut a piece of cheese, or sprinkle wheat germ into a dish. And this brings us to the sources of protein.

It is found in meat, eggs, seafood, dairy foods (milk including skimmed milk, cheese, yogurt), soya and soya products, nuts, seeds and pulses (peas, beans, lentils), wheat germ, wholegrains, brewer's yeast, sprouting seeds and grains. Because wholegrains contain the germ they have more, and possibly better, protein than refined grains.

Some proteins are more 'complete' than others. Animal origin foods are known as complete proteins because they contain all the EAAs in a pattern closest to what our cells need. The proteins in grains and pulses, on the other hand, have incomplete amino acids (more about this later). Soya beans and sprouting grains, both exceptions to this rule, are complete (SEE Table 4, page 53). The alga spirulina is also complete.

The part we can use
We have to remember that protein, before it can be used by the

4: Protein content in grams per 100g of some foods

Food	Completeness	Protein
Whole liquid milk	complete	3.3
Natural low-fat yogurt	complete	5.0
Dried skimmed milk	complete	36.4
Fresh eggs	complete	12.3
Cornflakes	incomplete	8.6
Oatmeal	incomplete	12.4
Cottage cheese	complete	13.6
Cheddar cheese	complete	26.0
Beef, cooked stewing steak	complete	30.9
Chicken, roast, light meat	complete	26.5
Tinned salmon	complete	20.3
White fish fillets	complete	17.4
Spaghetti	incomplete	13.6
Dried prunes	incomplete	2.4
Dried apricots	incomplete	4.8
Dry lentils	incomplete	23.8
Rice	incomplete	6.5
Wholemeal bread	incomplete	8.8
White bread	incomplete	7.8
Bacon rashers, cooked	incomplete	24.5
Roasted peanuts	incomplete	24.3
Marmite	complete	39.7

From MAFF Manual of Nutrition *(HMSO 1982).*

body, must be digested. The blanket term used to describe both a food's biological value and its relative digestibility is Net Protein Utilization, or NPU. The NPU of a food is the percentage of absorbed protein that your body can actually use. Here, we're in for a surprise.

Although steak is about one quarter complete protein, it does not rate first on the NPU scale. In other words, it does indeed contain all the EAAs we need, and in the right patterns too, but only about 67% of its protein can be used; it has therefore an NPU of 67. The highest scorer on the NPU scale (apart from human breast milk) is the egg at 94. This means that almost all the egg's protein will be usable when it is digested. Milk and yogurt come next, with an NPU of 82 (but remember that milk is only 4% protein in any case), and seafood follows with an NPU of about 80. (This figure does not apply to shark but I'm assuming you don't often eat it.) Cheese has an NPU of about 73. The NPUs for vegetable proteins are comparatively low, and I will say more about this later.

So we can look at protein in several different ways. First, is it complete or incomplete? Secondly, how much protein is there in the food? And lastly, how much of that protein actually goes where it needs to go inside us?

How much do we need?

How much protein you need is an individual matter and scientists can only give estimates. We in the West are more likely to be getting too much rather than too little. Are your skin, hair, nails in good condition, and do you heal quickly if you get a cut? If these parts of you are working well then you are probably getting enough.

If you want an estimate, things get more complicated. You should base your allowance of grams of protein per day on an NPU of 75% efficiency, which applies to a person eating half animal and half plant protein. Using this basis, a 58k (9st 2 lb) woman will need about 47 grams of protein a day, and a 70k (11st) man 57 grams. This would also apply to the person eating milk and other dairy foods but no meat. You can work it out yourself by multiplying your weight in pounds by .37 or by .8 for kilograms. Children need proportionately more; boys and girls of 7 to 8 years need about 45 grams a day, rising to 67 grams a day for boys from 15 to 17 years and 50 grams for girls between the same ages. A pregnant woman needs about 52 grams a day during the third to the ninth month of her pregnancy, and a lactating woman needs about 60 grams.

The situation is a little different if you are a vegan (a person who gets all his protein from grains and vegetables and eats no meat or dairy foods). Since, as we have seen, plant proteins have low NPUs (about 55) and are incomplete, we need more of them to make up the same amount of protein. An adult woman weighing 9st 2lb would need therefore about 64 grams (you can work this one out very simply by changing your weight into pounds and halving it), and an 11st man about 77. A pregnant vegan needs about 106 grams at 9st 2lb, and if she breast feeds her baby she will need, at the same weight, 93 grams. A vegan child needs, again, proportionately more.

These are averages and not minimums, and include a 30% safety margin for extra needs. For instance, if you are working in a hot climate where you sweat a lot, or if you are deliberately building muscle in an activity such as weight-lifting, then you will need extra protein, and this will also be the case if you are under any physical or mental stress. It is possible, too, that your individual make-up demands more protein.

In the unlikely event of your not getting enough calories (units for making energy), your body will use protein to make energy. Conversely, carbohydrates have a 'protein sparing' action, in that enough carbohydrates in your diet will free the proteins for the jobs they were meant to do.

Too much?

This is quite likely. Several nutritionists, particularly in America, have recommended very high protein intakes in the past – up to 200 grams – but these are now falling into disfavour. In the developed world we probably eat from 2½ to 3 times more protein than we need. All surplus protein leaves a residue which has to be eliminated by the kidneys and a high-protein slimming diet, for instance, can over-work them. Flesh foods create acidosis and help to form uric acid which can cause artery damage and rheumatic problems. When proteins are cooked, their structure is changed to a less digestible form and meat in particular makes putrefactive acids, putting a strain on the liver. Excess protein can lead to a calcium deficiency even though plenty of calcium is eaten, and possibly also to a shortage of vitamin B6. It can also be laid down as fat.

It has been established with laboratory animals that lots of protein for the youngsters – who need it – and much less for the adults results in longer lives and better health. Animals fed this way have better resistance to stresses including injuries, extremes of temperature, infections and strenuous activity. Researchers at the University of Minnesota say it may be possible to prevent cancer by restricting protein intake and Dr W.J. Visek of Cornell University comments that ammonia (a waste product of protein digestion) fills several criteria of a cancer-producing agent.

It seems, then, that lots of protein is needed by our children, and proportionately less by ourselves. We are also advised to eat a wide range of proteins.

Which brings me to my last point.

Complementary proteins

As we saw earlier, the NPUs of vegetable proteins are low compared with those of meat and dairy products, and their proteins are incomplete. This would appear to mean that, in order to get enough complete proteins from vegetable sources, we have to chomp our way through mountains of lentils and sunflower seeds every day; not an attractive prospect.

There are plenty of healthy people walking around who never eat meat – some cut out dairy foods as well. They don't need to stuff themselves to the brim with vegetables. How do these people get their proteins right?

People who use the cheaper proteins – grains, nuts, dairy foods – stay healthy because the proteins they eat complement each other. The essential amino acids in these foods combine, so that an EAA deficiency in one food is made up for by its presence in another without making it necessary to over-eat. Recent research, too, tells us that there are more complete proteins in some vegetables than we had thought. Some people can even live very healthily on just fruit and nuts only – but a change-over to this way of eating should be very gradual.

In fact, we can *boost* our protein absorption by a judicious combining of different foods whose amino acids balance each other. A molecule of the EAA lysine from a bean is identical to a molecule of lysine from a piece of beef. So 'by combining different proteins in appropriate ways, vegetable proteins cannot be distinguished nutritionally from those of animal origin. The amino acids and not the proteins should be considered as the nutritional units.'[1]

This combining has been done traditionally for centuries in many countries; rice and beans for instance are eaten together by many peoples. Look at the following table to see how these foods balance up their EAAs:

EAA	RICE	BEANS
Isoleucine	Low	High
Lysine	Low	High
Tryptophan	High	High

This is called Protein Complementation. We can make a list of the various ways we can arrange plant proteins so that they complement, and boost, each other:

1   Mix grains with legumes (e.g. pea/bean soup and a sandwich; rice and beans).
2   Mix legumes with seeds (e.g. legumes/seeds and nut loaf; sunflower/sesame meal in legume soup).
3   Mix milk, milk products or eggs with any or all plant proteins (milk and grains are especially good, e.g. wholegrain cereal with milk; bread and cheese).

To sum up, foods with no serious amino acid deficiencies are meat, seafoods and dairy products. These foods need no supplementation from other foods. But we can mix other, usually cheaper, sources of protein and, by eating a mixture of proteins, we can increase the nutritional value of the meal.

Recommended reading
Readers who want to know more are encouraged to read *Diet for a Small Planet* by Frances Moore Lappé (Ballantine Books, 1976). Also recommended is *Bean Feast* by Rose Elliot (White Eagle 1975).

Salt

There were once two daughters of a fairy-tale king. At a banquet, the king asked each of his daughters what was the most necessary flavouring for the food. 'Sugar' replied one of them and 'salt' the other. The king laughed at his second daughter, but soon changed his mind after he had ordered the banquet to be served without salt; no one would eat it.

Salt makes food come alive. It has always been considered valuable and it was once used as money; Roman soldiers once received a salt allowance, called a salarium, from which comes our word salary. The chemical name of the salt we use in our food is sodium chloride. This is a combination of sodium and chloride.

All salt is mineral, some occurring in liquid form – in the sea, of course, but in many lakes too. Traces of sodium are found in most crops and natural pasturelands; it finds its way into the cattle and from them into us. Sea creatures consume vast quantities of salt and this is passed on to us too.

Sodium helps muscle action, the transmission of nerve impulses and water distribution throughout the body. Our tissues and blood are salty, and we need about ½–1 gram of salt a day. We are not likely to run short of salt; rather the reverse. Occasionally however in very hot climates excessive salt is excreted with sweat and this can cause muscular cramps. (A severe deficiency, which can sometimes happen after diarrhoea and vomiting and certain hormonal and kidney disorders, will cause fatigue and mental apathy, nausea, dizziness, respiratory failure.)

Salt occurs naturally in foods. But we also add it, both during and after cooking. People add salt because it makes food more tasty, not because they need it. A normal diet, with salty foods, salt in cooking and on the table, gives about 10 grams a day. An enthusiastic salt-sprinkler can add another 10 grams a day to this intake. There is no such thing as a completely salt-free diet, but by not adding salt to our food we can achieve a low-salt diet.

In his book *This Nutrition Business*, John Yudkin makes the point that 'sodium is the only nutrient that we need but take in amounts so very much more than we need'. The first effect of too much salt is abnormal retention of liquids. Salt causes the cells to take in water and expand. The kidneys have to work extra hard to get rid of the excess salt and water, they become overworked and we get water-logged. This liquid retention (oedema) tends to rob tissues of oxygen, creating or contributing to circulatory problems, arthritis, and reduced visual, auditory and tactile sensations. This oedema is shown by an increase in weight. Joint and muscle stiffness in the morning can be caused by salt-induced oedema. There has to be an increase in heart action to increase the blood pressure and kidney action so that the extra salt can be excreted. Babies in particular have small kidneys which cannot cope with a lot of salt. Too much salt can form deposits inside the arteries and interfere with enzyme activity. It is also thought to displace calcium.

With some heart conditions causing oedema, a low-salt diet is prescribed (but please note that if you drink water filtered through a water softener, this alone will load you with sodium). As the excess salt is excreted, the oedema disappears.

Max Gerson (SEE *Cancer, The Gerson Therapy* pages 277–80) believes that a high salt intake is related to cancer and other diseases. People deprived of added salt for a time, or who have never used it, can react with toxic symptoms after taking it.

Research shows that in areas in Japan where lots of salt is eaten, there are many deaths from heart attacks, stroke and high blood pressure. Little of the mineral potassium is eaten in these areas too – more about this below.

The 1970 US report on Recommended Daily Allowances for nutrients states that adults should keep their salt intake down to 9 grams or less a day and infants under six months should have only 113 to 350 *milli*grams a day; this estimate is based partly on the salt taken in by breast-fed children. Elderly people in particular have lost some of their ability to deal with salt and should therefore keep down their consumption.

Salt . . . and potassium
Things, however, are not as simple as this.

Sodium does not work in isolation in the body. It has a special relationship with the mineral potassium. These two minerals must be in the right balance with each other and their relationship is made more effective by trace amounts of other minerals, notably magnesium. Potassium is critical to muscle contraction, notably the heart muscle; very low potassium can even lead to cardiac arrest. Extra potassium is needed by people who sweat a lot and potassium and sodium work together to keep the body's fluids in balance. Sodium is found mostly in the fluids circulating outside the cells, and potassium mostly inside the cells. These two minerals also help other substances to keep the right balance of acid and alkali in the blood and are essential parts of glandular secretions.

Too much salt is widely accepted to be linked with high blood pressure. Research has found that the ratio of potassium to sodium in the body has proved to be a more accurate index of blood pressure than just sodium alone.[1]

Dr Herbert Langford of the University of Mississippi states that potassium probably helps the kidneys get rid of excess salt, and the Canadian Medical Association *Journal*, as long ago as 1928, reported that potassium regularly produces a decline in blood pressure, while sodium just as regularly produces a rise.

This relationship between sodium and potassium is

5: Sodium and potassium in some processed and unprocessed foods

100 grams	mg of sodium	mg of potassium
Unprocessed foods		
Flour, wholemeal	3	360
Rice, polished	6	110
Pork, uncooked	65	270
Beef, uncooked	55	280
Haddock, uncooked	120	300
Cabbage, uncooked	7	390
Peas, uncooked	1	340
Pears, uncooked	2	130
Processed foods		
White bread	540	100
Rice, boiled	2	28
Bacon, uncooked	1400	250
Beef, corned	950	140
Haddock, smoked	790	190
Cabbage, boiled	4	160
Peas, canned	230	130
Pears, canned	1	90

From The Composition of Foods *by McCance and Widdowson (HMSO 1978).*

discussed in a letter from Dr Hugh Towell published in *The Lancet* for 22 July 1973. Dr Trowell asks for further research into the protection which potassium seems to afford against too much salt. He suggests that high blood pressure should be treated, not only by cutting salt, but by putting up the intake of potassium too.

Dr Trowell makes the point that when we were hunter/gatherers, we ate plenty of potassium in fruits, vegetables and whole cereals. The little salt we took was a natural part of our food.

Now, modern diets contain more sodium than potassium. A look at Table 5 (above) give striking proof that processed foods have a lot of salt added and a lot of potassium taken away. Cooking, too, leaches potassium away from vegetables into the cooking water. Some liquid slimmers' diets, which do not contain any potassium, can cause dangerous irregularities in the heartbeat, or worse.

So it's not just a question of avoiding too much salt. It also makes sense to include plenty of potassium-rich foods in our diet (SEE *Minerals* page 91 for a complete list).

Salt as a seasoning

Supermarket salt is refined. It has had all its minerals except sodium and chloride processed out, and usually an anti-caking agent added, such as magnesium carbonate. Iodized salt contains between 430 and 700 micrograms of iodine per ounce and half a level teaspoon supplies enough for half our estimated daily needs of iodine.

Rock salt and sea salt have more minerals, besides sodium, than ordinary refined salt. Recent work from the Brookhaven National Laboratory has, however, cast doubt on the purity of some sea salt – not surprising with our increasingly polluted oceans. Both rock and sea salt lack their original iodine, which evaporates in natural light.

It is sensible to buy your salt, or salt substitute, from your health food store. 'Ruthmol' contains no sodium; it is made up of potassium chloride. 'Biosalt' is a biochemically sound combination of minerals, including both potassium and sodium. Other substitutes include vegetable salt and ground kelp. (Potassium salt substitutes must be avoided on the low potassium diets used for some kinds of kidney disease.)

Books mentioned in this section
This Nutrition Business by John Yudkin.

Sugar

Sweet and High

We nibble our way through mountains of sugar. Between 1900 and 1970, world sugar production rose to 70 million tons. Indeed, sugar is replacing starch in our diet; since 1880

consumption of wheat and potato has fallen by half and that
of sugar doubled – a bonanza for Mr Cube. Since the early
eighteenth century, when sugar was an occasional treat, our
use has multiplied nearly 25 times, and we now eat a hefty
110lbs (about 50kg) per year *each*.

'Impossible,' you may think. 'I've given it up in tea and
coffee!' But it's not as simple as that. For in addition to the
sugar in chocolates and other sweets, there is also sugar in
cakes, biscuits, soft drinks, sauces, many 'quick' dinners, fruit
yogurts, jams and breakfast cereals. Tomato ketchup is 22.9%
sugar, dairy ice cream 22.6%, sweet pickle 32.6%, supermarket muesli 26.2% . . . there is even sugar in some tinned
and frozen vegetables, salad dressings and dried soups.

One of the reasons for our sweet tooth may be that, when
we were living in trees, the sweetest fruits were the ripest. But
the big difference now is that the sugar we use has been
separated from its natural source, so that we just spoon sugar
on to our strawberries instead of getting it by munching sugar
cane or sugar beet (the only two plants used today for the
manufacture of sugar). Sugar is also widely distributed in other
foods, especially in fruit.

What is sugar?

'Sugars' are the basic chemical units of all carbohydrates and
the most fundamental of all foods. Plants make simple sugars
in changing sunlight into food. Wood, the oil in a peanut, the
protein in a grain of wheat, the perfume of a rose all begin,
one way or another, as sugar.

Sugars include glucose, fructose, maltose, lactose, and
sucrose (composed of glucose and fructose). This last is the
one that concerns us most.

Raw sucrose from sugar cane and sugar beet goes through a
long process of purification before it reaches your sugar bowl.
In the first stages, impurities are removed and the molasses
(SEE pages 124–5) taken out – to feed cattle or perhaps turn
up in your local health food store. Later in the process, raw
sugars including Barbados, Muscovado and Demerara are also
extracted, and at the end of the process we are left with the
familiar white sugar.

Sugar cane sap, at the beginning of the refining process,
contains some vitamins and minerals. Also present in crude
sugar cane juice is a factor which protects the teeth from the

fermenting materials which cause decay. This factor is destroyed early in the processing, but the mineral and vitamin content remains up to the raw sugar stage and can be found in Barbados and other less refined sugars. (London Demerara, however, is made by simply colouring white refined sugar with molasses or syrup.) Thus the refining process removes not only dirt and other impurities but also the few nutrients that unrefined sugars can boast about. Maple syrup does a little better – it contains calcium, phosphorus, potassium and sodium – and golden syrup has a trace of B vitamins. But molasses, raw cane sugar and other crude sugars still contain sucrose, too.

The browner the natural colour of the sugar, the more easily digestible it tends to be. In his book *Sports Injuries*, Dr Christopher Woodard, honorary consultant to the British Olympic teams in 1948 and 1952, says 'the best forms of sugar in order of digestibility are brown sugar, honey, treacle and white sugar.'

At the end of the refining process we are left with white sugar, according to Tate and Lyle one of the purest foods known. In fact it is so pure that, as John Yudkin says in *This Nutrition Business*, 'Sugar is the only one of our foods that is absolutely and entirely free of nutrients.'

How to be fat, toothless – but sweet

Sugar is a boon to the food manufacturing industry. It is extensively used in food processing not only as a sweetener but as an activator, preservative, anti-coagulant, in fermentation, frozen food manufacture and in bulking (i.e. ice cream). Additionally, heavy sucrose syrup provides, according to the British Sugar Bureau, an 'attractive mouth feel to the product'.

In reply to scientists who say that sugar is just empty calories, the sugar manufacturers' claim that 'the expression "empty calorie" is a derogatory phrase used by those who attack white sugar because they say it provides the body with energy alone. This, however, is an oversimplification which assumes that the omission of white sugar from the diet would lead to the consumption of other foods containing more essential nutrients.' But if we omit the empty calories in sugar we can then eat a smaller amount of more useful calories which contain the nourishment we need. Since a calorie is just a way of measuring heat, *all* calories (including those in sugar) give you heat – i.e. energy. Sugar gives you nothing else.

Because it doesn't fill you up, refined sugar encourages you to overeat. Your body needs B vitamins and chromium in order to metabolize sugar and too much sugar can induce a deficiency of these, notably vitamin B1 (thiamine). In experiments a sugar-rich diet tended to cause digestive upsets, and the *British Medical Journal* has pointed out that pure sugar is an irritant that often causes eczema on the hands and arms of those handling it. This does not happen with unrefined sugar.

Perhaps the researcher best known for his forthright views on sugar is John Yudkin. He found that sugar increases the amount of uric acid in the blood, which can lead to gout. He repeated the assertion, made 30 years before by Sir Charles Best, that an excess of sugar can have the same effect as alcohol on the liver, making it fatty; it has also been linked to hyperactivity in children. But Yudkin's main interest has beem the relationship between sugar and heart disease.

This is the subject of a great deal of argument; different researchers blame different factors (SEE *Heart and Artery Disease* pages 309–24). Evidence has been put forward by Yudkin and his team that excess sugar consumption is statistically associated with atherosclerosis (artery disease) and heart attacks. These results have been duplicated by others, which means this must be considered a strong possibility.

Another strong case has been made for a relationship between sugar consumption and diabetes. When we eat sugar or starch, glucose is released during digestion and passes into our bloodstream. The level of blood sugar, therefore, goes up with the entry of the glucose. At this point the pancreas releases insulin, which lowers the blood sugar to normal again, chiefly by changing the glucose into glycogen and storing it in the muscles and liver for later use. The sucrose in sugar is absorbed into the blood very rapidly and easily – much more so than starch and proteins. (Incidentally, this rapid rise in blood sugar levels is parallelled by similar rises in blood fat and blood pressure levels.)

When someone eats large quantities of sugar, the pancreas is constantly asked to produce more insulin and becomes overworked. This results in a 'trigger-happy' pancreas, followed by pancreatic exhaustion and eventual failure. This, broadly speaking, is one road to diabetes.

People can of course be addicted to sugar and, less commonly, to refined starches. The sugar you eat gives you a quick lift, but then the insulin lowers your blood sugar, you feel hungry and depressed again, and you want more sugar.

Lastly, there is the effect we all know about on our teeth. Sugar combines with salivary bacteria to form plaque, a sticky white substance coating the teeth. An acid is produced in the plaque which attacks the teeth, and this acid production is made easier by a substance, dextran, which forms very readily from the sucrose in sugar.

The sugar we eat in processed foods is not necessary to health, and that applies to brown sugar as well as white. There are natural sugars in the fruits and vegetables we eat, and starches such as cereals and starchy vegetables are changed to sugar during digestion. Even meat contains some starch, which is turned into sugar by the body. In fact, about 65% of the food we put into our mouths is turned into sugar – full quota for anyone without ever going near a sugar bowl.

Books mentioned in this section
Sports Injuries by Christopher Woodward
This Nutrition Business by John Yudkin

Tea and Coffee

We take tea and coffee for granted. Factory workers down tools with relief when the tea-break comes – and they will strike to keep it. Teachers retire to the staffroom in playtime, leaving their charges to exchange blows behind the sports shed while they gratefully sip the cup that cheers. In an office where I worked once, the coffee machine broke down. 'Is it mended yet?' haggard people would ask, supporting themselves in the doorway.

So tea and coffee seem to be necessary to us. 'It's so lovely', said an overworked friend, 'just sitting in a coffee bar doing nothing.' For it's not just the drink that matters. It's the break from work, the chance to put your feet up and talk, or just think things over. While the world continues to rush by outside you are safe, idle, licensed to relax.

Most people have the good sense not to sip all day. Try downing several cups of coffee at once and – unless you're a hardened case – you will probably find that your heart is beating more quickly and you feel nervous. Gallons of tea aren't good for you either.

Coffee contains a drug, caffeine, which is a strong stimulant. Caffeine causes an increase in blood sugar, a small rise in blood pressure due to spasm of the small arteries and a slight heart contraction. It also stimulates the brain so that we feel more alert and can think more quickly. But after this initial boost the effects wear off as the blood sugar falls again and we are back where we started. This can create a vicious circle as the fatigue temporarily lifted by the coffee clamps down again, and we need another cup.

Tea has much less caffeine, but it also contains tannin, another stimulant, which can interfere with the absorption of iron. Coffee and tea – indeed too much of any liquid – produce more urine, and this will wash away essential nutrients. The chlorogenic acid in coffee burns up vitamin B1 (thiamine), and tea can also cause a mild B1 deficiency. Both contain oxalic acid, which can damage the kidneys and rob the body of calcium.

There are some illnesses during which coffee and tea should not be taken.

One cup of coffee causes a rise in blood fats, including cholesterol. Because of this, and its stimulating effect on heart action, it should not be taken by people with a heart condition. Tea has no effect on blood fats and little on heart action.

Weak kidneys are adversely affected by the alkaloids in tea and coffee. Coffee has more effect on kidney action, stimulating circulation in the kidneys and, because it increases urine flow, it is harmful to those suffering from irritations of the bladder and prostatic enlargement. An article in the *British Medical Journal* (May 1976) indicates that too much coffee drinking may increase the risk of bladder and kidney cancer.

Sufferers from high blood pressure should not take either tea or coffee. The caffeine causes a rise in basal metabolism (the rate of 'resting' body processes) and is harmful to the circulation. In people with hardened arteries, the effects of caffeine on the circulation are stronger and longer-lasting.

Coffee dilates the blood vessels in the skin, so it should be avoided by those with inflammatory skin conditions because it may make the irritation worse. Since it affects the blood vessels in the eyes, too, it should also be cut out by those with glaucoma.

Both tea and coffee stimulate the secretion of gastric juices, so they should be avoided by sufferers from stomach complaints, especially ulcers. Too much tea also delays the digestion of starch, and many migraine victims have found that coffee can trigger off an attack.

Coffee poisoning occurs more often than tea poisoning because coffee is stronger. A cup of brewed coffee contains between 100 and 150mg of caffeine; instant coffee contains less – between 86 and 99mg. Tea trails behind with 60 to 75mg, and cola drinks have 40 to 60mg per glass. Decaffeinated coffee comes in last with 2 to 4mg. An intake of over 250mg a day is considered harmful.

The American Food and Drugs Administration in an announcement dated 4 September 1980 advises pregnant women to limit the amount of caffeine they consume. A link is suspected between caffeine consumption and birth defects and this is being investigated.

Symptoms of coffee poisoning include insomnia, nervousness and irritability, an oversensitive skin. When the coffee addict gives it up he may get withdrawal symptoms – lethargy, nervousness, headaches. These unpleasant things rarely happen even with large quantities of tea.

Finally, Dr Richard Mackarness, a pioneer of food allergy in this country, has found that coffee is one of the main foods causing an allergic reaction in vulnerable people. High doses of caffeine can cause feelings of panic and anxiety.

Before you fling this book aside and plant geraniums in the coffee-pot, however, remember that many healthy people drink both tea and coffee in moderation without coming to any harm. Dr E.K. Ledermann puts the whole thing in a nutshell, 'moderate drinking of tea and coffee is clearly an acceptable social habit for healthy people, but the taking of excessive cups is something different.'

Readers might like to visit their local health food store to have a look at the herbal teas, grain coffees and so on, which offer harmless alternatives to their usual brew.

Vitamins and Minerals

Introduction

Vitamins and minerals are essential in varying quantities for life, growth and health. In some cases vitamins can be built up by the body, but minerals can never be produced by living cells, and have to come from our food.

Vitamins are mostly catalysts in a wide range of functions. Minerals influence chemical substances passing into cells, control the distribution of water and influence the action of glands, muscle responses and the transmission of nerve impulses. Vitamins and minerals work together, and they need each other. For instance, a deficiency of one may mean that some others are incompletely absorbed and cannot be properly used by the body. A person whose diet is rich in vitamin E will be able to use more of the vitamin A he gets – and so on.

There is still a lot of argument about how much of each vitamin or mineral we actually need. Recommended Daily Allowances are the amounts thought to be needed to satisfy the requirements of an average individual in good health, but we are all different in our nutritional needs, which vary as much as our finger-prints do. 'Some individuals, in the case of specific nutrients, may need from two to ten times as much as others. Each individual has a pattern of his own. . . . The information that is available with respect to calcium and several amino acids (proteins) for example, points clearly to the conclusion that five-fold variations are by no means uncommon.'[1]

The problem, therefore, is how to assess the actual amount of each nutrient which is needed for each person in order for him to be in the best possible health. These needs are also affected by body weight; generally speaking, the bigger you are, and the more you eat, the more you need. Needs also go up for children, pregnant or lactating women, the elderly, athletes and others involved in strenuous activity, and people getting over illness.

Doctors usually say that if we follow a 'good mixed diet' we don't need any additional supplements. This phrase is one of the most useless that we have around at the moment. What is 'a good mixed diet'?

It is true that if we eat a wholefood diet we are less likely to need vitamin or mineral supplementation (SEE *Whole Foods* section, pages 101–6). But even this is not certain. Whole foods are often hard to get and can be expensive. Storage and cooking can destroy nutrients.

So supplements have their place. But they are no substitute for the best eating we can manage. It is no good living on doughnuts and coffee and gulping down supplements, expecting them to do the job for you. Vitamins and minerals work as a team, as we have seen. Even a complete range of supplements, making you rattle like a pillbox, won't supply the trace elements and still unrecognized factors present in whole foods.

However consultant Alex Forbes said to me, somewhat despairingly, 'there are some people who are never going to follow a wholefood diet; they just won't. For them, if you're going to help them, supplements are needed.' Added vitamins and minerals, if you are healthy, are an extra bonus, an extra insurance; the icing on the cake. If you are ill, they can – hand in hand with a good diet – work near miracles in bringing you back to health.

Vitamins are measured in grams, milligrams, micrograms and International Units (g, mg, mcg, I.U.). The United States Pharmacopeia Units (USP) is sometimes used, but any other ways of measuring vitamins are very rare. The gram measurements are used when the vitamin's strength is always the same. This is a measure of quantity. International Units are used when there may be variations in the vitamin's potency. Mineral dosage is calculated in milligrams.

A natural vitamin is analysed in the laboratory and a synthetic counterpart can sometimes be built up; much argument rages over whether it is in fact identical to the natural substance. Vitamins are not found in nature in a concentrated form, so that large doses can often only be supplied by using the synthetic version. Synthetic minerals do not exist.

Some mineral supplements have the word 'chelated' on the label. This means that the inorganic mineral has been wrapped in a protein molecule, building a fence round the mineral and protecting it from chemical reaction within the intestinal tract. This is thought to increase absorption and utilization of the mineral within the body.

Once opened, vitamins should be kept in the fridge. Their effectiveness tends to decline with age, so it's better not to stockpile them. Vitamin preparations with a shelf life of less than three years must declare the expiry date on the label. Most last longer than this. Minerals are stable and do not deteriorate. Usually all supplements should be taken during or after a meal.

Finally, you must take your nutritional supplement for several months to give it a chance to work.

Throughout this section
1   *Wholegrains* include all unrefined cereals, wholemeal flour and brown rice.
2   *Seeds and nuts* also include the *unrefined* oils which are pressed from these foods.
3   Research continues into *sprouting seeds and grains*, and I have listed them as a natural source of vitamins and minerals only where their content has been established and published in the *Journal of Food Science* 1975. This does not mean that they do not contain some, or all, of the other vitamins and minerals listed here (SEE *Sprouting Seeds and Grains* pages 133–5).

Vitamins

Vitamin A
A fat-soluble vitamin. Can be stored by the body. Works with zinc and vitamin E. The pre-formed version retinol is found in eggs, milk fat, fish liver oils and organ meats especially liver.

A precursor of this vitamin – carotene – is found in carrots and green vegetables. It is converted by the body into vitamin A.
Functions Promotes growth, healthy skin and mucous membranes, good eyesight, good hearing and sense of smell, healthy teeth, gums and bones. Needed for reproduction, production of nucleic acid. Helps protect against cancer, air pollution. Works with C to heal wounds; applied directly alone will help to heal wounds.

Deficiency signs Night blindness, sore itching eyes, dry mouth, dryness of other mucous membranes; skin troubles, colds and other respiratory troubles, susceptibility to other infections, possibly excessive menstrual bleeding.

Needs raised by Cold weather. High-protein diet. Pregnancy and lactation, growth. Diabetics can be deficient.

Destroyed by Food processing, which can destroy about 40%. The food chemicals nitrates and nitrites. Air pollutants.

Natural sources Milk, butter, eggs, liver, fish, fish oils, carrots, watercress, spinach, the darker outer leaves of cabbage and lettuce, kale, broccoli, corn, cherries, watermelon, apricots, peaches.

Recommended daily allowance (Doses of 50 000 I.U. daily incur the danger of vitamin A poisoning if continued over prolonged periods in adults; children react to less than this. Please consult your practitioner.)

Babies – about 1400 I.U.

Children – about 1800 I.U.

Teenagers – about 4000 I.U.

Adult men and women – about 4000 I.U.

Pregnant and lactating women – about 5000 I.U.

The B Vitamins

The commonly known B vitamins work hand-in-hand (this excludes B13, 15 and 17). So, if you are taking a single B vitamin supplement, it should be taken with a diet especially rich in B vitamins in general – this means plenty of wholegrains, wheat germ, brewer's yeast and organ meats. B vitamins are water-soluble and cannot be stored by the body. So we need them every day. If you drink too much fluid – particularly too much coffee – they can be washed away. They are often thrown away in the cooking water.

If you suddenly start eating a lot of vitamin-B rich foods, you may suffer from flatulence for a while, but this will disappear. It is a sign that you have been deficient. Because of their fragility, widespread deficiencies of these vitamins are probably quite common. Most of the B vitamins are used up by the body in the digestion of refined carbohydrates; unrefined carbohydrates bring their own B vitamins with them.

Vitamin B1 – Thiamine

Functions Helps to use carbohydrates, turn glucose into fat, produce energy. Nourishes nerves, brain, maintains mental alertness. Controls stomach secretions, maintains muscle tone in digestive tract, heart. Essential for growth, healthy cells, healthy red blood cells. Has been used to help alcoholics.

Deficiency signs Poor memory and concentration, weakness, appetite and weight loss, bad nerves, depression and mental confusion, constipation, digestive problems, insomnia, dizziness, palpitations, discomfort in feet and legs. Deficiency may contribute to over-active thyroid, liver disease, glaucoma, cancer, low blood pressure, neuritis. Notably lacking in heart patients. Severe deficiency causes beri-beri.

Needs raised by Ageing, alcohol, sweating, stress, strenuous exercise, pregnancy and lactation, growth, eating a lot of refined sugars and starches, smoking.

Destroyed by Antibiotics, food processing and grain and rice refining, coffee, air, water, heat, alkalis such as baking powder. Partly destroyed by the chlorine in tap water.

Natural sources Whole grains, bran, organ meats especially liver, beef, ham, molasses, brewer's yeast, split peas, soybeans, sunflower seeds, wheat germ, skimmed milk, pulses, nuts, eggs; sprouting seeds and grains.

Recommended daily allowance

Babies – about 0.4mg

Children – about 0.9mg

Teenagers – about 1.4mg

Adult men and women – about 1.3mg

Pregnant and lactating women – about 1.6mg.

Vitamin B2 – Riboflavin

Functions Helps thyroid function, oxygen transport, conversion of fats, proteins, sugars into energy. Essential for growth, tissue maintenance. Detoxifies. Essential for healthy bodylining tissue. Helps protect against cancer.

Has been used for pregnancy cramps, to help cataracts, to reduce cancer in laboratory animals.

Deficiency signs Blotchy, purplish tongue, inflammation of mucous membranes, tiny wrinkles round mouth, 'twilight blindness', intolerance of eyes to light, blurred vision, bloodshot smarting eyes, scaly oily skin eruptions, oily hair, tiny blood vessels near skin, fatty deposits like whiteheads under skin; shaking, muscular weakness, dizziness, fatigue, appetite loss, bad nerves, possibly liver damage.

Deficiency can produce anaemia, will also reduce amount of folic acid available to liver, can cause personality disturbances.

Deficiency has produced malformed offspring in laboratory animals.

Needs raised by The Pill, pregnancy and lactation, growth, sweat, tears, stress, illness, alcohol.

Destroyed by Tranquillizers, antibiotics, heat, light. Destroyed in milk irradiated to produce vitamin D and in milk left on doorstep.

Natural sources Organ meats and muscle meats, wholegrains, milk, wheat germ, brewer's yeast, bran, eggs, cheese, yogurt, green leafy vegetables, tomatoes, potatoes, apricots, fish, peas, sprouting seeds and grains.

Recommended daily allowance

Babies – about 0.5mg

Children – about 1.0mg

Teenagers – about 1.5mg

Adult men and women – about 1.6mg

Pregnant and lactating women – about 2.0mg.

Vitamin B3 – Niacin

(Nicotinic acid, niaminamide, or nicotinamide)

Functions Helps brain function, utilization of fats, proteins, carbohydrates.

Nicotinic acid dilates blood vessels and can cause flushes and prickling; this is not the case with niacinamide. Nicotinic acid has been used to improve circulation in the elderly.

Has been used to treat schizophrenia, migraine, alcoholism, arthritis, and to lower high blood cholesterol.

Deficiency signs Blotchy skin, inflamed fissured tongue, appetite and weight loss, digestive problems, sore gums and mouth ulcers, depression, tension, hostility, instability, anxiety, forgetfulness, insomnia, headaches. May help to cause diarrhoea.

May contribute to hyper-activity or retardation in children.

Severe deficiency causes pellagra.

Needs raised by Eating a lot of refined sugars and starches, the Pill, pregnancy and lactation, alcohol, illness, stress, ageing, growth.

Destroyed by Cooking, heat, antibiotics, water.

Natural sources Organ and muscle meats, wholegrains, fish, brewer's yeast, wheat germ, nuts, bran, eggs, sunflower seeds,

sprouting seeds and grains, some in fruit and vegetables.
Recommended daily allowance
Babies – about 6mg
Children – about 12mg
Teenagers – about 17mg
Adult men and women – about 16mg
Pregnant and lactating women – about 19mg.

Vitamin B5 – Pantothenic Acid
(calcium pantothenate)
Human muscle has about twice as much as that of other
animals, and we can make a little in the gut.

It is argued that we need a lot, and that there is probably
widespread deficiency. Although this vitamin is widely
distributed in foods, it is easily destroyed.
Functions   Normal working of intestinal tract. Needed by the
adrenal gland for resistance to stress. Spreads throughout
body, vital to every cell; changes sugars, fats into energy, uses
PABA (SEE page 77) and choline. Helps create antibodies
against infection, with B6 and folic acid. Moderates allergic
reactions.

Has been used with calcium to treat tooth grinding
(bruxism). Has been used for arthritis and to protect against
stress.
Deficiency signs   Bad nerves, skin itching and burning, faulty
sense of balance, vomiting and weakness, insomnia, colds,
rapid heartbeat, cramps, headaches, dizziness, lowered
resistance to infection and stress, constipation.

Deficiency can contribute to low blood sugar, appears to
influence growth of hair, may cause birth abnormalities.
Needs raised by   Stress, convalescence, surgery, alcohol,
probably pregnancy and lactation, growth.
Destroyed by   Heat, canning, cooking, freezing, processing.
Natural sources   Organ meats, wheat germ and brewer's
yeast, bran, egg yolks, whole milk, royal jelly, wholegrains,
leafy green vegetables, soybeans, sunflower and sesame seeds,
peanuts, cod ovaries, sprouting seeds and grains.
Recommended daily allowance
Not specified.

Vitamin B6 – Pyridoxine
Functions   Helps the use of amino acids, fats, substances

essential for brain and nerve function, formation of blood, muscle operation. Essential for building tissues, synthesizing lecithin, controlling blood cholesterol. Works with magnesium to maintain magnesium level in body. Activates many enzymes. Helps the body to use iron.

Affects hair growth, colour and texture, condition of skin; may help to prevent dental decay, cancer. Has been used to treat asthma, skin allergies, seborrhea (oily skin), mild diabetes; also (with potassium) heart troubles, (with magnesium) teenage acne. Has been used in treatment of piles, migraine, radiation sickness from cobalt therapy, travel sickness, morning sickness, palsy, rheumatism and as a diuretic.

Deficiency signs (World-wide studies show that artery disease sufferers have low levels; the Pill leads to a B6 deficiency in *over 75%* of the women using it.)

Cardio-vascular troubles, dizziness, bad nerves, insomnia, depression, poor balance, headaches and fatigue, eczema, anaemia, neuritis, leg cramps and nausea in pregnant women, brain disfunction.

A deficiency causes in turn a shortage of niacin, contributes to some forms of liver damage, and to kidney stones of oxalic acid; may encourage tooth decay.

Needs raised by   Pregnancy and lactation, growth, the Pill, a high-protein diet, stress, drugs, alcohol, smoking, pollution, the menopause.

Destroyed by   Cooking, canning, light, long storage.

Natural sources   Bran, wheat germ, brewer's yeast, molasses, wholegrains, organ and muscle meats, egg yolks, bananas, fish, pulses, nuts, soybeans, sunflower seeds, raw peanuts, avocados, prunes, raisins, sprouting seeds and grains.

Recommended daily allowance

Babies – about 0.3mg

Children – about 1.0mg

Teenagers – about 1.8mg

Adult men and women – about 2.0mg

Pregnant and lactating women – 2.5mg – but many researchers now believe that 4–10mg a day could be needed (*Nutrition and Health*, Vol. 1, No. 2, 1982).

Vitamin B12
Unusual in that, although it is water-soluble, this vitamin can be stored in the body.

A complex vitamin; needs an 'intrinsic factor' produced by the stomach in order to be absorbed.

Some people can make their own B12 in the gut; this vitamin is made during fermentation.

A fraction only is needed.

Functions Works with folic acid to form blood cells, utilize fats, proteins, carbohydrates. Influences growth, fertility, resistance to infection. Protects myelin (protective sheath) covering spinal cord and other parts of nervous system; protects eyes from damage from tobacco smoke. The remedy for pernicious anaemia.

Has been used to treat heart disease, blood vessel disease, skin conditions, displaced spinal disc, asthma, some cancers, confusion in elderly people, night cramps. Some visual defects yield to it.

Deficiency signs (Vegans are sometimes deficient.) Damage to blood formation and nervous system, weakness, diminished reflexes and sensory perceptions, grooved and fissured tongue, weight loss, poor memory, stomach and chest pains, depression, fatigue, pins and needles in legs, breathing problems.

Needs raised by Stress, illness, the Pill, other drugs, alcohol, pregnancy and lactation, growth.

Destroyed by Light, strong acid/alkali solutions.

Natural sources Raw liver, other raw organ meats (some in cooked meats too), milk, some raw fish, raw eggs. Spirulina (a form of alga), obtainable at your health food store, contains a lot. Dulse (a form of seaweed) can contain some.

Many health food manufacturers offer foods containing B12. Please consult your local health food store.

Recommended daily allowance

Babies – about 0.3mcg

Children – about 1.5mcg

Teenagers, adult men and women – about 3.0 mcg

Pregnant and lactating women – about 4.0mcg.

Folic Acid

(folate or folacin)

Functions Essential for division of body cells and production of substances carrying our hereditary patterns, growth, utilization of sugars and proteins, working of nervous system. Helps make antibodies. Needed before pantothenic acid can be used. Works with B12, C and zinc.

Deficiency signs (Deficiencies thought to be widespread.) Increased susceptibility to infection, insomnia, memory lapses, loss of weight, irritability, depression and fatigue, paleness, shortness of breath, headaches, a type of anaemia (can mask a deficiency of B12), 'restless legs'.

A deficiency can worsen low blood sugar. Severe deficiency causes megaloblastic anaemia, mental retardation and can contribute to a difficult labour, weak baby.

Has been used for schizophrenia, circulatory problems.

Needs raised by Lactation, pregnancy (especially the last three months of term), lactation, growth, alcohol, stress, illness, old age (elderly people are often less able to absorb it); antibiotics, some infections.

Absorption may be blocked by the Pill.

Destroyed by Light, air, heat, storage, cooking, processing.

Natural sources Organ and muscle meats, dark green leafy vegetables (especially spinach), citrus fruits, wheat germ, brewer's yeast, soybeans, lima beans, nuts, wholegrains, orange juice, bran, turnips, potatoes.

Recommended daily allowance

Babies – about 50mcg

Children – about 200mcg

Teenagers, adult men and women – about 400mcg

Pregnant and lactating women – about 700mcg.

PABA
(Para-aminobenzoic acid)

One of the components of folic acid; can be made by intestinal bacteria. Little research has been done on this vitamin.

Functions Essential for growth, health of skin and intestines. Helps utilize proteins, produce blood cells. Protects against sunburn, helps heal eczema. Needed by folic acid, pantothenic acid.

Deficiency signs Digestive problems, bad nerves, depression. Said to be associated with greying hair and fatigue.

Has been used to treat skin cancer and as a sunscreen.

Needs raised by Alcohol.

Destroyed by Sulpha drugs.

Natural sources Liver, brewer's yeast, wheat germ, molasses, eggs.

Recommended daily allowance Not specified.

Choline
Little research has been done on this vitamin.
Functions Helps nerves to communicate with muscles, helps to insulate nerve fibres, helps control blood pressure, works with inositol to prevent fatty liver. Essential for synthesis of nucleic acid in every cell. Helps resistance to disease. May be necessary for kidney function.

Has been used in the treatment of diabetes, gall bladder disease, muscular dystrophy, glaucoma, artery disease, headaches, constipation.
Deficiency signs Hard to spot. Usually associated with gall bladder trouble, cirrhosis of liver, hardening of arteries, poor memory, weakness. May cause rise in blood pressure.
Needs raised by High intake of saturated fats, refined sugars, alcohol, probably pregnancy, lactation and growth.
Destroyed by Not established.
Natural sources Organ and muscle meats, fish, eggs, wholegrains, green leafy vegetables, seeds, peanuts, soybeans, wheat germ, brewer's yeast, lecithin.
Recommended daily allowance Not specified.

Inositol
Little research has been done on this vitamin. There is a high concentration in the brain, heart, lens of eye. It can be manufactured by the body.
Functions Helps control cholesterol levels and elimination. With choline, breaks up fat in the liver.

Has been used, with vitamin E, to treat nerve damage as a result of muscular dystrophy; with niacin, has been used in the treatment of mental illness. May be useful for hardened arteries; is being used to treat anxiety; has a mild inhibitory effect on cancer.
Deficiency signs Baldness in some men.

Said to contribute to constipation, eczema, eye troubles, loss of hair, digestive problems.
Needs raised by Alcohol, possible pregnancy, lactation and growth.
Destroyed by Not established.
Natural sources Organ meats especially beef brains, muscle meats, fish, molasses, green leafy vegetables, wholegrains, nuts, wheat germ, brewer's yeast, seeds, citrus fruits, lecithin, soybeans.

Recommended daily allowance   Not specified.

Biotin
(sometimes called vitamin H)
Appears to be produced by intestinal bacteria. Little research has been done on this vitamin.

Functions   Involved in utilization of carbohydrates, proteins and fats, (especially unsaturated fatty acids), helps to form blood and glycogen. Necessary for growth, healthy skin, hair, sebaceous glands, nerves, bone marrow, sex glands.

Deficiency signs   Deficiencies are rare. Muscular pains, appetite loss, dry skin, disturbed nerves, fatigue.

Needs raised by   Not established. Probably pregnancy, lactation and growth.

Destroyed by   Cooking, refining, antibiotics. Raw egg white prevents absorption, but this is not likely to have a significant effect unless you almost live on raw eggs.

Natural sources   Wholegrains, meats (especially organ meats), molasses, wheat germ, bran, brewer's yeast, egg yolks, milk, peas, nuts, fish, sprouting seeds and grains.

Recommended daily allowance   Not specified.

Vitamin B13
(orotic acid)
Some researchers say it does not qualify as a vitamin at all. Can be made by the body.

Functions   Has a central role in the production of the basic body constituents, RNA and DNA. These control cell regeneration, repair and growth as well as determining heredity.

Has been used to treat multiple sclerosis, liver disease, and gout. May increase growth rate in children.

In laboratory animals, has been shown to accelerate wound healing, prevent heart damage, act against inflammation; with vitamin D3 will strengthen bones in rats; may help to prevent liver damage in laboratory animals.

Deficiency signs   Not established.

Needs raised by   Not established.

Destroyed by   Not established.

Natural sources   Milk, whey, root vegetables.

Recommended daily allowance   Not specified.

Vitamin B15
(pangamic acid, or pangamate)
This substance has been widely researched by the Russians. In the West, however, opinion varies from attributing to it almost all the characteristics of health to saying that it does not exist at all and therefore has no therapeutic effects. In other words, it is at present fashionable.

Has never been proved to satisfy the criteria for vitamin status, so it is more correctly termed the B15 factor, or preferably pangamic acid.

Functions Stimulates oxygen transport and improves the body's efficient use of oxygen. Because cells operate more effectively with more oxygen, and their life is prolonged, it is thought to delay ageing.

Stimulates body's protection against viruses and bacteria, helps to neutralize toxins. Keeps fat from infiltrating the liver to excess, helps to destroy toxic free radicals.

Because of its action in helping the production of anti-stress hormones it has been used by Russian athletes. It is also claimed to remove wastes from the blood more quickly, maintain normal blood sugar levels, promote building of muscle, restore reflex time, improve stamina and wind, increase tolerance for hard work.

Has been used by Russian doctors for treatment of heart disease, artery disease, high blood pressure; with A and E for treatment of intermittent claudication (a circulatory disease), alcoholism, emphysema. Research is taking place on its use for diabetics.

Deficiency signs   Not established.
Needs raised by   Not estabished.
Destroyed by   Not established.
Natural sources   Brewer's yeast, bran, whole cereals including rice, wheat germ, liver, sunflower and pumpkin seeds, other seeds, apricot kernels.
Recommended daily allowance   Not specified.

Vitamin B17
(also known as laetrile, or amygdalin)
Only provisionally labelled a vitamin.

This controversial substance 'contains powerful cancer-destroying agents which are only released when in contact with an enzyme that is found mainly in cancer cells' (Leon Chaitow,

An End to Cancer?). For a discussion of this vitamin and its place in cancer treatment, please SEE *Cancer – Laetrile* (page 275).

Vit...
(as...
Ca... , or stored to any
sig...
Fr... e universal anti-toxin;
h... lead, mercury, food
a... side-effects of drugs,
c... for immune system, is a
... anti-viral, anti-bacterial
... low temperatures and
... ls to work. Works with
... ro-adrenal system; with
... olism.
... vels. Essential for health
... d healing (has been used
... rayed on burns.
... of collagen (intercellular
... and for cell activity.
... High Density Lipoproteins,
... e heart to heal itself after a

... k and to reduce risk of clots in
... nt of diabetes, arthritis, deep
... *cer and Vitamin C* page 272).
... lay to prevent backache and
... xercise. May protect against
... ay protect against gallstones.
May ... luction. Much argument over
whether it prevents ... ds.
Deficiency signs Deficiency thought to be widespread, especially in the winter. If your gums bleed and you bruise easily you are probably low in vitamin C. Deficiency will affect the efficiency of all body tissues; is thought to be a cause of artery and heart disease. Blood fats tend to rise when the body is low in this vitamin.

Fatigue, weight loss and shortness of breath, rapid respiration and heart beat, anaemia, tooth decay and gum disease. Severe deficiency causes scurvy.

Needs raised by Growth, adolescence, old age, intense mental, emotional, physical activity – *any* stress, alcohol, smoking, pregnancy and lactation.

Destroyed by Cooking, light, heat, air, drugs.

Natural sources All fruits, particularly citrus fruits, blackcurrants, strawberries, papaya, tomatoes. All vegetables, particularly green peppers. Fruit and vegetable juices, watercress, milk, chicken livers, sprouting seeds and grains.

Recommended daily allowance Dr Richard A. Passwater in his book *Cancer and its Nutritional Therapies* states, 'I have found that some people reach their supernutrition point (optimum health) at 500–750mg, whereas a few need more than 4000mg.'

Linus Pauling and Ewan Cameron in their book *Cancer and Vitamin C* state, 'We believe that the officially recommended dietary intake of about 45mg of vitamin C per day is so much less than the optimum as to constitute in itself a significant cause of cancer. It is our opinion that to keep the age-specific incidence of cancer and other diseases low it is necessary that the daily intake be at least 250mg, and for most people a daily intake between 1g and 10g per day may lead to the best of health.'

200mg a day is recommended by Dr E. Ginter, PhD, in *Nutrition and Health*, Vol. 1, No. 2, p.66.

The following RDAs were suggested by the US Food and Nutrition Board in 1973

Babies – about 35mg

Children – about 40mg

Teenagers, adult men and women – about 45mg

Pregnant and lactating women – about 60mg.

Vitamin D

A family of nutrients. Fat-soluble, can be stored by the body.

Functions Vital for a healthy heart, nervous system, eyes, bones, teeth. Needed for the absorption of calcium and phosphorus, controls the enzymes which deposit minerals in bones and teeth. Helps to increase the loss of salt in the urine, helps energy release. Works with vitamin A and affects every function of the body that needs calcium.

Has been used in the treatment of arthritis, conjunctivitis, distended cornea of the eye.

Deficiency signs Bone weakness, backache, nervousness,

twitching, muscular cramps and spasms, unstable heartbeat, cramp, insomnia, nose bleeding. Severe deficiency causes rickets.

Needs raised by Pregnancy and lactation (babies need extra), growth, ageing.

Air pollution can block sunlight; people who do not get enough sunshine may lack this vitamin.

Destroyed by The Pill.

Natural sources This vitamin is formed by the action of sunlight on the skin, so go out in the sunshine, and don't wash everything off directly afterwards.

Food sources are fish liver oils, sunflower seeds, eggs, fish, margarine and butter, milk.

Recommended daily allowance High doses (between 10 000 and 50 000 I.U.) daily over long periods of time are harmful, and children react to less than this – please consult your practitioner.

Babies, children, teenagers, adult men and women, pregnant and lactating women – about 400 I.U.

Vitamin E
Composed of seven kinds of tocopherols; alpha tocopherol is the most active.

Fat-soluble; can be stored by the body.

This vitamin is still not fully understood.

Functions Reduces the cells' need for oxygen. Has been shown to reduce the heart's need for oxygen and in large doses has been extensively used to relieve heart conditions; will reduce the danger of unwanted clots, restore permeability of capillaries, speed up opening of additional (collateral) circulation round damaged veins; therefore valuable after a heart attack. Has been used, with selenium, to reduce angina pectoris, and helps intermittent claudication (a circulatory disease). Has been used in high doses for varicose veins, for night cramps and 'restless legs', for pain in osteoarthritis; has been used for eye problems and in diabetes.

Acts as an anti-oxidant, protecting the cells against the harmful effects of oxidation, and this probably explains its reputation as a delayer of ageing. Stimulates immune system, moderates allergic symptoms. Often effective in relieving menopausal symptoms; with C has successfully treated hot flushes. Sometimes recommended for a healthy pregnancy/birth. Protects the lungs against air pollution; moderates allergy symptoms; involved in the transport of energy and boosts athletic performance; has been used with vitamin A in treatment of acne, has been used in treatment of asthma. Said to help enzymic reactions, some hormone reactions, increase alertness/learning ability.

When applied directly to the skin, helps to prevent and lessen wrinkles, heal burns and other wounds; can be effective this way against warts.

May help to protect against radiation.

Has been shown to reduce cancer formation in laboratory animals. Very dependent on other nutrients, e.g. selenium. Protects vitamins A and C from oxidation in the body.

Deficiency signs Not well established in humans. Pigmentation and anaemia may be signs of mild deficiency.

Signs noted in animals include nutritional muscular dystrophy, testicle shrinkage and blood-vessel disorders.

A deficiency in laboratory animals causes irreversible sterility, which does not respond to subsequent doses of the vitamin.

Needs raised by Vitamin E is needed by the body when using polyunsaturated fats and oils. Unless these fats and oils are unrefined, vitamin E is processed out of them. Pregnancy, lactation and growth. Menopause.

Destroyed by The Pill is an antagonist of vitamin E, and more E is therefore needed by Pill takers.

Inorganic iron (such as is often given in supplements) combines with E and destroys it to some extent. This does not happen with the iron in food.

Natural sources Unrefined oils and wholegrains, parsley, mature broccoli, asparagus, spinach, outer cabbage leaves, almonds, walnuts, seeds, wheat germ, meats, corn, carrots, eggs, sprouting seeds and grains.

Recommended daily allowance (People with high blood pressure, heart disease or diabetes should not take high doses of vitamin E at first. Start with 100 I.U. per day and increase only under medical supervision; it can put up your blood pressure slightly for a time. In general, the more E you take the less you absorb, so the actual absorption of very high doses is probably less than expected.)

Babies – about 4 I.U.

Children – about 9 I.U.

Teenagers – about 12 I.U.
Adult men and women – about 14 I.U.
Pregnant and lactating women – about 15 I.U.

Vitamin F
The name sometimes given to the Essential Fatty Acids – (SEE *Fats*, pages 23–35) because its lack can cause a fat deficiency disease.

Vitamin K
A fat-soluble vitamin; some is made by bacteria in the intestines.
Functions   Helps the blood to clot.
Deficiency signs   Bleeding that will not stop.
Needs raised by   Ageing; babies, too, can be deficient.
Destroyed by   Antibiotics, anti-coagulants, aspirin, sedatives, some illnesses involving a defect in liver function or fat absorption.
Natural sources   Spinach, cabbage, lean meat, pork liver, peas, cauliflower, carrots, tomatoes, soybeans, potatoes.
   It is not advisable to take vitamin K as a supplement.
Recommended daily allowance   Not specified.

Vitamin P
(A group of vitamins also called the bioflavonoids, or vitamin C2)
Functions   Helps to strengthen capillaries, helps to reduce inflammation, may be involved in defences against cancer. Has a direct effect on platelet clumping, reducing it, thus increasing ease of blood flow; a natural anti-thrombotic factor. Has been used to strengthen capillaries, to control retinal bleeding in diabetics, for menstrual problems, varicose veins, piles. Almost any problem involving bleeding has been alleviated by bioflavonoids. Has been used as part of treatment for arthritis.
Deficiency signs   Not established.
Needs raised by   Not established.
Destroyed by   Water, cooking.
Natural sources   Citrus fruits (most in the white pith), green peppers, tangerines, grapes, apricots, cherries, tomatoes, papaya, broccoli, cantaloupe. Is found in nature together with vitamin C.
Recommended daily allowance   Not specified.

Minerals

Calcium

Comes in many forms. Can pass through the body – does not dissolve easily. The most abundant mineral in the body; 99% is found in the teeth and bones. Is stored in, and released from, the bones, and these deposits are completely replaced about every five years.

Functions Needed for muscle contraction including heart action, normal growth, strong bones and teeth, blood clotting, transportation of nerve impulses, control of fluids passing through cell walls, function of parathyroid hormones.

Helps to excrete blood fats, including cholesterol, from the body.

Relaxes nerves, induces sound sleep, decreases sensitivity to pain.

Needs oestrogen to hold itself in the bones. At the menopause therefore, when oestrogen production diminishes, calcium is released from the bones.

Works with phosphorus, magnesium, sodium, potassium. Works with vitamin C to strengthen collagen, the intercellular cement; works with vitamin C to form scar tissue after wounds and to heal bone breakages.

Is vitally connected with vitamin D; unless D is taken in the diet or absorbed from the action of sunlight, calcium is poorly absorbed and will be excreted.

Blocks cadmium (a poisonous mineral) absorption in laboratory animals. Competes with lead for storage in the bones in humans, therefore blocking it. Enough fat, not too much, helps calcium absorption.

Has been used for menstrual cramps, the relief of pain (i.e. with B6 for migraine; with B6 for leg cramps in pregnant women), for jaw shrinkage (SEE *Teeth and Food* pages 202–9).

Deficiency signs Cramps, irritability, bone-softening diseases such as osteoporosis in older people, rickets.

Deficiencies can occur at the menopause, when a lack of oestrogen allows calcium to be excreted. Deficiencies probably widespread, however, in all age groups. Calcium deposits in soft tissues can become *worse* with a calcium deficiency. Blood calcium levels drop just before menstruation.

Needs raised by Growth, pregnancy and lactation, strenuous exercise, the few days before menstruation, menopause. Concentrated refined carbohydrates decrease calcium absorption.

Destroyed by Prolonged bedrest (is excreted), some laxatives, water softeners. The boiling of vegetables leaves it in the water.

Natural sources Milk an especially good source, because absorption is helped by the milk sugar, fat, phosphorus and magnesium present.

Skimmed milk, bread, wheat germ, bran, nuts especially almonds, seeds especially sesame seeds, cheese, yogurt, soybeans, molasses, sardines, spring greens, seaweed and kelp, sprouting seeds and grains (particularly alfalfa). It is also present in hard water.

Recommended daily allowance

Babies – about 500mg

Children – about 600mg

Teenagers – about 1200mg

Adult men and women – about 800mg

Pregnant and lactating women – about 1200mg.

Iodine

Functions Iodine is needed by the thyroid glands. They produce a hormone called thyroxin, which needs iodine for its manufacture. Thyroxin has a profound effect upon growth, mental and physical development, and the maintenance of health.

Works with vitamin E.

Deficiency signs A mild deficiency is associated with the incidence of thyroid cancer, high blood cholesterol, heart disease.

A marked deficiency results in an enlarged thyroid, or simple goitre.

Needs raised by Not known. Probably pregnancy, lactation and growth.

Destroyed by Light.

Natural sources All seafoods including fish, shellfish, seaweed and kelp; nuts and unrefined oils, spinach. Also added to iodized salt; contained in Biosalt, a balanced salt obtainable from health food stores.

Recommended daily allowance
Babies – about 40mcg
Children – about 80mcg
Men – about 130mcg
Women – about 110mcg
Pregnant women – about 125 mcg
Lactating women – about 150mcg.

Iron

The body can save iron and use it again and again.

Functions Essential for the manufacture of haemoglobin, a protein in red blood cells. Takes oxygen to every cell in the body. Works with folic acid and in many enzymes; probably helps muscle function.

Deficiency signs (According to a World Health Organization report, at least one-fifth of the world's population is deficient. When the body runs short, the level of haemoglobin drops and the system does not get enough oxygen. This results in iron-deficiency anaemia. Blood donors are sometimes deficient, women are often deficient.)

Irritability, depression, confusion, apathy, fatigue, clumsiness, dizziness, paleness, sore tongue, appetite loss, hammering pulse after short bout of exercise, heartburn, nausea after meals, itching, headaches, brittle ridged nails, hair loss, scanty or over-heavy menstruation.

A deficiency may lead to pica – eating unnatural substances, i.e. lead, soil, etc.

Needs raised by Women need almost twice as much iron because they lose it during menstruation; they also store less than men.

More is needed during periods of growth, repeated pregnancies, pregnancy and lactation, ageing (incidence of iron-deficiency anaemia increases with age). Babies are born with only a small iron store and can easily be deficient.

People with the following illnesses may need more iron: kidney disease, ulcers, colitis, infections, cancer, infected teeth, gums and tonsils, ear infections, chronic nose-bleeds, bleeding piles, diverticular disease, hiatus hernia.

Regular use of aspirin can cause irritation and bleeding of the stomach lining, putting up the need for iron.

Natural sources Organ meats (the best source), other meats, fish, wholegrain cereals, wheat germ, bran, dried fruit especially apricots, raisins, prunes, molasses, green leafy vegetables and their juices, legumes, brewer's yeast, nuts and seeds, sprouting seeds and grains, some in egg yolks.

Absorption of iron There are two kinds of iron: haeme iron and non-haeme. Haeme iron is more easily absorbed by the body. It comprises about one-third of the iron present in meats and fish. Non-haeme iron is present in cereals, vegetables, beans, etc. – all the plant sources. It is also present, with haeme iron, in meats and fish.

The greater a person's need for iron, the more he will absorb. Absorption of iron is greatly increased by vitamin C foods at the same meal in, for instance, orange juice, salad or fruits. Meat, containing haeme iron, also helps the absorption of non-haeme iron contained in other foods and eaten at the same meal – for instance, steak (some haeme iron) and vegetables (non-haeme iron).

Absorption is helped by the presence of the B vitamins and proteins, acid fruits (citrus fruits) and yogurt. Copper in very small amounts is also essential for the absorption of iron.

Ferrous gluconate, ferrous fumerate, peptonized iron or iron lactate are preferable sources for iron supplementation because they are organic, and more easily absorbed. If you are also taking vitamin E, do not take iron supplements containing *inorganic* iron unless you take them, and the E, eight hours apart. Inorganic iron can destroy vitamin E in the gut.

Destroyed by The pollutants lead and cadmium inhibit iron absorption; to some extent so does the tannic acid in tea.

Foods 'enriched' with iron are supplying hardly any. This is because the better, more easily absorbed kind may shorten shelf-life, discolour the product, and decrease the baking qualities of flour, so it is used less often. 'Enriched' foods may also contain EDTA, a preservative which reduces iron absorption by about half.

The phosphates used as additives in soft drinks, ice cream, baked goods, sweets, beer, also reduce iron absorption.

Recommended daily allowance
Babies – about 12mg
Children – about 12mg
Teenagers – about 12mg
Adult men – about 12mg
Adult women – about 18mg.

Magnesium

Functions Magnesium sparks off more chemical reactions in the body than any other mineral, and helps many enzymes to work, nerves to react.

Helps muscles contract, helps maintain healthy heartbeat, helps production and transfer of energy, synthesis of proteins and fats, use of calcium, potassium and sodium. Involved in storing sugar in the liver and releasing it into the blood.

Is associated with potassium so that a magnesium deficiency will encourage a potassium deficiency.

Deficiency signs A deficiency of magnesium puts a strain on the heart. Low magnesium levels have been found in the heart muscles of people dying from heart attacks, and heart spasms and artery spasms can be associated with a deficiency.

Signs range from fatigue, depression, irritability, muscle tremors, poor memory, to depression, heart spasms, difficulty in walking. Found often in alcoholics and those with cirrhosis of the liver.

Deficiency may cause painful uterine contractions at the end of pregnancy and may be related to premature births. (Laboratory animals made deficient have given birth to small, damaged litters. They also have damaged heart cells.)

Many soils are deficient, thus producing deficient crops. Dietary deficiencies are probably widespread.

Needs raised by Alcohol, high-protein or high-fat diet, high intake of calcium, excess sugar, illness (kidney disorders, diabetes) and other stresses, diuretic drugs, pregnancy, lactation and growth.

Destroyed by Refining of foods: wheat loses almost all its magnesium when refined, and refined sugars and fats have almost none. Water softeners. Boiling of vegetables (leaves it in the water). The use of chelating agents in the preparation of frozen foods results in a lower magnesium content.

Natural sources Wholegrains, bran, wheat germ, brewer's yeast, soybeans, molasses, green leafy vegetables and their juices, milk nuts and seeds, some in seafoods. Also found in hard water.

Recommended daily allowances (An excess is very rare, but can be toxic.)

Babies – about 65mg

Children – about 200mg

Adult men – about 350mg

Adult women – about 300mg
Pregnant and lactating women – about 450mg.

Phosphorus

With calcium, the most abundant mineral in the body, present in the bones, teeth and all other tissues. The average Western diet is very rich in phosphorus, and when phosphorus is a great deal in excess of calcium it is excreted in the urine, unfortunately as a calcium salt, which takes more calcium out of the body with it.

Functions Performs many functions; combines with calcium for bones and teeth and influences the intake and distribution of calcium.

Helps in the working of muscles, the use of carbohydrates, fats and proteins, the health of nerves and blood: Is partly responsible for transporting fats around the body.

Also works with vitamin D, potassium and magnesium.

Deficiency signs Muscle weakness, anaemia, increased susceptibility to infection. A phosphorus deficiency can contribute to a low level of potassium, and will also upset the balance between itself, magnesium, calcium and potassium.

Needs raised by Ageing – is absorbed less effectively by some older people. Vitamin D deficiency.

Destroyed by Alcoholism, antacid medicines and barbiturates, food refining, prolonged bedrest (is excreted).

Natural sources Brewer's yeast, wheat germ and bran, whole cereals, honey, soybeans, lentils, liver, nuts especially almonds, seeds especially sunflower, sesame and pumpkin seeds. There is some in dairy products and muscle meats.

Recommended daily allowance

Babies – about 270mg
Children – about 800mg
Teenagers – about 120mg
Adult men and women – about 800mg
Pregnant and lactating women – about 1200mg.

Potassium

Functions Closely inter-related with sodium chloride or salt. Generally speaking, potassium is inside the cells and sodium is outside them. Sodium and potassium must be in balance with each other (SEE *Salt* pages 57–61).

With sodium, keeps a normal fluid balance passing in and

out of the cells; with sodium, works to keep the acid-alkali balance of the blood; with sodium, is an essential part of glandular secretions, influences all muscles including the heart muscle, is essential for nerve responses, transport of nerve impulses to muscles.

High blood pressure has been successfully treated with large amounts of potassium chloride.

Deficiency signs (Excess of sodium leads to a shortage of potassium; shortage of potassium leads to an excess of sodium. A junk diet, high in sodium, leads easily to a potassium deficiency.)

Fatigue, constipation, apathy, muscle weakness.

High blood pressure has been produced by a potassium deficiency as well as from excess sodium.

The greatest harm from a deficiency of potassium is its effect on the heart.

Needs raised by Illness, alcoholism, strenuous exercise, sweat, long bedrest, diabetes, high blood pressure, liver disease.

Destroyed by Diuretic drugs, some drugs for high blood pressure, food refining; thrown away in vegetable cooking water.

Natural sources Our bodies excete potassium very wastefully in urine and sweat. There is plenty of potassium, however, in *whole, fresh foods* – wholegrains, bran, wheat germ, nuts and seeds, soybeans, red kidney beans, lentils and other vegetables and their juices, honey, dates, prunes, fruits (especially bananas), fruit juices, milk, brewer's yeast. Other sources: Biosalt, Ruthmol (both are salt substitutes from your health food store). Potassium pills can have serious side-effects.

Recommended daily allowance Not specified.

Sodium

Can cause illness if taken to excess. Sodium and potassium are closely inter-dependent. For a full discussion of sodium chloride, or salt, please SEE *Salt* (pages 57–61).

Functions Helps muscle action, the transmission of nerve impulses, water distribution throughout the body.

Deficiency signs (Uncommon – we are much more likely to take in too much salt.) Cramp. Severe deficiency can lead to fatigue, mental apathy, nausea, dizziness, respiratory failure.

Needs raised by Copious sweating, urination.

Destroyed by Not known.
Natural sources In almost all foods, especially seafoods.
Recommended daily allowance Not specified.

Zinc

Concentrated in eyes, sperm.
Functions Essential for good vision, appetite, sense of taste and smell, bone growth.

Mobilizes body's stores of vitamin A and works with A to resist infection and inflammation.

Essential for enzyme action – there are over 80 enzymes containing zinc. Works with the essential fatty acids, vitamin B6 and folic acid, helps good circulation, works with copper to control blood cholesterol levels.

Has been used to treat impotence, some skin diseases, mental exhaustion, body odour, rheumatoid arthritis, borderline diabetes, angina pectoris, artery disease.

With other vitamins has been used for schizophrenia, mouth ulcers, prostate problems. With vitamin A has been used for night blindness. With B6 has been used for pregnancy sickness.

Has been used to treat pica (craving for unnatural foods such as earth, coal, lead).
Deficiency signs Badly growing nails with white marks, poor hair, stretch marks on skin, acne, late menstruation, impotence, retarded healing of wounds, lowered resistance to infection, loss of sense of taste, possibly retarded growth and loss of fertility. Deficiency may be associated with anorexia nervosa.

Severe deficiency causes birth defects in laboratory animals.
Needs raised by (Zinc uptake possibly impaired by phytic acid which is present in whole cereals and bran, but this is debatable.) Growth, sexual development, pregnancy, lactation, pre-menstrual tension, the Pill, wounds, fractures, surgical operations – any other kind of stress.
Destroyed by Saturation of farming land with chemical fertilizers. Plants cannot take up the zinc and it cannot get dissolved; soil thus produces zinc-deficient crops. Also destroyed by food refining.

Thrown away in vegetable cooking water, excreted when excess liquid, particularly alcohol, is taken, absorption blocked by coffee. Too much phosphorus hinders absorption,

6: Composition per 100 g (raw edible weight except where stated)

Food	Calcium mg	Iron mg	Vitamin A (retinol equivalent) µg	Thiamin mg	Riboflavin mg	Nicotinic acid equivalent mg	Vitamin C mg	Vitamin D µg
Milk								
Milk, liquid, whole	120	0.1	46[1] / 32[2]	0.04	0.19	0.9	2	0.03[1] / 0.01[2]
Milk, dried, skimmed	1,190	0.4	0	0.42	1.60	9.7	6	0
Yogurt, low fat, natural	180	0.1	10	0.05	0.26	1.2	0	0.01
Yogurt, low fat, fruit	160	0.2	22	0.05	0.23	1.1	2	0.01
Cheese								
Cheese, Cheddar	800	0.4	412	0.04	0.50	6.2	0	0.26
Cheese, cottage	60	0.1	41	0.02	0.19	3.3	0	0.02
Meat								
Kidney, average	9	6.0	120	0.39	1.90	10.7	10	0
Liver, fried	14	8.8	19,010	0.26	4.30	20.4	12	0.38
Fish								
White fish, filleted	16	0.3	0	0.08	0.07	4.9	0	0
Eggs								
Eggs, fresh	52	2.0	140	0.09	0.47	3.7	0	1.75
Fats								
Butter	15	0.2	985	0	0	0.1	0	0.76
Margarine, average	4	0.3	900[3]	0	0	0.1	0	7.94[3]
Preserves, etc.								
Honey	5	0.4	0	0	0.05	0.2	0	0
Marmite	95	3.7	0	3.10	11.00	67.0	0	0
Vegetables								
Beans, broad	30	1.1	22	0.28	0.05	5.0	30	0
Beans, runner	27	0.8	50	0.05	0.10	1.3	20	0
Brussels sprouts, boiled	25	0.5	67	0.06	0.10	0.9	41	0
Cabbage, green, raw	57	0.6	50	0.05	0.05	0.8	53	0

Cabbage, green, boiled	38	0.4	50	0.03	0.03	0.5	23	0
Cauliflower	21	0.5	5	0.10	0.10	1.1	64	0
Celery	52	0.6	0	0.03	0.03	0.5	7	0
Lettuce	23	0.9	167	0.07	0.08	0.4	15	0
Mushrooms	3	1.0	0	0.10	0.40	4.6	3	0
Onions	31	0.3	0	0.03	0.05	0.4	10	0
Peppers, green	9	0.4	33	0.08	0.03	0.9	100	0
Potatoes, boiled	4	0.3	0	0.08	0.03	1.1	5-18[4]	0
Potatoes, roast	10	0.7	0	0.10	0.04	1.9	6-21[4]	0
Spinach	70	3.2	1,000	0.12	0.20	1.3	60	0
Tomatoes, fresh	13	0.4	100	0.06	0.04	0.8	20[5]	0
Watercress	220	1.6	500	0.10	0.10	1.1	60	0
Fruit								
Apples	4	0.3	5	0.04	0.02	0.1	5	0
Bananas	7	0.4	33	0.04	0.07	0.8	10	0
Blackcurrants	60	1.3	33	0.03	0.06	0.4	200	0
Dates, dried	68	1.6	10	0.07	0.04	2.9	0	0
Figs, dried	280	4.2	8	0.10	0.08	2.2	0	0
Grapefruit	17	0.3	0	0.05	0.02	0.3	40	0
Oranges	41	0.3	8	0.10	0.03	0.3	50	0
Peaches, fresh	5	0.4	83	0.02	0.05	1.1	8	0
Pears, fresh	8	0.2	2	0.03	0.03	0.3	3	0
Plums	12	0.3	37	0.05	0.03	0.6	3	0
Prunes, dried	38	2.9	160	0.10	0.20	1.9	0	0
Raspberries	41	1.2	13	0.02	0.03	0.5	25	0
Strawberries	22	0.7	5	0.02	0.03	0.5	60	0
Sultanas	52	1.8	5	0.10	0.08	0.6	0	0
Nuts								
Almonds	250	4.2	0	0.24	0.92	4.7	0	0
Peanuts, roasted	61	2.0	0	0.23	0.10	21.3	0	0
Cereals								
Bread, wholemeal	23	2.5	0	0.26	0.06	1.7	0	0

1 summer value   2 winter value   3 fortified   4 vitamin C falls during storage   5 Feb, 27; May, 14; Aug, 20; Nov, 21 (mg per 100g)

as does too much copper. The poisonous mineral, cadmium, is a zinc antagonist and hinders zinc absorption.

Natural sources   Organ meats especially liver, other meats, fish and shellfish especially oysters, lima beans, lentils, chick peas, green leafy vegetables and their juices (especially spinach), wholegrains, wheat germ, bran, soybeans, brewer's yeast, cheddar cheese, eggs, nuts and seeds especially sunflower and sesame seeds, sprouting seeds and grains.

The zinc from animal and dairy products is more easily absorbed than that from vegetables and cereals.

Recommended daily allowance

Babies – about 3mg

Children – about 10mg

Men and women – about 15mg

Pregnant women – about 20mg

Lactating women – about 25mg.

Trace Minerals

(Recommended daily allowances of trace minerals are not known.)

Chromium

Functions   Helps the body use proteins, sugars and fats; helps to control the cholesterol levels in the blood; is needed by the eyes.

Has been found essential for growth and longevity in laboratory animals.

May help low blood sugar levels.

Has been used to lower insulin needs in diabetics.

Deficiency signs   Deficiency inhibits the use of protein.

Needs raised by   Ageing, pregnancy, lactation. A diet containing lots of white sugar.

Destroyed by   Is processed out of raw cane sugar and whole cereals.

Natural sources   Some brewer's yeast, wholegrains and bran, wheat germ, beans, fresh fruits and juices, vegetables and their juices, cheese, mushrooms, liver.

Cobalt

Function Essential as a vital part of vitamin B12.

Deficiency signs There is no evidence of cobalt deficiency in human beings. It can, however, be lacking in certain soils.

Needs raised by Not known.

Destroyed by Refining of cereals.

Natural sources Whole cereals, wheat germ and bran, green leafy vegetables and their juices.

Copper

Plays a role in many enzyme systems, is essential to the production of the cell nucleus, helps the development of bones, brain, nerves, connective tissue, the function of nerves and brain.

Helps to prevent anaemia, is concerned with hair colour.

Is essential in small amounts for the production of haemoglobin.

Toxicity In excess can be toxic.

Excess copper may be a factor in hyper-activity in children.

Blood levels are higher with the use of the Pill, also in smokers, those with high blood pressure, those with a deficiency of zinc.

Environmental factors can cause copper overloading – for instance it can be in the drinking water coming through copper pipes.

Deficiency signs Some soils are deficient, and so are some farm animals. Many authorities consider that a deficiency in human beings is almost impossible, but this is debated.

It is thought possible that a deficiency cuts iron absorption and shortens the lifespan of red blood cells, thus contributing to anaemia. Deficiency seen in protein starvation disease, kidney disease. Copper is associated with zinc so that a high intake of zinc can mean a lower absorption of copper.

Needs raised by Not known.

Destroyed by Refining of cereals.

Natural sources Lamb's and calf's liver contain more than that of full-grown animals. Organ meats especially liver, fish, cheese, milk, nuts, whole cereals, bran, wheat germ, brewer's yeast, root vegetables, seeds, especially sunflower and sesame seeds.

Manganese

Can be toxic in industries where manganese-containing dust is inhaled.

Functions Needed for good bone structure, is involved in dealing with sugars and fats, reproduction, healthy nerves. Has an important role in brain function; is associated with vitamin K, has a role in blood clotting, is needed to activate various enzymes, works with choline.

Has been used to treat schizophrenia, to help diabetics, as part of treatment for myasthenia gravis (muscle disease).

Has a relationship with iron so that a lot of dietary iron reduces manganese absorption and a lot of manganese reduces iron absorption.

Deficiency signs Not proved, but may be common among older men; may be a cause of artery disease; may be involved in diabetes.

There are many manganese-deficient areas of soil, and therefore many manganese-deficient crops.

Needs raised by Not known.

Destroyed by Food processing.

Natural sources Whole cereals, wheat germ, bran, root and green leafy vegetables especially spinach, parsley and broccoli and their juices, legumes, fresh fruits and their juices, organ meats, nuts, unrefined oils.

Molybdenum

Functions Appears to help prevent dental caries, may help to prevent some kinds of cancer.

Deficiency signs May lead to impotence.

Needs raised by Not known.

Destroyed by Food refining.

Natural sources Whole cereals, wheat germ, bran, molasses, sunflower seeds, coconut, cocoa, lima beans, lentils, liver, kidney.

(Fruits, vegetables, muscle meats and dairy products contain very little.)

Selenium

Research on this mineral is relatively recent. An excess of selenium can be toxic. The human heart muscle contains a lot of selenium.

Functions Is an anti-oxidant; i.e. it prevents oxygen from reacting with other substances and damaging the cells. Helps to protect liver. Related to vitamin E, and increases this vitamin's effectiveness. Helps to activate immune system, may help body to produce the anti-viral substance interferon, may help to protect against cancer. Necessary for protein synthesis. Protects against the toxic effects of cadmium, arsenic, silver, mercury and copper.

Essential for normal growth of laboratory animals and may be connected with human growth. In laboratory animals, it is concerned with eye health, fertility, and normal muscle function.

Has been used, with other supplements, to treat cystic fibrosis.

Deficiency signs   Soils vary in their selenium content and this is partly due to geographical factors such as erosion. Soil deficiencies may relate to cancer incidence. May be concerned with some heart disease.

It is thought that a deficiency, perhaps together with a lack of vitamin E, could be connected with cot deaths. With a deficiency of vitamin E, may be connected with cystic fibrosis.

Needs raised by   Men probably need more than women.

Destroyed by   Food processing. Brown rice has 15 times more selenium than white rice; wholemeal bread has twice as much selenium as white bread.

Natural sources   Whole cereals, wheat germ, meat (especially organ meats), some brewer's yeast, vegetables and their juices, fruits and their juices, milk, garlic, nuts and unrefined oils, a little in eggs. Human milk has six times as much as cow's milk.

Sulphur

Found in every cell in the body, concentrated mostly in the skin, hair and joints. It is contained in four amino acids – cysteine, cystine, taurine and methionine.

During the last century sulphur was used to treat many ailments, including constipation.

Deficiency signs   Not known.

Needs raised by   Not known.

Destroyed by   Many soils are deficient in sulphur, and commercial fertilizers seldom restore it. Crops, therefore, will be deficient. A deficiency in humans has not been shown.

Natural sources   Eggs, meat, soybeans, onions and garlic, horseradish, nuts and seeds, bran.

Little-known and little-researched trace minerals

Other trace elements are nickel, tin, silicon, vanadium. These elements are believed to be essential to health.

Orthomolecular Therapy or Megavitamins

'Orthomolecular therapy' is a term coined by Nobel prize-winner Linus Pauling. It is from the Greek *ortho*, meaning right, or correct, and describes treatment which consists of providing the body with what it needs for optimum health. This may mean eliminating one substance or supplying moderate, or more often large, quantities of another. The point is that orthomolecular treatment uses only substances – usually vitamins and minerals – which are naturally present in the body.

In recent years, this therapy has come more and more to be associated with large doses of vitamins, or megavitamin therapy. But megavitamin therapy is only a part of the original concept. The definition of a megadose is at least ten times the recommended daily allowance.

The first great testing ground for megavitamin treatment was mental illness. Niacin and vitamin C were used for schizophrenia, and niacin, pantothenic acid, vitamins B6 and C have been used for another serious mental condition, autism. Recently Linus Pauling and Ewan Cameron have been using massive doses of vitamin C for cancer – SEE *Cancer and Vitamin C* (pages 272–5).

When there has been a nutritional deficiency over many years, it may take enormous doses to put matters right. Older people do not absorb nutrients very well, so a high dosage may be necessary, and the greater the concentration of a vitamin, the more efficient and faster it crosses from the bloodstream into the tissues. Everyone has nutritional needs which are different, too. These points may go some way towards explaining the undoubted success of megavitamin therapy for many illnesses.

When taken in enormous quantities, vitamins behave differently. For instance, large amounts of vitamin C cause the kidneys to work harder, taking water from body tissues so that the excess C can be excreted. In this way, the vitamin is acting as a diuretic.

Some vitamins – A and D for instance – can be toxic in very high doses. Research has shown that the vitamin pantothenic acid, in doses reaching the human equivalent of about 20 grams a day, can cause liver damage in animals. Further, megadoses of vitamins may have to be produced synthetically because the natural versions in pill form would be too big to swallow, and some people are allergic to synthetic vitamins. Some researchers have said that megadoses of vitamin C can cause the body to excrete valuable minerals such as calcium, magnesium and potassium, as well as the harmful lead, cadmium and mercury, and that over a long period this will encourage mineral deficiencies.

By taking vast doses of a nutrient, we may be creating needs for other substances to balance matters up. And in concentrating on one nutrient, or a few nutrients only, we are ignoring the naturopath's plea for an all-round approach to healing.

On the other hand, to compare the use of high doses of vital substances already needed by our bodies, the adverse effects of which are easily controlled, with the destructive, suppressive action of drugs, is to put all these objections into perspective. No doubt those lucky people who are still alive today as a result of massive vitamin C treatment for cancer, and those formerly mentally ill people who are now able to lead normal lives because of niacin can see these arguments in perspective too.

Megavitamin therapy is a relatively new area, and each case must be treated differently and by a qualified naturopath or other practitioner who understands it.

Books mentioned in vitamins and minerals sections
An End to Cancer? by Leon Chaitow (Thorsons 1978)
Cancer and its Nutritional Therapies by Richard A. Passwater
Cancer and Vitamin C by Limis Pauling and Ewan Cameron.

Whole Foods

What are whole foods?

'We should eat only those foods which rot, grow mouldy and

decay – and we should eat them before they do.'   ROBERT
McCARRISON

Let's be clear at the start – it's almost impossible nowadays to
live entirely on 'whole foods' unless you are Robinson Crusoe.
But what we can do is understand the principles behind whole
foods and try to follow them as much as we can.

Ideally, whole crops are grown on soils which have been
spread with compost and manure and not unbalanced by too
much artificial fertilizer. They have not been sprayed with
pesticides and other chemicals which linger on the crop and
finish up inside us. They are preferably eaten raw, or short-
cooked, and as fresh as possible.

The wholefood ideal for meat is that it should not come
from animals doctored by antibiotics and hormones and
penned in unnatural conditions. Eggs should not come from
hens trapped in battery cages. Hard evidence comparing the
nutritional value of the battery and the free-range egg is
scarce, but Dr Michael Crawford, of the Nuffield Laboratories
of Comparative Medicine, states that a battery egg has twice as
much saturated fat as a free-range one. The difference in taste,
at any rate, is clear enough.

It is difficult to get certified raw milk and, although
pasteurization destroys a certain proportion of vitamins,
minerals and enzymes in the milk, pasteurized milk is still a
nourishing food. (Enzymes are catalytsts which help chemical
changes to take place in the body. According to biochemist
Roger J. Williams, they are produced within our bodies and
are not necessary food ingredients.) Ultra heat-treated (UHT)
milk is heated at a very high temperature for a short time and,
if it is kept sealed, it will last almost indefinitely. Research at
the National Institute of Research and Dairying at Reading has
established that UHT milk is nutritionally inferior to both
pasteurized and certified raw milk. [1] Skimmed milk has had the
fat, and also the fat-soluble vitamins, removed, but these
vitamin losses are small. Goat's milk is digestible and high in
vitamins and minerals, but can interfere with thyroid function
and should not be used for babies and very young children. It
should be pasteurized or boiled to avoid the possibility of
disease. [2] Soya milk is very good, and there are several brands
on the market now.

I have covered the subject of wholemeal versus white bread

in the section on *The Modern Food Industry* (pages 42–51). Readers interested in switching to wholemeal bread should make sure that it is in fact *wholemeal* and that this is stated on the label. Some breads are just dyed with caramel to make them look brown.

Readers might like to turn to the *Vitamins and Minerals* section (pages 68–101) where they will read, with tedious regularity, that vitamins and minerals are found in greatest abundance in whole grains and fresh, raw fruits and vegetables, nuts and seeds. This applies particularly to the vulnerable – and essential – B vitamins and vitamin C, which are so easily destroyed by heat and other processing.

As far as meat is concerned, it used to be the case that unless you moved in huntin', shootin' and fishin' circles, you were unlikely to get meat which had not been artificially reared. 'Organically reared' meat is available now, however (SEE *Information* at end).

If you have a garden, then you can – and probably do – grow your own food, using home-made compost; the results are delicious, rewarding and healthful. Some health food stores sell fruit and vegetables grown without artificial chemicals. All fruit and vegetables from an ordinary greengrocer should be thoroughly washed or scrubbed.

Wholegrain breakfast cereals and wholemeal bread are widely available now, but at your supermarket the grain used will of course have been sprayed.

Getting all these different whole foods must seem like a tall order for many of us, and it's no good trying to do the impossible. But to do the best we can, and stop worrying about the rest of it, is a better idea than to turn into cranks and make ourselves ill from anxiety!

Why whole foods?

Since virtually the whole of this book is devoted to answering this question, I would like here just to give a couple of examples out of the vast amount of research and writing available.

In the 1920s a young doctor, Robert McCarrison, went to live and work among a tribe of people called the Hunzas. These poor peasants live in north-west India, 8 000 feet up in the Himalayas. McCarrison spent seven years among them and served as doctor there to 10 000 people. *He did not see a single case of our Western degenerative diseases during all that time; cancer was then unknown to the Hunzas.* (They have to some extent come under Western influence since then and have started to share our diseases.)

The Hunzas at that time worked hard, with plenty of strenuous exercise. They were eating wholemeal chapatti, plenty of vegetables which they usually ate raw, cheese, lots of apricots, yogurt; meat was an occasional treat and their drinking water came from a mineral-rich glacier. They were frugal eaters.

Intrigued by the excellent health, long lives and splendid physique of his patients, McCarrison set up a laboratory and carried out nutritional research.

In one of his experiments, McCarrison used two colonies of young rats.[3] One group ate white bread, with a margarine substitute and tinned jam spread on it, vegetables thoroughly cooked in water with bicarbonate of soda and salt added, tinned meat, sweet tea and water. The rats acquired an extraordinary liking for the tea, so they got plenty of it. The second group ate a whole diet, with plenty of raw vegetables and fruit, sprouting grain, dairy products, wholemeal flour made into chapattis, with occasional fresh meat. The experiment was continued for six months.

The mortality in the first group was 45% and in the second 15%. The first rats were ill-grown, with poor fur and little energy. The second group were well-grown, sleek and strong. 30 of the rats in the ill-fed, first group were killed and eaten by the others; this did not happen at all with the well-fed rats. Two litters were born to the ill-fed rats but none survived. 20 litters were born to the well-fed colony and all the babies survived. Post-mortem examination of the ill-fed rats found many signs of damage and deterioration.

From both McCarrison's observations of the Hunzas and their diet, and his controlled study using rats, it is obvious that a diet of fresh, whole foods is essential to freedom from illness, positive health, and a long and vigorous life. In a diet of whole foods, it is not one vitamin, or mineral, that encourages health, it is the *whole complex of vital nutrients*, working together.

For an ideal diet – used to treat illness – please SEE the *Food Therapy* section (pages 396–401).

Are health foods a swindle?
There is little doubt that many 'health foods' are very
expensive. The manufacturers explain this by saying that foods
produced without artificial chemicals most more to produce
and that they are in any case retailed in smaller quantities.

Bran and wheat germ, however, are not expensive, and
whole cereals such as Weetabix and Shredded Wheat (not
organically grown) can be bought in a supermarket. If you
decide to cut down on meat, this will save you a lot of money.
Fresh vegetables and fruits *in season* cost less than the
preserved versions, and lentils and pulses are not expensive.
You will probably find free-range eggs, brown rice and some
kinds of honey rather expensive, but you save on cream, white
sugar, convenience and preserved foods.

It is probably easier to live, like McCarrison's rats, on white
bread, jam, tinned meat and tea. And cheaper. And –
eventually – fatal. . . .

To summarize then:
1   Get organically-grown foods if you can. If you can't, then
don't get neurotic about it.
2   Read the *Bonus Foods and Supplements*, and *Vitamins and
Minerals* sections of this book.
3   Use wholemeal bread and other whole cereals including
brown rice, fresh raw salads, fresh and dried fruits, dairy
foods, nuts, pulses and lentils. Sweeten sparingly with honey,
molasses or dark brown sugar. Cut down on salt and all fats.
Meat is expensive and not essential to health.
4   Chew your food well – and enjoy it!

Recommended reading
The Real Food Cookbook by Vivien and Clifford Quick
(Thorsons 1981)
The Natural Foods Primer by Beatrice Trum Hunter (Unwin
paperbacks 1979)
The Natural Foods Cookbook by Beatrice Trum Hunter
(Faber paperbacks 1977)
Salads the Year Round by Joy Larkcom (Hamlyn Paperbacks
1980)

Information
There are now several organizations devoted to the organic

food movement. The Soil Association, for instance, awards its circular symbol (SEE diagram) to farmers and growers who produce food according to high standards laid down by the association. Producers carrying the symbol are regularly inspected by the Association's field officers. Broadly speaking, the Soil Association demands proper care of the soil without artificial chemicals with biological crop protection, humane care of livestock without drugs or antibiotics, and dairy foods from approved animals, produced without synthetic additives; there are similar rules for other foods.

ADDRESS
The Soil Association,
Walnut Tree Manor,
Haughley, Stowmarket,
Suffolk
Telephone: Haughley (044970) 235

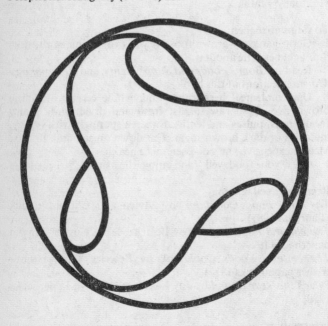

BONUS FOODS AND SUPPLEMENTS

Biochemic Tissue Salts

Biochemic tissue salts are the innovation of Dr W.H. Schuessler of Oldenburg, Germany, who in the 1870s developed the idea that disease can be contributed to or brought about by an imbalance of mineral salts in the body.

The life of your body depends on the work of its cells. Inside these myriads of cells, living protoplasm is created, serves its purpose, and dies. This continuous building up and breaking down is fuelled by materials from the blood, including the essential minerals. These inorganic elements, therefore, although present in minute quantities, are vitally important. Germs only succeed in making us ill if the conditions inside us permit them to do so and one of these conditions is the balance of mineral salts. The number of cells rendered ineffective or diseased may be very small.

Dr Schuessler incorporated the principal minerals in his remedies to correct biochemically any deficiencies interfering with cell function.

The remedies, prepared in accordance with the homoeopathic principle of using extremely small quantities, are finely sub-divided and combined with lactose (milk sugar). Because they are treated in this way, they are rapidly absorbed into the bloodstream when placed on the tongue and do not need to be digested; it is believed, therefore, that they are particularly suitable for people with poor digestion.

Again following homoeopathic principles, the particular salt or combination of salts chosen will vary according to the *symptoms*, and not the disease; there are, for instance, three different combinations for three different kinds of digestive trouble. (The salts can also be obtained singly.)

Dr E.P. Anshutz, in his *Guide to the Twelve Tissue Remedies of Biochemistry* says that 'the brilliant success that has attended their use lends colour to the claims of Scheussler;

whether they are "all-sufficient" therapeutically is a question that must remain open.'

Schuessler, however, believed in their efficacy for many conditions when used alone and as such they are widely used today. They are also frequently prescribed as part of a whole treatment by naturopaths and homoeopathic physicians.

Their manufacturers stress that 'serious diseases should always be treated under medical supervision' and advise people to seek medical advice if the symptoms persist, adding 'a homoeopathic physician should be consulted whenever possible.'

Books mentioned in this section
Guide to the Twelve Tissue Remedies of Biochemistry by E.P. Anshutz.

Recommended reading
A Guide to Biochemic Tissue Salts by Dr Andrew Stanway (Van Dyke 1982).

Brewer's Yeast

Brewer's yeast is a by-product of the brewing industry. It is skimmed off the head of the liquid during the beer-making process and the residue dried into a powder and sold as a supplement. It is in fact a tiny one-celled plant, about the size of a human blood corpuscle, and is one of the most nutritious foods you can buy.

'The use of yeast alone', says American nutritionist Adelle Davis, 'could correct the majority of the world's nutritional problems; the proteinless meals of China and India; the B-vitamin needs in the Orient and the tropics; the iron starvation of women the world over; and the trace mineral deficiencies of both sexes of all ages of every nationality.'[1]

Richard Doisy and his team of researchers tried giving brewer's yeast to diabetics on insulin. After taking the yeast, some patients were able to lower their dosage. This was due to the chromium in the yeast, which helps to keep blood sugar levels normal. This chromium (part of the GTF, or glucose tolerance factor) also helps to lower blood fats when they are too high. Experiments with animals have shown that if they are fed a high cholesterol diet together with brewer's yeast, their blood cholesterol is lower than without the yeast. In another study a group of volunteer women taking brewer's yeast containing chromium also experienced a cholesterol drop.

Selenium is another mineral sometimes found in brewer's yeast. In parts of the world where this trace mineral is abundant, there is less cancer, and it is believed that selenium increases resistance to illnesses in general. A selenium deficiency has a bad effect on the heart muscle.

Because it contains almost no fat or sugar and only 22 calories per tablespoonful, brewer's yeast is a very useful supplement for slimmers. It is helpful as a gentle natural laxative, too, because of its B vitamin content.

But perhaps the most useful way in which we can use brewer's yeast is to nourish and strengthen the nerves, particularly if we are under stress. Like liver, it is believed to contain an 'anti-stress' factor and, because its plentiful B vitamins are together, they work well.

If you have not tried brewer's yeast before, then please go carefully. Should your digestion be a little below par, yeast can cause a lot of gas – and be warned, it tastes pretty peculiar. So start by adding half a level teaspoon to a large glass of fruit juice, or see the section on *Fatigue* and try the energy drink described there. Indeed, if you are deficient in B vitamins you are more likely to get gas from yeast and the only way to avoid this vicious circle is to take just a little to start with. Brewer's yeast can also be used in bread mixes, brown rice, casseroles and soups. Please note that *baker's* yeast is not the same thing at all and should not be taken uncooked in any case because it absorbs the B vitamins instead of supplying them.

Brewer's yeast is about 35% to 50% complete protein (with about 18 amino acids) and has nearly all the B vitamins, some varieties even boasting B12. It has about 14 minerals, including twice as much potassium as sodium (an excellent balance), with phosphorus, iron, magnesium, calcium, copper, manganese and a very little cobalt. Not all brewer's yeast contains chromium or selenium, so look on the packet. It can

be taken in tablet form, but if you decide to do this you will
need about 16 tablets to equal the nutrients in 1 tablespoonful
of powder.

Cider Vinegar

Apple cider vinegar takes the manufacture of cider a step
further. The apple juice is squeezed from the crop and the
sugar in the juice is changed by yeast into alcohol, making
cider. After the cider has matured the alcohol is changed by
bacterial action into acetic acid; this happens in all vinegars.
Sulphur dioxide – or preferably vitamin C – is then added to
stop the cider vinegar from oxidizing.

Chemical analysis of cider vinegar shows that it contains
high levels of the essential mineral potassium. This mineral is
crucial to health and it may be that, in association with the
many other minerals found in cider vinegar, it is potassium
that is responsible for its therapeutic effect.

For cider vinegar is a puzzle. It has been credited with many
benefits to health but 'the great mystery is why these changes to
cider that transform it to cider vinegar also create such a
remarkable aid to health for so many people'.[1]

An early cider vinegar enthusiast, Dr D.C. Jarvis, used it for
arthritis, along with a wholefood diet and supplements. It has
been successfully used for rheumatism, gout, coughs, colds
and laryngitis, asthma and hay fever, digestive troubles,
constipation, and is recommended for improving the condition
of the hair, skin, nails and eyes.

Different cider vinegars contain different proportions of
minerals; calcium, phosphorus, sodium, with traces of iron,
zinc, copper, etc. Sometimes there is a little vitamin B2 and, if
vitamin C has been added to preserve the vinegar, then of
course this will be present too. It also contains acetic acid, a
very little protein and small amounts of invert sugar. The most
remarkable ingredient however is the potassium, present in
very large quantities, in the order of between 100 to 120 mg per
100 ml.

Evening Primrose Oil

The pale yellow flowers of the evening primrose bloom at night and die out the next day. The plant originated in the eastern USA and the American Indians used its extracts to heal wounds and skin inflammations. Brought to Europe, it was dubbed the 'King's Cure-All'. The evening primrose has long been known to medical herbalists in England, who use the leaves and bark for their astringent and sedative properties.

The composition of the seed from which the oil is produced varies enormously with the many different types of plant. This oil was first investigated in 1919, when its vital component – GLA (Gamma Linolenic Acid) – was first identified. Studies recommenced in the 1940s and now evening primrose oil is the subject of hundreds of current trials and papers.

GLA

To appreciate the benefits of evening primrose oil, we must understand the action of GLA.

Essential fatty acids (EFAs) are crucial to health (SEE *Fats* pages 23–35). The most important EFA, linoleic acid, must be changed into GLA before it can be used by the body. Otherwise it is virtually useless. Most of the GLA thus formed is changed again into an intermediate substance, DGLA (dihomogammalinolenic acid). DGLA is converted in its turn into substances known as prostaglandins (PGs), which form the last link in the chain. (Another EFA, arachidonic acid, can also be changed into prostaglandins.)

Prostaglandins, therefore, depend for their manufacture on the original supply of fatty acids, which must be changed into GLA as part of the conversion chain.

What do prostaglandins do?

Writing in *Medical Hypothesis*[1] leading researcher David Horrobin states 'prostaglandins play major roles in many and perhaps most tissues of the body'. This family of hormone-like substances have been labelled like vitamins – A, B, C and so on. The most important is PGE1. They were originally found in high concentrations in the prostate gland; hence their name. It is better to help the body manufacture its own PGs than to give them orally, although they have been injected.

PGs regulate cell function second by second, and the same PG may have different functions in different tissues. They are involved in combatting pain, inflammation and fever. They can dilate blood vessels, stop thrombosis and slow down the manufacture of cholesterol, thus exerting an influence on the heart, arteries and blood pressure. They have a beneficial effect on the menstrual cycle and the brain, and on the immune system's reaction to disease. In a wide variety of disease states, now being researched, they are found to be either in excess or deficient.

It is clear that while the essential fatty acids in their original state are vital as nutrients, their role in prostaglandin manufacture is equally important.

Breaks in the prostaglandin chain
It is thought that many, or even most of us, are unable to manufacture PGs efficiently. The following factors prevent this process:
1   A diet rich in saturated fats.
2   A diet rich in refined oils and fats. When oils are processed to make salad and cooking oils or margarines, much of the original EFA, linoleic acid, is changed into an artificial transfatty acid. Transfatty acids, plentiful in refined oils and fats, cannot be converted by the body into PGs. Further, transfatty acids raise blood cholesterol levels and increase the need for linoleic acid which means that less is available for conversion into prostaglandins. David Horrobin estimates that the hydrogenation of processed vegetable oils converts up to 40% of the natural EFAs into trans-fatty acids (SEE *Fats* pages 23–35).
3   Plenty of alcohol.
4   Diabetes.
5   Ageing. The loss of the ability to manufacture PGs may be a major factor in the ageing process.
6   Deficiencies of the nutrients needed to help the body make PGs – zinc, magnesium, selenium, vitamins B6, E and C, with possibly niacin and folic acid.
7   Viral infections, radiation and cancer.

PGs and evening primrose oil
This oil contains a high proportion of GLA, part of the PG

conversion process. The best oil now produced contains about 9% GLA and the rest is about 72% linoleic acid.

Research into evening primrose oil and the prostaglandins

There is a lot of current interest in this field. Research is going on in many countries and several projects have been set up in the UK.

Evening primrose oil can be effective against rheumatoid arthritis[2] and eczema.[3] It is thought that several illnesses which can be due to allergy, including eczema, rhinitis (runny nose) and asthma may be due to defective PG formation and a possible link between this process and several human diseases of inflammation and defective immunity is being researched.

PGE1 caused weight loss without deliberate dieting in about half of a group of volunteers who were more than 10% overweight. It can protect laboratory animals from fatty liver caused by alcohol,[4] and evening primrose oil is being researched for its effects on alcohol withdrawal symptoms. The oil is currently being given to hyper-active children and improvement has sometimes been dramatic, particularly when it is rubbed into the skin.[5] These children may be unable to absorb essential fatty acids or to form prostaglandins effectively.

Dr Kenneth Vaddadi, a psychiatrist at Leeds University, is using evening primrose oil for schizophrenic patients; they have very low levels of PGE1. The oil has an effect on the brain, producing a sense of well-being. The Schizophrenia Association recommend that it should be taken with vitamins B6, B3, C and zinc.

Most researchers are using evening primrose oil encapsulated under the name 'Efamol'. A pilot study at St Thomas's Hospital in London, using Efamol on women with intractable pre-menstrual symptoms, shows that over 60% of these women report an improvement, including the relief of breast pain. The oil has been researched for its effect on benign breast lumps at the Universities of Wales and Dundee. (Large amounts of PGs are found in women during natural childbirth, and some PGs are able to induce labour in women at full term.) Evening primrose oil is being increasingly used as part of the nutritional treatment for Multiple Sclerosis (SEE *Multiple Sclerosis*, pages 353–63). It can potentiate the effect of insulin.

David Horrobin believes that failure to produce PGs is one of the factors responsible for heart disease. He has found that prostaglandins regulate blood pressure, stop thrombosis, increase cardiac output, improve circulation and dilate blood vessels. They also lower cholesterol levels and can prevent the unnecessary clumping of platelets, thus acting as anti-clotting agents. PGE1 can relieve angina pectoris[6] and evening primrose oil has been successfully given to heart patients.

Finally, there is a strong possibility that prostaglandins may help the body fight against cancer. Many cancer cells cannot make PGs. In laboratory tests on animals, PGs have stopped the growth of some kinds of cancer cells.

Producers of evening primrose oil capsules

Britannia Health Products Limited (under the name Efamol). With added vitamin E.

Bio-Oil Research Limited (under the name Naudicelle).

The Evening Primrose Oil Company Limited.

Associated Health Foods (under the Healthcrafts label, Gamma Formula).

Evening primrose oil takes from twelve weeks to several months to have an effect.

Garlic

If there is a miracle plant, it's probably garlic.

Man's use of this odiferous little bulb is nothing new. In about 2600 BC, the slaves building the Great Pyramid of Cheops went on strike when they were deprived of their garlic rations. The athletes of Ancient Greece used it for strength and stamina in their Olympic Games.

In recent years scientists all over the world have been researching into the curative properties of garlic. In *The Lancet* (11 September 1976) researchers describe an experiment establishing, not for the first time, that garlic and onion in the diet protect against the high blood fat levels (including cholesterol) which figure in heart and artery disease. The component in garlic which exerts this effect is, like the component in onion, heat-stable and can be cooked without losing its virtue.

Several researchers, including a scientist at Geneva University, have found that garlic reduces high blood pressure, and it has been suggested that this effect is partly due to dilation of the blood vessels. It could also be due to the protection afforded by garlic against high blood fats. An accumulation of cholesterol lining the arteries can narrow them, thus putting up the blood pressure.

Garlic is also a purifier, having one-tenth the strength of penicillin and no side-effects. In the USSR it is called Russian penicillin and has been widely used to treat the wounded in two World Wars. It can chelate – or grasp – harmful additives and metals like mercury and lead, excreting them from the body.

American studies suggest that it may be a good treatment for tubercolosis and even typhus. Because of its powerful anti-bacterial action it can be used against intestinal disorders and it can be effective against rheumatism. It has been found, too, to lower the blood sugar in diabetics and is good for the nerves and digestion.

Experiments in 1957 showed that garlic protected mice injected with cancerous cells, in some cases delaying tumour formation and in some actually preventing it.

Garlic is better known in the UK for its action in respiratory disorders and is useful in coughs, colds, bronchitis and asthma. It is an excellent additive to any medicine chest, but please remember that, like many natural substances, it will in most cases work only slowly.

Many researchers are puzzled by the many benefits of garlic and feel that the vitamins and minerals in it are not enough to explain its wide-ranging beneficial effects. They conclude that the allyl disulphate in the odiferous 2% of the herb may be responsible, and that garlic, by its purifying effect, helps the body to heal itself of many disorders.

Garlic consists of several combined cloves and its active properties depend on an essential oil which can be obtained by distillation. It contains some protein and calcium, a lot of potassium and phosphorus, selenium, some of the B vitamins and C, together with allyl disulphate. Some of its ingredients can be destroyed by heating.

Ginseng

Panax Ginseng is a shrub with a large, tendril-covered root which grows in moist, shady forest places. The word ginseng means 'manlike' and is a reference to the shape of the root, which is the part used. Panax comes from the Greek word for 'all healing', as does panacea. People expected too much of the goddess Panacea, however. She found not a cure for all diseases, but a remedy for maintaining the health of the people. Perhaps this applies, too, to ginseng.

The herb has long been cultivated in Korea, China, Taiwan, Canada and the USA. The Asian stock, Panax Schinseng, contains a lot of the alkaloid ephedrine while the American, Panax Quinquefolium, has none; the Oriental root is held in higher esteem. The Mandarin ginseng, or Imperial grade, was assiduously cultivated by the Chinese emperors and it is recommended in a herbal which dates from the first century BC.

Known as the Miracle Root, the Root of Life, and the King of Herbs, ginseng has given rise to many legends and is even mentioned in the Bible. In the USA the Cherokees asked forgiveness of the earth each time they pulled up a root and the Pawnees prized it as an aphrodisiac. In Chinese Imperial times, a properly cured, best quality old root would fetch much more than its weight in gold.

Ancient traditions say that it will lengthen life, maintaining vitality and sexual activity; modern research has been more concerned with its effects on stress.

The Russians have done a lot of research into the herb. Professor Brekhman, head of the Institute of Biologically Active Substances in Vladivostok, has established that mice given ginseng will swim nearly twice as long as those without. Professor Petkov of the Institute of Advanced Medical Training in Sofia finds that it increases cerebral efficiency, staving off mental fatigue. It appears to take over the work of certain adrenal hormones so that the relevant area of the brain can work less hard.

Physical vigour and stamina, too, are improved by ginseng, as Professor Brekhman found when he gave it to soldiers in training, and early Russian astronauts were given the root to chew in orbit.

Concerning dosage, an attempt was made at the University of Paris to give some mice an overdose, but this just resulted in a lot of fat, but otherwise healthy, mice. Clinical trials on human patients have thrown up no ill effects.

Evidence shows that ginseng both stimulates and sedates. These apparently contradictory findings stem from the fact that it contains two groups of glycosides, one of which energizes while the other depresses. One raises blood pressure while the other lowers it and the same thing happens with levels of blood sugar. It would seem, moreover, that these glycosides only work when required, acting to normalize body functions. This has led Professor Brekhman to suggest that ginseng is one of a new class of substances, Adaptogens, which are passive in the absence of stress, but which act in its presence to bring the body back to normal.

Professor Shellard, Professor of Pharmacognosy at the Chelsea College, University of London, states that 'there can be little doubt today that ginseng may be considered as a true tonic'. No serious claims, however, are made that it will cure any specific illness.

Ginseng contains glycosides, amino acids, essential oils, fatty acids, ginsenin, phytosterin, mucilaginous resins, enzymes, vitamins, sugars, certain unknown alkaloids, minerals, silicic acid and not more than 13% moisture; research continues into this intriguing herb.

Eleutherococcus
This plant with the jawbreaking name is a close relative of ginseng, and has in recent years been the subject of some new research which claims that the two plants have similar properties.

Like ginseng, it is adaptogenic, and many researchers maintain that its effects are more marked and longer-lasting than those of the more familiar Root of Life.

Honey

Our first taste of honey dates far back to our earliest ancestors who scooped it out of a bees' nest. Since then honey has always been part of our history and mythology. The original Bardic name for Britain was Honey Isle of Beli; we were great beekeepers in those days. The ancient Greeks regarded honey as an elixir of youth, and the father of medicine, Hippocrates, recommended honey (presumably unfiltered) to his patients.

This sticky miracle, made by bees from nectar and other plant substances, was at one time the only concentrated sweetener available and was highly prized as a great delicacy.

Honey is mostly natural sugars. About 95% of it consists of two simple sugars, glucose and fructose, both quickly and easily absorbed by the body. Among the 24 or so other natural sugars present in minute quantities is trehalose, a major source of essential fats.

Fructose (fruit sugar) does not need insulin for absorption, so a little honey can be taken by diabetics. Our muscles can use fructose for immediate energy and it is therefore useful for athletes. (Fruit sugar can now be bought separately.) With vitamin C, it will prevent or alleviate a hangover, and it helps the body to absorb iron. Honey's great sweetness comes largely from the presence of fruit sugar.

The saccharase in honey helps to prevent dental decay; those prone to caries have been found to carry very little of this enzyme in their saliva. The calcium and phosphorus in honey

7: What 100 grams of honey contain

(Average sample)

Calories	288	Copper	0.07mg
Protein	0.25 – 2.75g	Iron	0.4mg
Fat	trace	Manganese	0.2mg
Fructose	27.25 – 44.26g	Phosphorus	17mg
Glucose	22 – 40.75g	Vitamin A	trace
Sucrose	0.25 – 7g	Vitamin B1	2 – 12mcg
Maltose	2.7 – 16g	Vitamin B2	7 – 145mcg
Higher sugars	0.13 – 13.2g	Vitamin B6	1 – 480mcg
Water	14.4 – 22.9g	Pantothenic acid	9 – 360mcg
Potassium	51mg	Nicotinic acid	4 – 590mcg
Sodium	11mg	Vitamin C	0.5 – 6.5mg
Magnesium	6mg	Biotin	3mcg
Calcium	5.3mg	Folic acid	trace

are essential minerals for healthy teeth. On the other hand, both fructose and another sugar in honey, sucrose, will encourage tooth decay.

Acetylcholine, another substance present in small quantities, increases the blood flow to the heart and decreases the blood pressure and heart rate; honey has also been used to regulate the heart rhythm[1] and German research has isolated a factor encouraging growth. Honey has probably been used in healing for as long as it has been a food. It contains a bacteria fighter, inhibine, and can be used for wounds, burns, mouth infections and so on. It is a mild sedative – honey with lemon juice is a traditional cough remedy – and it has a gentle laxative action.

There are many vitamins in honey and the vitamin C content is protected and not easily destroyed as it is in fruits and vegetables. Honey also has plenty of minerals but the mineral content depends on the soil in which the nectar-bearing plants have grown. If the soil is mineral-deficient then the honey will be, too.

Honey is pure. An EEC directive brought into English law in the Honey Regulations of 1976 lays down that nothing must be added to honey sold within the EEC and also limits its heating to a level at which the honey will not be damaged. (Most commercial honey is pasteurized to delay crystallization.) Any honey not meeting these requirements cannot be sold within the EEC. Industrial honey, for instance, has been overheated and is used in food manufacture. It cannot be sold separately.

It is interesting to note that there is no EEC directive concerning the filtering of honey. It is possible to filter out most of the pollen (SEE *Pollen*). Probably the easiest way to get unfiltered honey is to buy a comb yourself, although primary, or virgin, honey has been simply allowed to drip out of the comb.

Honey with a high moisture content is very runny. If it solidifies, or 'granulates' (caused by the action of two of its sugars) it will be just as good. Rock-hard honey will soften if you warm it for a short while.

It is sometimes impossible for the bees to replace all the honey taken from the hive before they hibernate. So their keeper feeds them sugar syrup (he may have to do this in the spring, too). The bees are fed white sugar syrup; apparently they cannot tolerate the less refined brown. It has been found, not surprisingly, that bees reared on the nectar and pollen they have gathered themselves are better specimens than those given sugar syrup. No studies have been done, however, to compare the honeys produced in these two ways.

The contents of honey are affected by its source and age, whether it has been heated and how much pollen has been removed, and even by its container. Its colour is affected mainly by its source, and paler honeys are milder in taste.

One last word: although as we have seen honey is a delicious and nourishing food, it is *very* high in calories. A little of its strong sweetness will go a long way.

Kelp

The word kelp describes now one particular branch of the seaweed family. Earlier it meant the actual plant itself, and originally it referred to the ash left from dried, burnt seaweed from which soda was extracted. Kelp supplements are made from dried, ground seaweed.

Seaweed itself has always been a valuable food and the Japanese, who eat it a lot, are developing underwater seaweed farms; it is also used as a fertilizer. Seaweed is a sea vegetable, but without true leaves, stems or roots. A marine alga, it has a leaf-like blade, a stipe instead of a stem and a holdfast which does duty as a root. Seaweed takes nutrients from the sea through the entire surface of its blades, and perhaps this is why it is one of the most nutritious plants there is, having in particular a very high mineral content. Unlike land plants, it can sometimes manufacture vitamin B12.

Many seaweeds have antibiotic properties, and one variety can apparently turn saturated fats into unsaturated oils in the body. Tests at the Medical College of Pennsylvania seem to indicate that large amounts of seaweed can protect against goitre and breast cancer and this is supported by the geographical pattern of these diseases when compared with the places where it is eaten. It is also claimed to help control weight, lower blood fats and regulate bowel action. Seaweed acts as a tonic and blood cleanser and is good for the accumulation of toxins called catarrh; one variety, carrageen moss, is a traditional remedy for coughs, colds and other respiratory conditions. In a Philadelphia test kelp supplements improved the quality of hair and nails and were thought to help those with skin complaints and arthritis.

You can get dried seaweeds – agar, dulse, nori, kombu, hiziki, wakame – at your health food shop, and kelp tablets too.

Seaweed used to make kelp tablets contains protein (sometimes as much as 25%), plenty of vitamins A and C, vitamins D, E and the B vitamins B1, B2 (and occasionally B12), pantothenic acid, niacin and folic acid, with vitamin K. The many minerals include large quantities of calcium, iron, iodine, potassium, sulphur, magnesium and sodium, with phosphorus, manganese, zinc and trace elements, together with a little fibre and some fat. All these constituents vary according to the type of seaweed and where and when it is gathered.

Lecithin

Lecithin is a natural food of enormous value. It is found in soya beans, unrefined vegetable and seed oils (and of course seeds), nuts, wheat germ, egg yolk and liver. It is also widely distributed in animal and plant cells. Although it occurs in so many unrefined foods, it is destroyed by food processing and is not present in refined flours and hydrogenated (hard) fats.

It was discovered in 1850 by Maurice Gobley, who noticed that it enabled him to mix oil and water together. Its name derives from *Lekithos*, the Greek word for the source of his first extract – the yolk of an egg.

In supplement form, it is usually isolated from the soya bean rather than the egg. From crude liquid lecithin, a drying process produces granules with added vitamin E to keep them fresh and these are the best source. Capsules contain too little lecithin to be effective.

An essential part of body cells, lecithin is found everywhere in the body. About 25% dry weight of the brain is lecithin and it helps to make up the myelin sheaths protecting the nervous system. Its main function is to emulsify fats, breaking them up into small particles and suspending them in the blood. It is also needed to help the body make use of Vitamin B6 and the mineral magnesium. As well as helping to absorb and carry fats, lecithin is an extremely rich source of the essential fatty acids, helps with the transport of the fat-soluble vitamins A, D, E and K and feeds the skin with these nutrients.

The liver can produce lecithin, using sugars, fats, the B vitamins choline, inositol and B6, magnesium, an amino acid, (methionine) and an essential fatty acid (linoleic acid). But it can only do this when the diet is adequate.

There has been a good deal of research into the therapeutic uses of lecithin. Because of its ability to emulsify fats, it can reduce the plaques forming on the insides of the arteries by dissolving the cholesterol part of them. Two tablespoonfuls of granular lecithin taken at each meal have been shown to reduce patients' high blood cholesterol levels within three months, and it has been used to treat psoriasis, a skin complaint associated with high levels of cholesterol.

Those taking a lot of saturated fats in their diet risk an excess of blood fats, a condition where blood cells called platelets – needed to plug the bleeding when you cut yourself – clump together. (In this form they are commonly found in sufferers from heart attack and stroke, and in some women who take the Pill.) Platelets are discouraged from such unhelpful behaviour by the polyunsaturated fatty acids, and lecithin contains two – linolenic and linoleic acid. It has been suggested, further, that people with atherosclerosis and victims of heart attacks have low levels of lecithin in their blood. Recent research shows that lecithin will put up the proportion of HDLs (beneficial high-density lipoproteins) in the blood, and HDLs are strongly tipped to protect against atherosclerosis. Lecithin, therefore, can offer protection against heart and artery disease.

Lecithin deficiency affects the kidneys and *The Lancet* reports[1] 'a combination of cholic acid and lecithin does lower the cholesterol saturation of bile and may promote gallstone dissolution.' If the liver is short of the materials needed to make lecithin, fatty liver (a secondary symptom of diabetes) can result. But taken in therapeutic amounts, lecithin will emulsify deposits and start production up again. Lecithin, therefore, or its constituents, is essential for a healthy liver. One study states that it also reduces insulin needs in diabetics. It is claimed to act as a diuretic, helping the kidneys to get rid of excess fluid.

Perhaps it is best known in the UK for its action in helping the correct metabolism of fats, and its consequent value in weight reduction (although it is fairly high in calories – 3.5g contains about 35 calories). In fact all the essential fatty acids, in which lecithin is so rich, are involved in this.

In Germany lecithin is widely used for the protection it is believed to give against both mental and physical stress; many people have found that it helps them recover from exhaustion. Indeed another *Lancet* report describes a study where it improved the impaired thinking and learning ability of patients with pre-senile dementia.[2]

Lecithin is a mixture of phospholipids, made of fatty acids linked to phosphorus and combined with choline and inositol.

Liver

Many primitive peoples, including the early Eskimos, would give the organ meats of their kill to the successful hunters, and the muscle meats would be shared among the underlings struggling along behind.

The habit of lashing out on a huge steak, confident that we're getting not only the most expensive meat, but the best, is a modern one. The superiority of steak is a myth. The organ meats – brains, heart, kidney and liver – are the most nutritious parts of an animal. Of these, the best food is liver.

Liver is complete protein and contains an astonishing range of vitamins and minerals. For instance, about three ounces of liver will have 40 000 to 45 000 units of vitamin A – most meats have little or none. It has vitamins D and K and plenty of C. It is an excellent source of all the B vitamins, especially pantothenic acid, folic acid, and B12.

Before 1926, a diagnosis of pernicious anaemia usually meant death. In that year two doctors treated pernicious anaemia with liver and their patients recovered. Later on, in 1948, the factor in liver responsible for this was isolated and named – vitamin B12. Liver is the richest natural source of this vitamin.

Liver has valuable minerals, too; copper, zinc, chromium and phosphorus. It is enormously rich in iron, containing about 7.5mg in a three-ounce serving. This iron, unlike that from vegetables, is easily assimilated by the body, and it even helps the vegetal iron to be absorbed too.[1] This high iron content is particularly good for women, who often have iron-deficiency anaemia.

Also found in liver are lecithin (SEE *Lecithin*) which dissolves unwanted fats and polyunsaturated fatty acids in a natural, unprocessed form.

Research by Dr Benjamin Ershoff has established[2] that liver contains a factor which helps laboratory animals to resist stress. His experiments showed that animals resist intense cold, toxic drugs and even radiation better when they are given liver. This anti-stress factor, however, has yet to be isolated.

Choose lamb's liver. Sheep are still free-range and not as subject to the battery of chemicals used on intensively reared stock. These chemicals are processed by the animal's liver and we can do without them in our food.

Molasses

When sugar cane is harvested, it is crushed and the juice is concentrated by boiling. The refined sugar crystallizes out during this process and is removed by spinning the juice in a machine rather like a spin drier. After several more boilings and spinnings most of the sugar has been extracted and the syrup that remains is blackstrap molasses (molasses cannot be made from sugar beet).

There are other grades of molasses which are less concentrated, and which have been obtained after less processing, but these contain more refined sugar. Some people prefer these grades to the very strongly-flavoured blackstrap.

Molasses is rich in the B vitamins and in minerals, particularly iron. The iron content of blackstrap molasses is more, weight for weight, than in liver, and it is one of the richest vegetable sources of iron. It also acts as a mild, natural laxative.

The American nutritionist Adelle Davis tells us a cautionary tale, however, about a child of three who had been given large quantities of molasses and whose teeth were 'decayed to the gum margin'.[1] Perhaps he had never been taught to clean them.

Although nutritionists tell us that we do not need to add sugar extracted from cane or sugar beet to our diet because it occurs naturally in so many foods, most of us have a yearning sometimes for something sweet. So it makes sense to use, in moderation, sugars such as molasses which have not been robbed of their vitamin and mineral content.

Blackstrap molasses contains between 18% and 20% sugar, and most of that is glucose and fruit sugar, with some sucrose. There is also 3% protein and it has small amounts of the B vitamins B1, B2, pantothenic acid, niacin and plenty of inositol and B6. 10% of molasses is made up of iron, copper, calcium, chromium, phosphorus, potassium, magnesium, zinc and a variety of trace elements.

Muesli

Dr Bircher-Benner was one of the pioneers of modern nutrition. When he qualified in his native Switzerland in 1891, nothing was known about vitamins and minerals and the subject of nutrition did not exist. People boiled their food to keep it 'uncontaminated' and the young Bircher-Benner began by treating his patients in the orthodox way. One of his patients, however, was a woman suffering from a gastric disorder which he was quite unable to treat, and she went from bad to worse until a friend suggested a diet of raw vegetables and fruit. Bircher-Benner accepted this suggestion (perhaps the most astonishing part of this story) and the woman recovered completely.

This started him on a five-year course of private study which led him to explain this cure – the first of many – in terms of nutrition, and led eventually to the founding of the Bircher-Benner Clinic in Zurich, a source of healing for patients and a powerhouse of ideas for doctors from all over the world.

As a major part of his dietary treatment Bircher-Benner developed his Bircher Muesli, used so often at his Clinic that it was known simply as 'The Dish'. It had been an old Swiss custom to eat for a light evening meal a kind of fruit porridge consisting of cereals with fruit in season and milk straight from the cow, the whole delicious dish crowned with a few nuts. But this habit had fallen into disrepute and people were doing their best to avoid fruit. So Bircher-Benner, believing in fresh raw foods, softened the blow by serving fruit to his patients with a little cereal underneath.

This recipe – one level tablespoonful of oatflakes or other cereal grains, with a preponderance of fresh fruit and milk or yogurt – is a far cry from the rather sugary packets of mixed cereals that we can buy nowadays.

Muesli is better eaten at the beginning of a meal, usually breakfast, because the raw fruit does more good on an empty stomach. Fresh fruits which make a delicious muesli are apricots, peaches, strawberries, blackberries and all the soft fruits, and apples can be grated into the mixture (but please do this at the last moment or you will get a discoloured mush). You might like to add a little fresh lemon juice or perhaps a little honey. I always pour some wheat germ on to a little wholegrain muesli and, if I have any, top up with a few sprouting grains.

Packet muesli or Swiss breakfast food contains oats, and in nearly all processing some or all of the soft bran, or skin, of the oat is removed. This does not seem to be, however, the ruthless stripping of many nutrients that happens with the wheat grain, but is an incomplete process. Although they may be pretty sugary, therefore, supermarket mueslis based on oats are often not a completely refined food, although those from a health food shop are probably better.

You can buy an interesting mixture of whole grains and

make your own muesli, adding lots of fruit for a superb and
nourishing breakfast dish.

Pollen

Pollen originates from the male element of the flower. A very
fine powder of various colours, it appears on the stamens and
is carried by the bees in cross-pollenation so that the flowers
may produce fruit and seed. The honey-gathering bees search
for pollen to give to their larvae. A hive gathers 30 to 40kg of
pollen a year and by using a special apparatus the beekeeper is
able to take 10% of this amount without disturbing the hive.

Pollen is a highly complex substance, and its constituents
vary according to its type. Analysis of the pollen used by the
Health and Diet Food Company for Pollitabs reveals that it
contains up to 21 different amino acids and all the known
vitamins except B12, with carbohydrates and lecithin. Other
research into pollen has identified the minerals sodium,
potassium, magnesium, calcium, aluminium, iron, copper,
zinc, manganese, silica, phosphorus, chlorine and sulphur and
it also contains rutin which strengthens the capillaries. Oddly
enough, it can be effective against hay fever if taken
continuously, starting well in advance of the pollen season.

Additionally, pollen is antibiotic, has a benign influence on
intestinal flora and contains a factor influencing growth.

Many scientists believe that it is the *mixture* of substances,
in very small amounts and working together, which creates the
proven beneficial effects of pollen. It could in fact be used as a
survival food if supplemented with fibre and water.

Early primitive peoples were aware of the value of pollen,
and the natives of India and the Maoris of New Zealand used it
to make cake. By eating unstrained honey, too, these peoples
would have been ingesting pollen.

Pollen grains are extremely small – you would need more
than 14 000 to make up a single gram. Almost indestructible,
pollen grains from plants growing millions of years ago have
been found in the earliest geological strata.

Many experiments have been carried out to test pollen, and its tonic effect on the nerves, the intellect and the muscles has been documented. Many sportsmen now take pollen to increase their stamina. It has been used during pregnancy, for menstrual/menopausal difficulties, for anaemic, sickly children, and for elderly people who are exhausted and confused. Research has also established that it reduces the unpleasant, sometimes disabling side-effects accompanying radiation treatment for cancer.

The way it works is unexplained at present.

Propolis

This sticky resinous substance is collected by bees from certain plants and trees, especially the poplar, and taken back to the hive. There, it is used to stop up any cracks and to cover over any insects which may have wandered into the colony and been killed.

Propolis (from Greek, meaning 'bee-glue') is a harmless anti-infective agent, known since the time of Aristotle, when it was used for bruises and strained muscles. A mixture containing propolis proved effective for wounds during the Boer War and recent research confirms that wounds, including burns, treated with it will indeed heal more quickly; this also applies to skin inflammations and even warts. People with acne or shingles should dab a little on to the skin several times a day. It can be applied to mouth ulcers, too, and some dentists now are using a propolis gel for gum disease.

Taken internally, it helped patients in the Austrian Klosterneuberg Hospital with gastric and duodenal ulcers by reducing pain in 70% of cases. American doctors are currently recommending it not only to fight infection but also to reduce the effects of stress.

Propolis is a natural antibiotic which awaits further research before we can fully document its healing applications. It contains resins, wax, etheric oil, pollen, minerals and vitamins, proteins and various microelements.

Raw Juices

In a Swedish experiment, twelve men aged 20 to 50 walked a distance of 50 kilometres (about 31 miles) per day for ten days on a diet of fruit and vegetable juices and bottled water, supplemented with vitamin and mineral tablets.

Not surprisingly, the men lost weight during their walk, but they finished the experiment in excellent health. 'The nutrients supplied by the raw vegetable and fruit juices were obviously fully adequate to meet most of the demands of the body in such circumstances.'[1]

Raw foods and their juices have long formed the basis of nutritional therapy given by many doctors and naturopaths and the raw foods themselves are fully discussed in the *Whole Foods* section, pages 101–6). The raw juice fast is used for many conditions and has a cleansing and rejuvenating effect (SEE *Fasting* pages 159–63).

Fresh juices contain all the vitamins, minerals and essential fatty acids of the plant in a balanced form – quite a different matter from some of the sugary, processed liquids in the shops. They are particularly valuable for old people who may find chewing salads and fruits laborious and difficult.

A warning however – fruits and vegetables are meant to be *chewed* and so their juices should be savoured in the mouth, too, and not knocked back in one gulp. Such unkindness to your stomach should be resisted.

There are many juice extractors on the market, including an inexpensive hand-operated wine press, and of course for citrus fruits you can use the ordinary squeezer shaped like a pointed hat. The juices, once made, can be frozen; this should be done as soon as possible.

When juicing citrus fruits, lightly cut away the coloured outside of the peel and juice the white pithy part. That way you are getting the bioflavonoids (vitamin P) as well as vitamin C in a natural combination. If you are putting fruits and vegetables intact into your juicer, please be sure to wash them very thoroughly first, unless of course they have been grown without artificial chemicals.

Raw foods are best taken at the start of a meal, so follow the traditional habit of serving your raw juices first, and use them as soon as possible after extraction.

8: Raw juices*

This chart lists some common fruits and vegetables which you can use for juicing, showing their main therapeutic uses:

Fruit or vetetable	Properties	Beneficial effects on
Apple	Minerals, vit C, B vits	Liver, digestion, kidneys, skin
Apricot	Vits A, C	Eyesight, mucous membranes
Raw beetroot	Minerals, amino acids	General weakness
Beetroot tops**	Minerals, vit A	General weakness; eyesight
Brussel sprout	High vit C	Colds, other infections
Carrot	Vita A (in the form of carotene, ready to be converted to A), B vits, minerals	Nursing mothers and infants, eyesight
Orange, grapefruit, lemon	Vits C, P	Colds, other infections
Parsley**	Lots of vits A and C	Digestion, rheumatism, colds, eyesight, water retention
Spinach	Many minerals esp. iron. Vits A and C, B vits	Expectant and nursing mothers, rheumatism general weakness
Tomato	Vits C, D, E and P, B vits, many minerals	Digestion, general fatigue
Water-cress**	Vits A (carotene), C and B vits, many minerals esp. sulphur, iodine	Digestion, liver, general fatigue.

* Commercial juices (not 'squashes') have some nutritional value, and should be unsweetened.
** Dilute with other juices; flavour very strong.

Recommended reading
The Complete Raw Juice Therapy by Susan E. Charmine
(Thorsons).

Royal Jelly

A lot of rubbish has been talked about royal jelly. Minute
amounts of it have been sold at outrageous prices, especially
on the Continent and 'in no circumstances whatever could
these tiny quantities do anybody any good' (E.C. Barton-
Wright). So let's first have a look at what it is.

The only apparent difference between ordinary worker bees
and the enormous immobile egg-factory called the queen bee
is diet. Royal jelly is fed to an ordinary infant bee and it turns
into a queen bee. This substance is rather difficult to produce
in large quantities, as the bees only make it when they need
another queen. So you have to take away their present queen
to persuade them to start making it again, and if you keep on
doing this you will probably end up with a lot of discouraged
and neurotic bees.

Royal jelly has been used by doctors to treat artery disease,
menopausal problems, fatigue and depression. It is said to
have a rejuvenating effect and to help underfed children to
recover good health. It has been used, too, for arthritis but
success appears to be limited. Because, like propolis, it is a
natural antibiotic, it will help to stop the growth of unfriendly
bacteria and works with the body cells in their fight against an
infection.

In small doses, royal jelly has a definite biochemical action
in man. It contains almost all the B vitamins, with a lot of
inositol and relatively enormous quantities of pantothenic
acid. It is thought that its effects may depend largely on the
quantities present of this last vitamin. It also has about 20
amino acids, enzymes and a trace of vitamin C. French
researchers have recently isolated vitamin E in it. Lastly it
contains high quantities of acetylcholine, which influences the
glands and nerves. The proportions of these nutrients, and its
potency, vary considerably.

Spirulina

Spirulina is a primitive single-celled alga, one of the oldest plants in the world. It has been used as a human food for many centuries and grows in salty or alkaline water and on land.

This highly nutritious plant has now been analysed. It is the richest natural source of complete protein yet discovered and contains 70% protein. It contains more than twice as much vitamin B12 as liver. Spirulina offers many minerals – plenty of potassium, calcium, phosphorus and iron, with some magnesium and several trace minerals. Its vitamins include B1 and B2, and it is particularly rich in the substance which enables the body to make vitamin A, beta-carotene. Spirulina contains gamma linolenic acid, a fatty acid which the body needs but usually has to make for itself (SEE *Fats*, page 23); the only other substances containing GLA are evening primrose oil and human breast milk. During processing, vitamin C is added to spirulina to prevent oxidation.

Because of its high B12 content, spirulina is useful for vegans who may be short of this vitamin.

Dr Sakai of Japan has found it helpful for slimmers too. It has plenty of the essential amino acid phenylalanine, which is believed to act directly on the mechanism controlling the appetite. Its protein is easily assimilated, so that blood sugar is constant, preventing sudden hunger pangs. It may also line the stomach, making the person feel satisfied and relaxed.

Some sportsmen are using it now to prevent cramp and increase stamina. In a hospital in Bichat, France, it was given to undernourished children and adults, with good results.[1] These results have been duplicated in Mexican research.

Because of its enormous potential, and the current world food shortage, it is being widely researched. There are two main varieties, Spirulina maxima from Mexico and Spirulina platensis from Chad. Most work is being carried out on the Mexican strain.

Spirulina is of course a food and therefore quite safe to take, but because it is very concentrated large amounts may make some people feel queasy. It is available in capsules, tablets, or in powder form.

Recommended reading
Spirulina: Nature's diet supplement rediscovered by Maurice Hanssen (Thorsons, 1982).

Sprouting Seeds and Grains

'The nutritive value of sprouting seeds and beans would be difficult to exaggerate.' Naturopath LEON CHAITOW, *An End to Cancer?*

To anyone really interested in their own health and in the health of their family, sprouting seeds are indispensable.

When seeds start to germinate they release enormous quantities of vitamins, minerals and proteins to feed the embryo plant. This is the only time when these large quantities of nutrients are present. We harvest the sprouts, therefore, after the seed has started to germinate and before the growing plant has used up all the nourishment.

The increase in vitamin content alone is staggering. Sprouting wheat seeds have been analysed and found to contain 200% more vitamin B2, 90% more niacin (vitamin B3), 30% more pantothenic acid; and 100% more biotin and pyridoxine (all parts of the vitamin B complex) than dormant wheat seeds. During germination, vitamin C is increased by 60% in cereals. Oats multiply their niacin and vitamin B6 content by five, and in some other seeds vitamin E increases threefold. Sprouting alfalfa, mung beans, lentils and buckwheat contain laetrile (SEE *Index*).

Protein content, classified as 'complete', is rendered more digestible in the sprouting process, and sprouts contain polyunsaturated fats, enzymes and natural fibre, with a little carbohydrate and plenty of minerals. Alfalfa, for instance, is so rich in calcium that the ashes of the leaves are almost pure calcium, and tests prove that it lowers blood cholesterol levels. (Protective factors, known as pacifarins, have been identified in sprouts.) In fact they could be used as a complete food and as such have nourished laboratory animals for generations. No doubt part of their value stems from the fact that the nutrients in them are all taken together.

Before you rush out to the shed to bring in that left-over packet of runner beans, however, please remember that just any old seeds won't do. Always buy your seeds for sprouting from your health food store – otherwise you are getting pesticides as well.

Seeds you can buy for sprouting include soy beans, mung beans, peas, lentils, wheat, alfalfa, rye, corn, millet, parsley, clover, liragold, fenugreek and adzuki. (N.B. *Sprouted potato and tomato seeds are poisonous.*)

Sprouting is very easy and can even be done if you live in a bedsit. Take an old jam jar and a piece of muslin with a rubber band to cover the mouth, or a large colander lined with gauze; or you can buy a special sprouter. Damaged seeds won't sprout, so discard them. Put about a tablespoonful of seeds into the jar (the seeds will expand to several times their own volume, and the smallest ones will expand the most) and pour in plenty of tepid or cold water. I use tepid water in the winter and cold in the summer. The smaller seeds like alfalfa will only need soaking for about 4 hours and the larger ones like beans and grains for 15 hours, but it's quite good enough to leave any seeds to soak overnight.

Seeds need air, warmth and water to sprout. So they may go mouldy if they are overcrowded. They need a temperature of between 13 and 18 degrees centigrade (55–65F), so they won't like either cold rooms or radiators. If you leave them in the direct sunlight they will taste rather bitter but a cupboard suits them very well.

After you have soaked them, they only need rinsing night and morning so that they are left just damp. If they smell less than fresh, rinse them more often and put them in a cooler place; they may need this treatment if the weather is very hot. Don't waste the rinse water; use it in soups and casseroles. Soya sprouts should be boiled for ten minutes before they are eaten.

Grains and sunflower seeds are best used when the sprout is about as long as the seed. Mung is ready at about two inches long, alfalfa at half an inch, lentil at one inch and peas and soybeans are good short or long. Don't let your seeds get too big. I grew some wheat sprouts once with roots all over the place which tasted, and felt, like coconut matting. If you are going to cook your sprouts, they just need to stay in the boiling water long enough to go limp – about 30 seconds, the quicker the better; or you can steam or stir-fry them.

Some people store their harvested sprouts in the fridge in a covered dish or a plastic bag, but it's really better to use them at once if you can. Eat them raw in a salad, scattered over your breakfast cereal, in soups and casseroles, and as a garnish on omelettes and toasted cheese and a filling in sandwiches.

Recommended reading
The Complete Sprouting Book by Per and Gita Sellman (Turnstone Press 1981)
Successful Sprouting by Frank Wilson (Thorsons)
The Sprouters' Cookbook by M.P. Blanchard (Dietmars).

Wheat Germ

A grain of wheat has three parts. Inside the protective skin – the bran – most of the grain is made up of a starchy substance called the endosperm. At one end of the grain is the tiny germ. Manufacturers of refined flour mill out both the bran and the germ, using only the endosperm.

Bran is discussed elsewhere in this book (SEE *Fibre*, pages 35–42). Although the endosperm contains a store of plant food to sustain the seedling while it sprouts roots, the germ – less than 3% of the total grain – is by far the most nutritious part.

Wheat germ is about 35% high quality protein, which makes it one of the best sources we have. It is also the richest natural source of Vitamin E and contains most of the B vitamins, with many other essential nutrients. It helps Vitamin C to go to work in the body and experiments have also shown that it carries a factor, as yet unidentified, which helps the body to resist stress. It has been used to heal eczema and is helpful for anaemic people. The oil from the germ has been researched too and it will reduce menopausal symptoms and improve athletes' strength and stamina.

You can buy untreated wheat germ in some chemists or in a health food shop. There is a particular enzyme in the oil which turns it rancid after a time, so keep the packet in the fridge. Or you can buy it 'stabilised', probably for a slightly higher price. This toasted version is not quite so good as the heating process may have destroyed some of the more fragile nutrients.

Wheat germ is ideal for breakfast, so mix it with some wholegrain cereal and bran for a good, sustaining start to the day. Half a cup contains 14 grams of protein.

Wheat germ contains Vitamins B1, B2, B3, B5, B6, Inositol, Choline, Folic Acid, PABA, Biotin, Vitamin E, some Vitamin A, proteins and essential fatty acids, calcium, iron, magnesium, sodium, phosphorus, zinc, trace minerals and other substances.

Yogurt

The name 'yogurt' is Turkish in origin; this rather sour, curd-like food has been eaten for centuries virtually all over the world. When Little Miss Muffet sat on her tuffet eating her curds and whey, she was eating a kind of yogurt.

Yogurt is made by allowing milk containing bacteria to ferment. The bacteria multiply rapidly, changing the properties of the milk and causing it to thicken.

Yogurt has long been recommended as a food which prolongs a healthy life because the Bulgarians, who are said to eat a lot of it, apparently live long and vigorous lives. Without asking these yogurt-eating – and mythical? – Bulgarians what else they get up to, it is impossible to test this idea.

Yogurt is, however, a very healthy food. The milk protein, or casein, has been changed by the friendly bacteria into a more digestible form and the sugar content slightly reduced during fermentation.

It is an excellent source of high quality protein and has lots of easily assimilable calcium. The bacteria which make the yogurt also make B vitamins in the process and yogurt has more vitamin B2, or riboflavin, than plain milk.

If yogurt is eaten in large quantities, it appears to discourage harmful bacteria in the gut, including many of the gas-forming organisms. The friendly lactobacilli thus encouraged to grow have been shown to act against harmful bacteria which can cause bowel infections. The L. Acidophilus bacteria in yogurt may inhibit the enzymes that activate bowel carcinogens.[1]

Yogurt can help constipation and can relieve gastro-intestinal disorders in both adults and children; it cures diarrhoea better than some antibiotics. Many doctors now recommend it after a course of antibiotics because it helps to restore the valuable intestinal bacteria which have been destroyed by the drug. An experiment where yogurt and prune whip were given to 194 elderly hospital patients resulted in improved bowel action, better skin condition, an improvement in those patients who had diabetic ulcers, and better morale all round.[2] Yogurt may help to protect against urinary infections; it also helps to reduce blood cholesterol levels.[3]

Many people who are allergic to milk or who cannot digest it can tolerate yogurt and it is thought that yogurt inhibits the production of histamine. (Presumably this is not the case with a fruity, sugary yogurt, which to an allergic person might be less disgestible.) For people who cannot take anything made from cow's milk, not even yogurt, goat's milk yogurt can be tried. Since this milk may carry disease, it should be pasteurized first.

Argument rages over whether supermarket yogurt is alive or dead – i.e. whether the beneficial bacteria in it are still working or whether they have been killed by the processes used to make the yogurt.

The best way to kill yogurt bacteria and thus give the product a longer shelf-life is to pasteurize the yogurt. According to Marks and Spencer, however, most yogurt sold in Britain is not pasteurized; it is a short-life food. A *Which?* investigation, reported in the issue for July 1971, 217, states that in both supermarket and health food store yogurt 'the two main bacteria were alive and well – hundreds of millions of them'. The *Which?* team tested many brands in their research. Unless it has been pasteurized, therefore, (not likely in this country) most yogurt is live, with active bacteria.

Supermarket yogurt may have additives such as colour, flavour, preservatives, thickening and jelling substances and emulsifiers. On the other hand the manufacturers of yogurt for health food stores and similar outlets take a pride in their unadulterated product. Losely state that 'we do not use artificial flavours, colours, purées, syrups or preservatives'. Any yogurt, wherever you buy it, which has fruit and sugar added will be course carry more calories.

Most supermarket yogurts have some milk fat taken out and skimmed milk added. There are three basic types:

Low-fat, which means containing less than 0.3% fat on average.

Partly skimmed – 1–2% fat.

Containing at least 3½% fat and the most calories.

Even plain supermarket yogurt is more nutritious than milk; from the nutritional point of view, a low-fat 'natural' yogurt, without fruit, sugar or other additives, is the best buy. Vitamins A and D are added to some yogurts.

You can make your own yogurt, even from soya milk. Yogurt makers, with full instructions, are now available from many stores.

PART TWO

Eating for Specific Purposes

Breast-feeding

'A pair of substantial mammary glands has the advantage over the two hemispheres of the most learned Professor's brain, in the art of compounding a nutritious fluid for infants.'
OLIVER WENDELL HOLMES

The giving of cow's milk to babies was first mentioned in 1772. Otherwise, a wet nurse was employed if the mother did not nurse the baby herself. Feeding our babies with a bottle and a proprietary feed right from the first wail is still widespread now, in spite of evidence overwhelmingly in favour of breast-feeding.

Almost every woman can breast-feed if she wants to and if she is given enough information and help (SEE end of this section, page 144). Most proprietary baby feeds are made from cow's milk (some are from soya), so let's look first at the differences between human milk and *unmodified* cow's milk.

Every mammal has very sensibly developed a milk to suit its own young. This takes into account the rate and type of growth, the kind of digestive tract the animal has, its natural illnesses and so on. For instance, a rabbit's milk is about 12% protein compared to the 1.2% in human milk, so that the baby rabbit can grow rapidly. Whale milk has a high fat content to help the infant whale form a layer of thick blubber against the cold.

Cow's milk also differs in many ways from human milk, containing far more protein (because the calf doubles its birth weight in 50 days), almost four times as much mineral content (and filtering all that is a lot to ask of a baby's kidneys) and more saturated fats. The antibodies in cow's milk, of course, are there to fight a calf's diseases.

The human baby grows much more slowly than a calf. The baby's fast-developing brain and nervous and vascular systems are vastly more complicated, and for this kind of growth it needs the generous helpings of polyunsaturated fatty acids present in human milk; these fatty acids are digested sooner, so they are more easily accessible to the baby too. A baby's growing nerve fibre coatings also need more lactose than is supplied in cow's milk. The essential mineral calcium, is treated roughly by cow's milk which causes an acid to be released during digestion, taking calcium out of the body. This does not happen with breast milk.

The iron in breast milk is absorbed more easily, helped by the higher levels of the vitamins C and E and the mineral copper. Until quite recently it was believed that breast milk contained so little vitamin D that babies needed extra. Recent work, however, has shown that there is indeed vitamin D in breast milk, but it is water soluble and did not show up in the earlier tests.

The 1.2% of protein in breast milk is made up of curd and whey proteins. Although the protein content is relatively small compared with many other mammalian milks, there is more of the two proteins cystine and methionine and these are especially valuable for premature babies. There are, too, more nucleotides (the building blocks for *making* protein) in breast than in cow's milk.

Cow's milk has six times as much tough, indigestible casein as human milk. Because breast milk passes quickly and easily into the small intestine from the stomach, the breast-fed baby will be hungry more often than the baby on cow's milk. But he will need less, because he uses all the proteins he can get, in contrast to the baby on cow's milk who uses only half and whose stools will therefore be bulkier. Bottle-fed babies' stools contain less water than those of breast-fed babies because cow's milk has a higher proportion of substances which dissolve in water and the bottle-fed baby will get constipated more often.

The milk produced during the first few days after birth is called colostrum. This special milk contains high amounts of vitamins A, E and B12, and lactoglobulin; these quantities are somewhat lower in the later breast milk. The lactoglobulin carries antibodies which protect the baby against illnesses – both bacterial and viral. When he is a few months old, the baby will make his own antibodies, and this early period during which he needs to be protected by the substances in his milk is known as the Immunity Gap. This early protection also takes in the illnesses which the mother has had or has been immunized against, and food allergies.

So babies resist illness better on breast milk, and it's easy to see why. Additionally, the proportions of lactose, phosphorus and protein in breast milk prevent the growth of certain unwelcome bacteria. A breast-fed baby's gut contains thousands of tiny helpful organisms which are quite different from those produced by bottle-feeding. This is why his stools are sweeter-smelling than those of a bottle-fed baby. One organism called the bifidus factor prevents the growth of many disease-producing bacteria, as does a protein called lacto ferrin. Cow's milk has beneficial live cells, too, in different quantities. But they are destroyed by processing. Breast milk on the other hand is a living fluid.

Figures show that breast-fed babies get fewer illnesses, and that there are fewer cot deaths among them. Many babies are allergic to cow's milk, and this can show itself in a wide variety of symptoms: diarrhoea, vomiting, failure to thrive, bleeding from the gut with consequent anaemia, colic, eczema, nettle rash, runny nose, cough, wheezing and rattling on the chest, asthma and bronchiolitis. Recent studies suggest that between ½% and 7% of bottle-fed babies are affected by this allergy. A single bottle of cow's milk can sensitize a baby, and the allergic symptoms can happen at once, or the next time he takes cow's milk, or even some time later. Breast-fed babies are less obese, too, and other advantages include better jaw and mouth development and even less dental decay.

What about modified cow's milk?

In 1974 the Department of Health and Security's report *Present Day Practice in Infant Feeding* recommended breast-feeding and stated that babymilks should be as close as possible to breast milk in their composition. In their report of 1977, *The Composition of Mature Human Milk*, the DHSS acknowledged the variation in breast milk's composition, but stated 'the more an artificial milk food departs from the average composition of human milk, the greater is the possibility of untoward effects in the infants to whom it is fed.' Babymilk manufacturers, therefore, base their products on the need to approximate to breast milk.

There are two types of babymilks, 'highly modified' and 'less modified' (your doctor or a dietician will tell you if your baby needs the latter). The highly modified milks have a casein/whey ratio to bring the milk more in line with breast milk. Most babymilks are composed of skimmed cow's milk, lactose, butterfat and vegetable oils; vitamins are added in accordance with DHSS recommendations and mineral content adjusted (sodium, potassium, calcium and phosphorus levels have been lowered and iron has been added). The protein

content is lowered to match that of breast milk. The following
table gives some comparisons:

	100ml Mature Breast milk	100ml Highly modified babymilk	100ml Cow's milk
Protein (g)	1.3	1.5	3.2
Fatty acids			
Saturated (%)	51.4	47.5	63.3
Unsaturated (%)	48.6	52.5	36.7

(based on figures supplied by Cow and Gate)

It is clear, therefore, that if you are unable to breastfeed your
baby, the proprietary feeds now available have been carefully
modified to provide a nourishing alternative.

If your baby cannot tolerate cow's milk in any form, your
doctor or local dietician will advise you on proprietary alternatives.

Following the dictum of an eminent nutritionist, that
cuddles are more important than calories, let's end the list of
advantages with probably the most important factor – the
attachment to mother. Not too easy to encourage, perhaps,
when he is left in his cot holding an unfriendly bottle. The
baby whose mother gives him her breast – or just a cuddle –
when he cries, surely has the best chance of growing up secure
in her love.

Information

Please also read the *Pregnancy, Lactation and Food* section
(pages 188–99) for good nutrition while you are nursing your
baby.

Mothers who doubt their ability to breast-feed should
contact The National Childbirth Trust, at 9 Queensborough
Terrace, Bayswater, London W2 3TB, telephone 01-221 3833
who have over 500 breast-feeding counsellors in Great Britain.
These counsellors are all mothers who had experience of
breast-feeding before their training. They are available 24
hours a day for telephone counselling and aim to give mothers
the support, encouragement and practical advice they often
need. The counsellors also give antenatal talks, visit hospitals
and offer a selection of literature for sale or loan. The NCT
sells nursing bras and hires out electric breast pumps and, in

some areas, donates breast milk to the hospital milk banks.

Another organization offering support to breastfeeding mothers is La Leche League of Great Britain, of Department A, B.M. 3824, London, WC1 6XX.

Recommended Reading
An excellent book is *Breast is Best* by Drs Penny and Andrew Stanway (Pan 1978).

Children and Food

'The evidence is slowly accumulating that all is not well in this "sugared" generation and that health does really derive from what we eat.' JAMES LAMBERT MOUNT, *The Food and Health of Western Man.*

Many of our children are inadequately fed. A Ministry of Health pilot survey among 430 children of pre-school age showed that intakes of calcium and vitamin D were low.[1] One-third of 4365 Scottish children between one and two years old were also short of vitamin D;[2] this can cause rickets. Iron deficiency is common in small children. A 1953 survey in *Paediatrics* showed that half the young children examined were short of this essential mineral. A more recent survey in 1972 established that one-third of 450 infants aged between six months and two years were actually anaemic.[3]

Obesity is a threat to health in the West and it often starts in childhood. 261 infants were examined and over half of them were putting on weight too fast and likely to be fat. Most were artificially fed, with too much cereal, sugar and prepared foods. These babies were only *six weeks old*.[4]

In another survey, 57% out of 4382 schoolchildren in England and Wales had inadequate diets. The food of 11% of these children was 'extremely poor'. About a quarter of our schoolchildren skip or skimp their breakfast and rely on buns and crisps from the school tuckshop to keep them going until lunch.[5] School lunches themselves are generally inadequate[6] and many schools are providing a snack counter now instead, where the children can stuff themselves with more junk foods. A 1972 survey in the *British Medical Journal*[7] showed that 41% of children ate school lunch then, 20% brought food from home and 31% bought snacks at school. 4% ate nothing at all. Since this survey was carried out the cuts in school meals services have made matters worse. Even an inferior school dinner is better than a bag of crisps and a can of fizz from the school snack counter.

A 1959 report in *The Teenage Consumer* stated that about 12% of a teenager's money is spent on snacks, sweets and soft drinks. Since then, the growth in the convenience food industry has probably boosted this figure.

Vitamin C deficiencies are widespread. In the winter months, more than half the households in the UK are probably short of vitamin C. During the entire year, 20% of UK households consume less than the British recommended daily allowance of this vitamin.[8] This allowance, 30mg, is in any case considered by some authorities to be far too low.

A diet can lack certain nutrients, or it can have too many additives – food chemicals, salt and sugar. It is true that the additives put into our convenience foods have been tested on laboratory animals for cancer and other cell damage. But to test one substance in isolation on laboratory animals for its ability to cause obvious, limited harm is not the same as testing several substances together (after all, they are eaten together) for long-term, insidious damage to human beings. Research is now going on, too, into the effects of some food additives on children's behaviour, and the results are disturbing (SEE *Hyperactive Children* pages 333–9). The vitamin and mineral destruction in our convenience foods, and the chemicals added to them, are more fully discussed in the *Modern Food Industry* section (pages 42–51).

'We (and the food industry) need to appreciate that for young children the "headstart" we give them educationally may be more than cancelled by the "hindstart" we give them nutritionally.'   ROGER J. WILLIAMS, *Nutrition Against Disease*

Each child must grow at his own rate; rapid growth is only a good thing when it is right for that particular person. Several nutrients are notably essential for healthy, natural growth.

Vitamin A is called the growth vitamin and a shortage is probably widespread. In 1968, the US Citizen Board of Inquiry into Hunger and Malnutrition reported that up to 40% of all Americans were short of vitamin A. The B vitamins riboflavin, biotin and pantothenic acid are also involved in growth and the *Journal of Clinical Nutrition* for September/October 1953 reported that B12 supplements given to growing children exerted a growth-promoting effect on them and improved their general health as well, helping them to resist infection. The minerals calcium, phosphorus and zinc are concerned with growth, and protein is of course vital in building new tissue.

Almost all nutrients are concerned in helping your child to throw off infection and stay well. If he is constantly catching cold and is usually laid low by the 'bug that is going around', then make sure that his diet has plenty of vitamin A, C and the B vitamins. Antibiotics have undesirable side-effects and may damage his health in the long run, but a child eating a wholefood diet (SEE *Whole Foods* pages 101–6) has a well-nourished immune system which is able to resist infections.

Vitamin B1, or thiamine, is sometimes called the 'morale vitamin' because of its effect on the mind. A deficiency can cause depression, nervousness and confusion, and a severe deficiency beri-beri. A shortage of the B vitamin niacin can also cause irritability, anxiety and bad memory, and a severe deficiency leads to pellagra. The B vitamins, in particular B1, are used by the body to metabolize carbohydrates. Unrefined starches and sugars bring their own B vitamins with them but refined carbohydrates – white sugar in particular – deplete the body of these valuable vitamins (thiamine and niacin are however added to white flour). It can be seen that white sugar is therefore the main culprit, and that the more white sugar you eat, the more B vitamins you need.

Many teenagers eat out a lot and their café diet, although not cheap, is very poor and loaded with sugar. Writing in *The Health Quarterly* nutrition expert Doris Grant links an inadequate diet, made deficient in the B vitamins by excessive sugar, with our rising incidence of juvenile crime and delinquency.[9] In the April 1958 issue of the journal *Science*, Nobel prizewinner Linus Pauling blames deficiencies of B1, niacin, B6, B12, biotin, folic acid and vitamin C for some kinds of mental illness. Current interest is focussing on the strong link between hyper-activity (SEE page 333) and food.

Our high intake of white sugar and white flour must also be blamed for the state of our children's teeth. We are becoming a nation of false teeth wearers, and tooth and gum disease in both children and adults are reaching epidemic proportions.

'Good nutrition fosters good nutrition.'   ROGER J. WILLIAMS,
Nutrition in a Nutshell.

To improve the health of the nation by improving the quality of its food, we must start with nutritional care *before conception*, during gestation (SEE *Pregnancy, Lactation and Food* pages 188–99), and through infancy and childhood to a healthy adolescence. Children brought up to eat properly will need no further prompting and will in their turn see that their own children are well-nourished. The prospective mother therefore is responsible for the sound eating which will do so much to guard her own and her family's health.

Weaning your baby
This is an individual thing. There is no advantage in weaning your baby on to solid foods earlier than is good for him.

There are three dangers for young babies who are being given their first solid food; too much salt, too much sugar, and the giving of cereals too early. Be very careful about introducing cereals until your baby is six months old; he may develop an allergy to them.

Start by giving your baby extra liquid, in very small quantities so that he can adapt to the new food. At two months he could have half a teaspoonful of freshly-pressed orange juice mixed with two teaspoonfuls of cooled boiled water or mineral water. Low-mineral waters such as Malvern, Evian and Aquapura are best. (Water from a water-softener contains a lot of sodium and lacks calcium and magnesium so it should not be given to babies.) This juice mixture should be given at least half an hour before a milk feed, and can be increased at the rate of about half a teaspoonful a week so that by the time he is eight months old your baby is taking the juice undiluted and in larger quantities. Give him also some freshly pressed carrot or celery juice; you can press carrots without an extractor by grating some into two or three thicknesses of muslin and then twisting it and squeezing out the juice.

At four to five months, baby can have small amounts of pureed steamed vegetables or raw fruit. He might like some cooked and sieved carrot, and some mashed fruit pulp – peeled and depipped grapes, apple, pear or ripe banana. Increase the amount you give him at the rate of half a teaspoonful every week. At four months your baby might also like some orange. Peel the fruit, pulp it and put it through a sieve or a blender; give half a teaspoonful to start with. (The pulp is nutritious too.) At this age you can also add just a taste – about a quarter of a teaspoon – of egg yolk, curd cheese, sieved potato or pureed beans with his sieved vegetables. These amounts can be gradually increased.

At five to seven months, breast feeds may be replaced by the bottle; some mothers however continue to breast-feed up to eight months. If the child reacts to cow's milk, Plamil or another suitable soya milk may be given. Goat's milk, if used, should be pasteurized. You might like to add a *small* pinch of brewer's yeast to the bottle feed. At six months baby may take a little whole cereal – for instance, Weetabix – with milk and some sieved prunes or grated raw apple. (Some babies find prunes rather laxative and in this case they should be left out until later on.) Give your baby a piece of baked wholemeal crust, or a piece of apple or scrubbed carrot to chew on, to exercise his jaws and help his teeth erupt. From now on he will be taking more solid foods and may start learning to drink himself. He may like to take a little yogurt or grated cheese at this stage, and some home-made soup made for instance with vegetables and a lentil base.

At eight months, your baby may be fully weaned on to cow or soya milk and a good eating plan would look like this.

On waking Freshly pressed orange or other fruit juice.

Breakfast A little whole cereal without added sugar and a half a teaspoon of wheat germ, a little grated apple or some other fruit, milk.

Mid-morning Fresh, diluted fruit or vegetable juice, or clear unsalted broth.

Lunch Sieved, steamed carrot or green vegetables, mashed baked potato, egg or grated cheese or a pulse dish; some fish or a little lamb's liver, cut into small strips and sautéed in unrefined oil.

Peeled, de-pipped grapes, or some sieved prunes or other

fruit; baked apple with junket, or egg custard, or plain yogurt with some milk.

Give baby water or milk to drink only if he wants it.

Mid-afternoon   A drink, as mid-morning.

Evening meal   Fruit or vegetable juice.

Squares of wholemeal bread spread with curd cheese, with some peeled, finely chopped raw carrot and tomato and a little chopped lettuce. Some mashed ripe banana in milk with perhaps a little cereal added.

Give baby water or milk to drink as well only if he wants it.

Note: Do not add either salt or sugar to your baby's food, either in cooking or on the plate.

Commercial baby foods

These are undoubtedly much better than they used to be. Salt and sugar are kept to a minimum but Boots tell me that they have to be careful not to add too little sugar since mothers may add more to sweeten the food to their own taste. Some manufacturers (for instance Heinz) do not use chemical additives at all. On the other hand, there must be vitamin destruction in these foods during preparation and storage. So keep them for a standby.

If you need any more guidance on diet and possible supplements for your baby, please consult a naturopath (SEE appendix), a nutritionally aware doctor, or your baby clinic.

Schoolchildren and food

A skipped breakfast is a bad way to start the day. Give your children fruit juice, followed by wholegrain cereal with wheat germ and milk; add to taste fresh fruit topped with honey, yogurt, dried fruit or unsalted nuts. Or scramble some eggs on wholemeal toast, with a scrap of bacon for added flavour, and some fruit to follow. A high-protein, sustaining breakfast will stop your child filling himself up with junk at the school tuckshop.

If school meals are unobtainable or awful, your child can take a lunch-box; wholemeal sandwiches of cheese or cold meat, with frest fruit and salad and some dates. For sandwich spreads, breads, cookies and other wholefood delicacies, see Beatrice Trum Hunter's *The Natural Foods Cookbook*.

Children are under a lot of pressure from their friends to conform, so when the gang comes to tea, soft-pedal your notions about food. It's better to give ground sometimes rather than be labelled a crank. The occasional can of coke isn't going to do your child any permanent damage. Hungry children will eat absolutely anything that you put before them, so when they come in give them fruit and cheese or nuts to keep them going until the main course; this way they will get something raw at the beginning of the meal. *The Natural Foods Cookbook* gives recipes for homemade ice-creams and other delicious foods which your children will enjoy.

Cow's milk can encourage catarrh, so if your child is very prone to coughs and colds, try replacing it with fruit and vegetable juices and soya milk. Children do not need added sugar, although they will probably like it. There is plenty of natural sugar in foods without your having to add any and sugar can be a menace to your child's teeth and waistline.

Give your child whole cereals including wholemeal bread, fresh raw fruits and salads, plenty of protein (for growth), with dried fruits, honey, molasses and dark brown sugar in moderation for sweetening – SEE the *Whole Foods* section (pages 101–6) for more information.

If you need any more guidance on diet and possible supplements for your child, please consult a naturopath (SEE appendix) or a nutritionally aware doctor.

Recommended reading
Let's Have Healthy Children by Adelle Davis (Unwin 1975)
Growing up with Good Food ed. Catherine Lewis (Unwin Paperbacks 1982).

Books mentioned in this section
Nutrition Against Disease by Roger J. Williams (Bantam 1978)
Nutrition in a Nutshell by Roger J. Williams (Dolphin 1962)
The Natural Foods Cookbook by Beatrice Trum Hunter (Faber 1977).

Compatible Eating

Digestion is one of the most important processes in the body.

Anything, therefore, that makes it easier and more complete has a tremendous influence on our health.

Although the young and strong can eat almost anything mixed with almost anything else, this is not true of us all. Several illnesses, including digestive troubles, may be helped by compatible eating and it is recommended by some naturopaths and nutritionally aware doctors.[1] It is, however, controversial.

This way of eating is basically a matter of not mixing high-protein foods or acid fruits with high-carbohydrate foods. In other words you don't eat bread with meat, and you don't eat sugar with oranges.

The demise of the ham sandwich (bread and meat) is a pretty shattering idea. Why are we recommended to eat like this, and what does it do for us?

Foods contain, of course, mixtures of proteins and carbohydrates in varying proportions. So it should be impossible to separate these two categories in any practical way. But let's take a closer look.

High-protein foods   This means foods containing not less than 15% protein – meat, fish, eggs, cheese, milk and yogurt fit into this category.

High-carbohydrate foods   These are foods made up of about 50% starches and sugars – cereals, bread, rice and potatoes.

Using this classification, any food containing relatively small quantities of protein, for instance grain, does not qualify as a high-protein food. Carrots, which contain a little carbohydrate, do not qualify as a high-carbohydrate food, either.

Acid fruits   These are all the citrus fruits (oranges, lemons, grapefruit, tangerines, satsumas, etc.) and acid-tasting berries.

In a nutshell . . .

To sum up, to eat compatibly you simply avoid taking any food from the high-protein group and eating it at the same meal with any food from the high-carbohydrate group. You also avoid combining acid fruits and high-carbohydrates at one meal.

The reasons

To understand the possible advantages of compatible eating,

we need to look at what goes on inside the stomach during digestion.

Proteins need an acid medium to be digested properly. When animal proteins pass into the stomach, hydrochloric acid is produced in exact ratio to the amount of protein eaten. This acid activates an enzyme, pepsin. Pepsin splits up and digests the protein. This process can only take place in an *acid* medium.

On the other hand, carbohydrates (starches and sugars) need an *alkaline* medium for digestion.

The whole process of carbohydrate digestion starts in the mouth where the enzyme amylase (formerly ptyalin) begins to split up the starches. This splitting process goes on further when the carbohydrates reach the small intestine; here they are thoroughly digested. Incidentally, it is easy to see from this how important it is to chew our food properly; not to do so impairs digestion.

What about acid fruits?

Acid fruits can cause indigestion when eaten with starches or sugars at a meal. So don't eat cake with oranges – or sugar with oranges, either. Acid fruits counteract the alkaline saliva in the mouth and the alkaline medium in the stomach which, as we have seen, are essential for the proper digestion of carbohydrates.

(Perhaps here is the place to explain that acid fruits do not in fact have an acid effect on the body. When completely digested, they change their character and leave behind an alkali residue. Their acid content is soon excreted.)

Going back again to proteins and starches, we can see that by combining high-protein foods (needing an acid digestive medium) with high-carbohydrate foods (needing an alkaline medium), we are asking the stomach to perform two contrasting functions at once. This puts a strain on the digestive organs and encourages indigestion.

Mixing high-proteins with high-carbohydrates at the same meal produces incompletely digested proteins, as the stomach tries to cope with both. These proteins are toxic, and some of them can manufacture histamine, the chemical which is released during an allergic reaction. Allergic patients who agreed to give compatible eating a try found in many cases that they lost their allergic symptoms and felt well for the first time in many years (SEE *Allergies to Food* pages 219–29).

As well as causing fermentation and decay of undigested foods, the wrong mixture leads to the development of irritants, with constipation and acidosis, a condition which lowers the body's resistance to disease. Discussing artery disease in a letter to *The Lancet* of 3 July 1971, Dr P.D. Newberry wrote, 'it is possible that the combination of foods *habitually eaten together* [my italics] may be no less, or more, important than the total quantity of any given food in the diet. . . .' Not surprisingly, this way of eating has been found helpful in many illnesses – indigestion, obesity, arthritis, and asthma.

There is one more point to make.

Each kind of protein, when it is eaten, demands a different reaction from the liver. When we eat meat, for instance, the liver supplies the right substances to help digest it. When we eat cheese, the liver adjusts its reaction to suit the cheese, and so on. Therefore it is better to eat only one kind of protein at each meal. The same rule applies to high-carbohydrate foods, which also demand help from the liver to be digested. Eat just one kind – either bread *or* potatoes – at one meal.

High-protein foods Meat, fish, eggs, cheese, milk, yogurt (17.5% protein), brewer's yeast (35% to 50% protein), wheat germ (35% protein), seeds (20% to 30% protein). *Combine with:* fats and oils, all vegetables except potatoes, all salads, sprouting seeds and grains, salad dressing, nuts, all fruits and dried fruits.

High-carbohydrate foods All cereals including rice, bran, all cereal products including bread, pastas, cakes, etc., potatoes. *Combine with:* fats and oils, all vegetables, all salads, sprouting seeds and grains, yogurt, salad dressing, nuts, all *sweet* fruits and dried fruits, sugars such as honey, molasses and dark brown sugars.

Try to eat one protein meal a day, one meal of mostly starch (unless you are young or very physically active), and thirdly fruit with milk or yogurt once a day. Eat your salads, vegetables and *sweet* fruit whenever you like.

In the case of legumes – peas, beans, lentils, peanuts – nature has boobed. High-proteins and high-carbohydrates are found together in these foods; this is why they can give you indigestion. If you sprout your legumes, however, you won't get any trouble (SEE the *Sprouting Seeds and Grains* section, pages 133–5, for advice on this).

It is important to allow an interval of at least four hours between meals of different character – i.e. between a starchy meal and a protein meal.

Recommended reading
Your Daily Food by Doris Grant (Faber 1973).

The Eyes and Food

The human eye is a marvellous, complex organ.

The eyeball is filled with a jelly-like fluid surrounded by tissue called the sclera. This sclera wraps right round the eye, and is seen at the front as the eye-white. The very front of the eye is also covered by the transparent cornea. Light enters the eye through the cornea and the lens behind it, focussing on the retina at the back of the eyeball. As the light enters the eye it is bent by the cornea and the lens, and as it is focussed on the retina it activates the optic nerve. This sends a message to the relevant part of the brain, and we see. The iris contracts and relaxes to adapt the pupil to the amount of light available and the distance of the object being looked at.

The retina at the back of the eye is made up of cones, which are sensitive to colour, and rods, which are sensitive to light and shade. The rods of the retina work by allowing the breakdown of a red pigment called rhodopsin; this breakdown is speeded up by high intensity light.

The list of vitamins and minerals needed by the eye is long. Deficiencies cause reading difficulties, fluctuations in eye refraction so that glasses have to be repeatedly changed, short sight, and intolerance to light so the eyes need sunglasses. Poor diet is a prime cause of squint. 'Approximately 50% of people who wear spectacles for distance or general purposes can be cured of ocular discomfort and given a higher lever of visual acuity by nutritional therapy.'[1]

Vitamin A   This is the most important nutrient for the eyes.

Vitamin A is essential for vision. Every year many thousands of children all round the world go blind as a direct result of its deficiency. Vitamin A is concerned with the rods at the back of the eye and the breakdown of rhodopsin. A deficiency – probably widespread in this country – results in difficulty in seeing in dim light ('night blindness') and itching, burning eyes with reddish eyelids and susceptibility of eye infections. The eyes will be tired and aching after close work such as reading, and there may be headache, pain and watering of the eyes, blurred or double vision and dizziness.

People working under bright lights use up plenty of vitamin A in their retinas and the eyes also need more in dim light. A severe deficiency can result in a damaged retina, causing blind spots in the visual field, clouding and ulceration of the cornea,

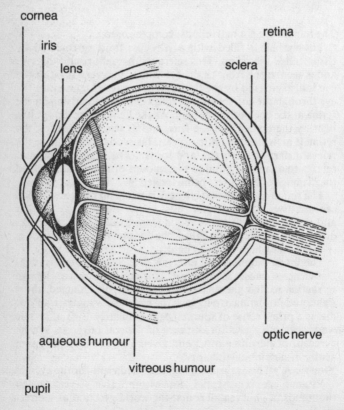

cornea

iris

lens

retina

sclera

aqueous humour

vitreous humour

optic nerve

pupil

and the eye can lose its ability to remain moist. This can end in blindness. With a less severe deficiency, the eyes look dull and the cornea is weakened. A healthy transparent cornea depends on this vitamin and so do normal eye movements, both reflex and controlled.

The B vitamins These vitamins have an enormous effect on eye function. Recent research in India found a significant association between different vitamin B complex deficiency signs and visual defects.[2] B vitamin deficiencies can damage both the sheaths protecting the nerve pathways and the nerves themselves, and blurred vision has been caused in volunteers by feeding them food lacking in vitamins B6 and pantothenic acid. Vitamin B2 works with A; a deficiency can cause oversensitivity to bright light and faulty vision in dim light; the eyes water, are bloodshot, and cannot focus sharply. A lack of B6 can cause muscle irritability and eye spasm; a deficiency of the B vitamin choline interferes with muscle action and will sometimes lead to eye haemorrhage. The vitamins B1 and B2 are necessary, like A, for a healthy transparent cornea.

Vitamin B1 has been studied for its effect on the eyes. Rats on B1-deficient diets suffered degeneration of the optic nerve, and four human patients experienced improved vision after thiamine was added to their diet.[3] Research at the University of Alabama found that nearly half a group of cataract patients were lacking in B2, and the report states that riboflavin deficiency may play a role in cataract development in man.[4] B-vitamin supplements given to 70 children resulted in improved vision in 56.[5]

Vitamin C Stress increases the body's need for vitamin C – and any eye trouble causes stress. The lens contains a high concentration of this vitamin. It is important for the transparency of the crystalline lens and a shortage is one cause of cataract. Vitamin C helps to heal eye inflammations and encourages a good blood supply to the eyes.

Vitamin E The absorption of the most vital nutrient for eyesight, vitamin A, depends partly on vitamin E; a shortage of E will make worse the damage done by a lack of A. Vitamin E also has a direct effect on the retina. Its lack can damage the nerve sheaths and lower visual acuity; it can cause muscle weakness and degeneration of blood cells and can weaken the capillary walls in the eye. Vitamin E works with C to heal injuries and eye inflammations. Experiments with animals indicate that it is probably concerned in the prevention of diabetic cataracts.

The Bioflavonoids Sometimes called vitamin P, these substances may help prevent cataracts in diabetics.

Zinc This is the most important mineral for good eyesight. There is a lot of zinc in the retina and it helps to mobilize vitamin A stored in the liver so that the vitamin can reach the eyes. Zinc has been successfully used, with vitamin A, to treat night blindness. Carrots by the cartload won't help the eyes without zinc.

Calcium Calcium is needed for the relaxation of a muscle after its contraction and a shortage can cause spasm and cramp in the eye. Vitamin D is needed for the proper use of calcium.

Potassium and magnesium A shortage of potassium can cause sluggish action of the eye muscles and a lack of magnesium can cause irritability of the voluntary muscles, possibly with muscle spasm.

Protein The crystalline lens in the eye is mostly protein, and any protein deficiency may predispose to cataract. Protein is also needed for eye muscle action.

Sugar Laboratory animals on a high-sugar diet developed short sight, and human volunteers eating a lot of sugar started to develop long sight.[6] It seems likely, therefore, that sugar interferes with normal eyesight. Nutritionist John Yudkin in his book *Pure White and Deadly* suggests that because sugar is involved in producing diabetes, which is so often accompanied by severe eye damage, it may also be involved in producing other, less serious, eye defects. Ophthalmic nutritionist Stanley Evans also recommends a reduction of refined sugars and starches.

Good food for good eyesight

The health of the eyes, like that of the rest of the body, depends largely upon good nutrition. This means a wholefood diet, with whole grains and cereals, raw or short-cooked vegetables, fresh raw fruits. Cut down on all fats and salt and use just a little dark brown sugar, molasses or honey for sweetening. Vegetables and fruit should form a high proportion of the diet; this ensures the right alkali/acid balance in the blood which is necessary for good sight. Please SEE *Whole Foods* (page 101) for more information.

Too much smoking and alcohol are bad for the eyes. Stanley Evans warns about this in his book *Nutrition in Eye Health and Disease.*

I have not written about eye diseases here, but it is interesting to know that veteran naturopath Stanley Lief recommends fasting for eye conditions, stating that many cases of eye trouble have been cleared up by fasting.[7]

Supplements should be taken under the guidance of a naturopath (SEE appendix page 405), a nutritionally aware doctor, or an ophthalmic nutritionist (SEE below).

Information
Readers seeking nutritional treatment for eye diseases will be interested to read *Nutrition in Eye Health and Disease* by Stanley C. Evans (Roberts Publications 1978). Mr Evans is a practising ophthalmic nutritionist and orthoptist.

The Bates method of eye exercises can ease or correct many visual defects. For the name of your nearest practitioner, please write to: Michael Ronan, Secretary of the Bates Association of Eyesight Training, 49 Queen Anne Street, London W1.

These two books will tell you more about the Bates method: *The Art of Seeing* by Aldous Huxley (Chatto & Windus 1943). *Better Eyesight without Glasses* by W.H. Bates, MD (Granada).

The eyes need natural light: please SEE *Health and Light* by John N. Ott (Watkins Publishing 1976).

Other books mentioned in this section
Pure White and Deadly by John Yudkin.

Fasting

Fasting has a long and honourable history.

The cave family would gorge themselves on a lucky kill and would then fast for a couple of weeks, until the next successful hunt. When we are ill, too, we have the same ability as many other animals to go for periods without food. Unfortunately we rarely use this ability now to get well, preferring to believe that regular eating is essential during illness to keep up our strength.

Fasting has long been used for religious and political ends. All the major world religions have at some time or another demanded it and pagan magicians often went without food before making magic.

Fasting for health was used in the time before Hippocrates by the priests of the Aesculapian order and the Greek physician, Athenaeus, praised it, saying that it 'cures diseases, dries up bodily humours, puts devils to flight . . . and raises man to the throne of god' – a reference no doubt to the bounding optimism and euphoria known as the 'fasting high'.

Fasting is a cornerstone of nature cure, or naturopathy.

The naturopath tries to restore to his patient the wholeness and balance which mean health. Naturopathy teaches us that the body will heal itself given the chance, and careful, controlled fasting offers it that chance. By giving the digestive organs a complete rest, fasting allows the body to throw off accumulated poisons. While the gastrointestinal system rests (30% of the body's energy is used for digestion), toxins from stress, poor living habits and adulterated food are discharged through the kidneys, bowels, lungs and skin. The cleaner and stronger the body is, the more healing vitality it can summon up to fight disease.

Fasting – emphatically – is not the same as starving. 'To fast is to abstain from food while one possesses adequate reserves to nourish vital tissues; to starve is to abstain from food after reserves have been exhausted so that vital tissues are sacrificed.'[1] During a fast the body turns over naturally to using stored nutrients as energy, and it is possible to live quite happily for a long time on these.

Don't listen, therefore, to well-meaning friends who tell you that you will collapse without regular meals. It just isn't true. The energy we get from eating has to be processed by the body before it can be used as energy. Water is the only thing – except air of course – we must have to survive over a few days.

Benefits
The first and most obvious result is weight loss. You should only believe your scales, however, after you have started eating

normally again, because this initial weight loss is probably just fluid that is easily replaced. Regular short fasts will bring your weight down over a period of time, and because it is easier for some of us to eat nothing at all than to eat less, many people use fasting to control their weight.

Fasting is a rejuvenating beauty treatment. As the body takes this opportunity to spring-clean itself, we look and feel younger; this is particularly noticeable on the skin. Fasting is a cure for digestive complaints, 'flu, diarrhoea, colds and catarrh.

If you are running a temperature, fast – but call your doctor under the following circumstances:
1   If the fever is greater than 103°F.
2   If it persists for more than 48 hours.
3   If it is accompanied by increasingly severe symptoms, particularly pain and dehydration.
4   If you are unsure of your diagnosis.

Fasting is prescribed by naturopaths for any acute condition, including attacks of bronchitis, cystitis, tonsillitis or any of the children's diseases such as measles. It is also part of the naturopathic treatment for arthritis and rheumatism, asthma and hay fever, varicose veins, high blood pressure and many other chronic diseases.

Perhaps the most valuable result of a fast is that it proves to us that we can do without food and crutches such as alcohol, tea and coffee for a while without falling apart. A fast can be the beginning of a psychological change for the better.

When not to fast
All this sounds wonderful, and it is. However, there are some important points to bear in mind when undertaking a fast.

The following people should not fast; pregnant and lactating women, very young children, teenagers and the very old. Do not fast if you expect to continue with a taxing job, if you are under inescapable stress, if you are physically weak, exhausted or depressed. Do not fast if you are receiving drug treatment, if you are anaemic, or if you suffer from high or low blood pressure (unless under medical guidance), heart trouble, gout, gastric or duodenal ulcers, cancer, a kidney or liver disorder or a chronic disease of the nervous system.

Extended fasts of up to thirty days are not unusual, but a

long fast, perhaps for a serious condition, should be undertaken in a health farm or some other place where you can be supervised by a practitioner *with an experience of fasting.* During a prolonged fast, symptoms of long-suppressed illness may reappear, and other profound and complex changes happen in the body; for instance, damaged tissues are destroyed and sound cells built up afterwards when the fast is broken with whole, unadulterated food.[2]

The short fast

A short fast is a period of from twenty-four hours to three days without solid food. You should have fruit juices, although you may find that citrus juices provoke a rather drastic reaction and are best avoided; take vegetable juices as well if you like but don't mix your juices too freely. These liquids contain vitamins, minerals, carbohydrates including fruit sugar, with alkalis to counteract the over-acidity of the stomach when it is empty. Fruit juices in particular give you plenty of potassium, an essential mineral that the body excretes during a fast, and the potassium and fruit sugar will help to stabilize your blood sugar level. Mix the juice half-and-half with bottled mineral water and add if you wish just a little honey. Start your fast day by sipping a glass of hot mineral water with a slice of lemon added and take your juices at normal mealtimes. If you are thirsty between these times, drink bottled mineral water. During a 24-hour fast you should take at least two pints of liquid.

Turn your fast into a relaxing holiday and spend it in comfortable familiar surroundings where you can switch off and just sleep, walk, read or listen to music. Your concentration will probably be diminished and your reactions slower and you should not drive a car. You will probably feel colder than usual, you may have a slight headache, and your tongue may be coated with a white fuzz – all this is quite normal. These symptoms show that your body is throwing off toxins, and you can help the process a little by taking warm – not hot – leisurely baths. Bowel action may slow down but it is not necessary to use an enema during a short fast.

Fasters often experience an ecstatic 'high', when the world is shining and wonderful and everything is possible. The late Sir Francis Chichester said that he always left any important decisions until a day or so after he had ended a fast, as he always felt so marvellous that his choice was over-optimistic and likely to be the wrong one!

'Any fool', said George Bernard Shaw, 'can go on a fast, but it takes a wise man to break it properly.' It must be emphasised that to break a fast with a gigantic meal is extremely harmful. There have even been a few cases of people who have died after breaking a prolonged fast because they were given the wrong food and too much of it. So even after a short fast, break it sensibly with a little fruit. Make the meal after that one a raw salad only.

The body is more sensitive to alcohol and coffee after a fast, too, and you may find your reactions to these stimulants very marked, so go carefully.

Those who are unable to relax at home and fast completely may like to try a fruit fast for one day once a week or so. By eating nothing but fresh fruit for 24 hours you are not, of course, fasting in the true sense, but fruit is cleansing and you will reap real benefits. Grapes in particular (thoroughly washed) are an excellent way to detoxify.

Apart from its almost miraculous effect on illnesses and its invigorating effect on the body and mind, fasting helps us to listen to our own bodies. We take time to reflect, to relax, to realize that we need only eat when we are hungry and not just as a habit, a reward or a prop. Everyone can develop his own intuitive knowledge of what he needs to eat, and when. Living in a society deluged with food and food advertisements, we learn to be less dependent on our food, to choose it more wisely and to enjoy it more.

Recommended reading
The Secrets of Successful Fasting, by Dr Hellmut Lützner (Thorsons 1978)

Hair and Food

You have about 100 000 hairs on your head. Hair protects the head from extremes of temperature and cushions it against injury. Hair is mostly keratin (a kind of protein) and each strand consists of three layers; the outer skin or cuticle, the cortex containing the pigment, and the innermost layer, the medulla. The root, lying beneath the scalp, includes the hair follicle in its sac and a storeplace for nourishment, the papilla. Sebum sacs are attached to the follicle, and blood vessels lead to the root. Your hair grows straight or curly according to the structure of the root.

Each strand grows, rests for a time, then falls out and is replaced. Hair grows at about half an inch a month, more slowly with age, and falls out most in the autumn and least in the spring. So don't worry about the few hairs you may find in your comb.

The hair, like every other part of us, depends on good nutrition and good circulation to stay healthy. A vitamin A deficiency results in dry, lifeless hair and often dandruff. The keratin which forms hair is a kind of protein so that a protein deficiency (unlikely in the West) can result in hair loss.

When your hair turns grey, the middle section of the hair shaft stops making pigments and fills up with colourless air bubbles. B vitamins thought to be especially associated with hair colour are folic acid, choline, pantothenic acid, para-aminobenzoic acid (PABA) and biotin. A deficiency of copper, too, can result in premature greying. Hair loss is often associated with deficiencies of certain amino acids and the B vitamins, especially inositol. Women, although apparently needing less inositol than men, are often deficient in iodine or vitamin B1, and this may impede scalp circulation and hold up the growth of new hair. The minerals calcium, copper and iron are needed for healthy hair.

Since vitamins and minerals are inter-dependent and work together, they are most effective when taken as part of a good diet. For instance, the nutrients I have mentioned above need vitamins E, C, the range of B vitamins and zinc in particular to work efficiently. For healthy hair, therefore, eat whole grains, wheat germ, brewer's yeast, liver if you eat meat, plenty of fresh green salads, raw and short-cooked vegetables, fresh fruit (SEE the *Whole Foods* section). Use Biosalt and include seaweed or kelp tablets in your diet, and for snacks try some seeds (SEE sections on *Salt*, *Kelp* and *Seeds*). Remember that hair grows and changes slowly and that the dietary approach will take time.

American dermatologist Dr Irwin Lubowe states that a diet unbalanced in favour of animal fats, white flour and white sugar and their products may affect the output of the sebaceous glands and cause greasy hair. So, if your hair is very oily, cut out refined and fried foods and follow the diet for healthy hair. Use four parts of water to one part of cider vinegar in a final rinse, pouring it over several times; the strong smell soon wears off.

Dry hair often signals not only a deficiency of vitamin A but a deficiency of essential fatty acids. These are found in nuts, beans, seeds, wholegrains, green leaves and unrefined oils. So take care to include these nutrients in your diet.

Your hair is sloughing off matured cells and waste through the pores of the scalp all the time. When the scalp cells start coming off in flakes, however, you have dandruff. (Make sure that it *is* dandruff and not just shampoo that has not been rinsed off properly.) Lubowe writes that 'the basic causes of dandruff are faulty diet, emotional tension, hormonal disturbances, infection due to disease, injury to the scalp and unwise or excessive use of hair cosmetics';[1] it is common in teenagers because of its connection with hormonal changes.

Anti-dandruff shampoos often contain powerful chemicals which can irritate the scalp. Although they temporarily remove the dandruff, they can force the sebaceous glands to make more oil as a protection. Some of these shampoos can even cause falling hair and allergic reactions as well. And – of course – they only control the condition. They do not cure it. The dietary treatment for dandruff is the best way of dealing with it in the long term, and the guidelines are the same as those given above for healthy and over-greasy hair. You could also take a vitamin A supplement and use a diluted version of the cider vinegar rinse recommended for greasy hair.

Hair can fall out as a result of stress, illness or pregnancy, or as a symptom of an under-active thyroid or anaemia. Antibiotics can harm your hair and you can help to counteract this effect by eating at least two cups of yogurt a day. Smoking, because it impedes good circulation, is not good for the hair and neither is a lot of alcohol. Pollutants such as exhaust fumes and cigarette smoke are easily absorbed into the hair, and permanent waving, harsh hair colours, too many sessions under the drier and heated rollers can all have a damaging effect.

Additional therapies
Biochemic tissue salts: K combination, for dandruff, falling
hair: SEE pages 107–8.
Deep breathing: SEE appendix, page 405.
Hair brushing and scalp massage.
Yoga: any inverted position: SEE appendix, page 405.

Macrobiotics

The word 'macrobiotics' comes from the Greek *makros* (large)
and *bios* (life), meaning a way of living life to the fullest to
develop both health and understanding. The macrobiotic way
of eating originated in the Far East some 4000 years ago and it
was first *described* as macrobiotic by George Ohsawa, a
twentiety-century doctor and philosopher from Japan who
brought it to Europe and the USA.

Macrobiotics is an attitude to life based on an understanding
of the importance of diet. Underlying it is the principle of
complementary opposites, antagonistic and yet united,
necessary to each other. These opposites are known as Yin and
Yang.

Yin represents the feminine, passive principle, cool and dark
like the night, slow, silent, cold, expansive, centrifugal. In
foods, Yin is said to be acid and includes drinks, fruits,
summer-grown tropical foods and foods of sweet and sour or
hot flavour, large expansive texture, purple, green or blue in
colour; the mineral potassium is Yin.

Yang is the masculine, active principle, bright, hot,
centripetal. Yang foods are alkaline and include cereals and
foods that are compact and hard, salt or bitter in flavour,
which mature in the autumn and winter, in northern lands.
Colours are red, yellow, orange; sodium (salt) is Yang. The
very few foods of animal origin eaten in this diet are Yang.

Followers of macrobiotics say that most illnesses can be
attributed to an excess of either Yin or Yang, and they try to
maintain a proper balance. They try to keep to a ratio of five
parts potassium to one of sodium, and to avoid complicated
mixtures of foods.

Macrobiotic eating centres on whole grains – mostly brown rice, with whole wheat, rye, barley, oats, millet, buckwheat and maize. These grains are supplemented with vegetable pulses such as soya, adzuki, mung and pinto beans. Whole vegetables including the outer skin are eaten as a secondary food; these are usually cooked and should be organically grown. In general, followers of a macrobiotic diet try to use only vegetables in season, and grown within a 500-mile radius of home. Potatoes, tomatoes and aubergines are virtually excluded because they are considered to be too Yin. Seaweeds are eaten as a vegetable. Fruits and nuts can be eaten occasionally – again when in season – and sunflower, sesame and pumpkin seeds too. Fish can form an occasional part of the diet, usually in cold weather. Natural unrefined sesame, corn, soya or sunflower oils are used for cooking. Any dried fruits should be free from sulphur dioxide (visit your health food store for these). Milk, cheese, butter and eggs are eaten very occasionally. The white meat of poultry is preferred, although meat is almost always avoided completely, as are all convenience foods.

Macrobiotic specialities include Miso purée, Tamari sauce, the soya bean cheese Tofu, Seitan (whole wheat gluten), salt pickled plums known as Umeboshi, the condiment Tekka, Bandua tea and Mu tea, which contains fifteen roots and herbs including ginseng. Gomasio, a sesame seed salt, is used, and a little honey instead of sugar to sweeten. Since there is plenty of liquid in the foods we eat, it is not considered necessary to drink more than about a pint of liquid a day. Drinks such as grain coffees and herbal teas are taken after meals.

Macrobiotic cooking is a high art, done quickly with very little salt. Thorough chewing is very important – in Gandhi's words 'drink your food and chew your drinks' – and you should stop eating before your appetite is satisfied.

Macrobiotic eating has been used both to enhance health and to heal. To cleanse the body and cure digestive disorders the ten-day rice diet is sometimes used, where the only food taken is brown rice with a little water. This is *not* to be practised regularly or kept up for any longer than ten days.

A while ago the newspapers reported that four babies of parents following 'extreme vegetarian diets' were found to be severely under-nourished and ill. An article later appeared in the British Medical Journal[1] stating that the babies were subsequently treated with diets which, in fact, complied with the dietary principles laid down by Ohsawa. So this kind of eating can be dangerous if not properly understood. For instance, to follow the brown rice and water diet all the time would virtually be a partial fast.

The British Nutrition Foundation Bulletin No. 26 comments that 'the original principles of macrobiotics have been mistranslated and misused' and that 'all in all, there is no reason why the diet should not be as nutritious as a standard vegetarian diet'.

Information
Readers interested in macrobiotics should contact The Community Health Foundation, 188 Old Street, London EC1, telephone 01 251 4076.

The Menopause

The menopause (climacteric, or change of life) is the time when a woman ceases to menstruate and is no longer fertile. The usual age for this is the late forties or early fifties, and women who begin their periods early in life usually have their menopause late. Some women sail through this time without any problems at all, and some have symptoms of varying severity for five years or more during the time leading up to the menopause. About 10% to 15% of women seek medical help. A very few women experience the menopause in their early twenties, perhaps because of a hysterectomy with removal of one or both ovaries. This is usually accompanied by very troublesome symptoms.

As a women's ovaries get older they respond less and less to the hormone FSH (follicle-stimulating hormone) which encourages egg production. This results in a decreased output of oestrogens and, for a time, an increased output of FSH. Another hormone, LH (luteinizing hormone) starts to under-produce, and ovulation fails to occur during some cycles. As the function of the ovaries decreases, ovulation stops altogether. Oestrogen and progesterone production fall off and in the end the periods stop completely. These and other hormonal changes may cause the unpleasant symptoms associated with the menopause.

The background cause, therefore, of menopausal problems is the decrease in hormone production and the ageing process in general. Your reaction to this profound physical change is also affected by social and cultural factors and – perhaps most important of all – the kind of woman you are.

Symptoms
There are many symptoms which a woman can experience during her menopause. These may be grouped as follows:

Physical Menstrual irregularities, hot flushes, sweats, palpitations, pins and needles, thinning of hair and ageing of skin, shrinking of breasts; pruritis (itching), dryness of vagina and thinning of its lining; constant desire to urinate, especially at night; shrinking of external genitalia and loss of tone in pelvic muscles; headaches, breathlessness, fatigue, dizziness, pains in joints and muscles.

Psychological Depression, insomnia, nervousness, anxiety, irritability, poor concentration; a significant number of women can be regarded as mildly neurotic at this time.

These symptoms can start several years before the actual cessation of menstruation.

Post-menopausal women tend to get osteoporosis, when their bones get porous, spongy, more liable to break. Calcium is lost from the body without being replaced.

After the menopause, women, who have been relatively protected from artery and heart disease, gradually catch up with men. At 44 a women is 14 or 15 times less likely to develop coronary heart disease than a man, but by the time she is 70 the risks are nearly equal. This may be partly due to the protective effects of oestrogen, and the post-menopause rise in blood fats, which can be up to 20% of the pre-menopause level.

The menopause is complete when your periods have stopped for 8 to 12 months; you should keep up contraception until they have ceased for at least 6 months. *See your medical practitioner* if you have bleeding between periods, irregular periods, flooding, or a watery discharge.

Social and cultural influences
It must be true that the way a women reacts to her menopause

is heavily influenced by surrounding attitudes. For instance, some African tribes promote a woman to full tribal equality when she has ceased to menstruate. Increased status replaces her ability to bear children and she is rewarded for the maturity that comes with advancing age. Women from the Rajput class in India look foward to the menopause, because they will no longer be contaminated by menstruation.

But we in the West take an opposite view. We are obsessed with youth, and a high value is placed upon a woman's ability to look not just attractive, but attractive *and young*. The woman whose beauty and femininity have been her main concerns and source of satisfaction is particularly vulnerable now and, although a modern woman can do much with nutrition, exercise and relaxation to extend her youth, eventually the signs of natural ageing will begin to appear.

The menopause comes at a difficult time for many women. Children have grown up and are leaving home so that the woman is faced with the challenge of adjusting to life, and a relationship with her husband, without children. Many women lose an elderly parent now. Others are widowed and have to come to terms with life alone. This is the time for the house-bound woman to find new activities and enthusiasms, but she may lack confidence and experience, and training for a new job can be difficult. On the other hand, the career woman without children will probably have reached her professional peak; disconcertingly, she may get very broody as she realizes that the comforting possibility of having children is slipping away. The mid-life crisis is on a woman now. Shades of the prison house close in on the middle-aged woman and she realizes that the time for doing all those wonderful things and exploring all those unopened rooms in herself is running a little short. Ageing – that thing that only happens to other people – is happening to her, too.

It has been shown, not surprisingly, that women who feel secure and important in their jobs and relationships do better at this time. Perhaps this is partly because they don't have time to worry about their symptoms, and partly because, no matter what their age, they feel valued as people.

A Swedish study shows that most women lose interest in sex to some extent as they grow older. But writer Alex Comfort thinks that people stop having sex for the same reasons they stop riding bikes. They are afraid of not being able to ride the bike, they are afraid of looking a fool, they haven't got a bike. Barbara Evans in *Life Change* puts it another way: 'few older women advertise their continuance of sexual activity because public opinion regards it as abnormal after the flush of youth has been replaced by the flushes of the menopause'.[1]

Orthodox treatments: hormones and drugs

Hormone Replacement Therapy is simply putting back deficient hormones, usually oestrogen, to counteract menopausal symptoms. (It does not of course prevent ovary shutdown and consequent infertility.) There are many drugs being used, combinations of oestrogens and progesterone or some containing male sex hormones in small doses. The oestrogen preparations are usually synthetic, although natural oestrogens are available.

There is no doubt that HRT works well on menopausal symptoms, improving hair and skin quality and banishing depression for many women. Some doctors believe in giving oestrogen to prevent osteoporosis, or brittle bones, developing after the menopause.

But HRT is admitted by doctors themselves to be a very tricky business. Few panel doctors have time for the close supervision of their HRT patients. The long-term effects of administering hormones, whether in the form of HRT or the Pill, are not yet known.

Greeted with much enthusiasm by some doctors when it was first developed, HRT has since been found to have risky side-effects. For example, oestrogen prescribed for a menopausing woman influences the blood fat levels in a complex way, reducing cholesterol and increasing triglycerides. Indeed many doctors now think that the danger of clotting disorders at the menopause if HRT is given is at least as great as the cancer danger which has received so much more attention. There is some evidence that the natural oestrogens which are sometimes prescribed do not cause this effect, nor do they apparently cause the rise in blood pressure which so often accompanies synthetic hormone treatment. I am told, however, of at least one patient who developed thrombosis as a direct result of taking natural oestrogen. High, continued oestrogen dosage prevents the body from adjusting to its own lower hormone level as it should.

Can hormone replacement therapy cause cancer?

The risk of a woman developing a cancer in the uterus after the menopause is about 1 in 1000. If she takes oestrogen continuously, her chance is increased to, at the worst, between 4 and 8 in 1000 and there is now little doubt that an association with cancer exists when the hormone is over-prescribed or the treatment insufficiently monitored. For instance, oestrogen blood levels reached during the hormonal treatment for hot flushes are often very high and can be five times or more the natural levels of oestrogen in the blood before the menopause.

But there is a lot of argument over the findings, and British work on this point is not as plentiful as American because British women take less HRT than American women. We are, it seems, doing our best to catch up however – in 1978 the UK figure for women taking HRT was nearly 200 000 and British prescriptions for oestrogens other than the Pill have more than trebled since the early 1970s. So we should soon have more British evidence one way or the other.

The list of conditions when HRT is not advisable is daunting. It includes obesity, high blood pressure, cigarette smoking, varicose veins, thrombosis, liver disorders; some breast tumours grow faster with oestrogen. Oestrogen-takers have an increased chance (1½ times) of getting gallstones needing surgery. Low risk factors indicating care in prescribing HRT are high blood fats and diabetes; side-effects include nausea, water retention and weight gain.

Other drug treatments
These include analgesics for painful joints, sleeping pills and sedatives, and diuretics for water retention. These drugs have possible side-effects and it is obvious that none of them does anything to improve the general health of the woman who is taking them. But it is the good health of the individual – decided partly by what she eats – which determines how she will cope with her menopause.

Nutritional and other drugless measures
As you approach your change of life, put yourself in the hands of a qualified medical practitioner, preferably a naturopathic practitioner or medical herbalist (SEE appendix page 405). If you decide to take HRT, make sure that your treatment is properly supervised and that you are having vitamin E as a supplement to lessen circulatory damage; see that you get regular cervical smears.

The menopause is a natural phase and not a horrible disease. Many women pass through it without any trouble and symptoms can be alleviated or cured by proper nutrition, including if necessary supplements and herbal medicine (for instance, backache often responds to 1g of vitamin C a day).

Many vitamin and mineral needs go up at this time (consult your practitioner). When the oestrogen output goes down, more calcium is lost in the urine than before and not replaced. As well as encouraging bone weakness and shrinking, this deficiency can cause nervousness, insomnia, headaches and depression. Many menopausal problems are believed to be due to magnesium and protein deficiencies, too, or a greater need for the vitamins A, D, C, and the B complex, including pantothenic acid, B6, B5 and B3. Vitamin E is needed in much greater amounts now; 500 units a day can be prescribed for hot flushes, but do not go above 100 units a day without checking with your practitioner first. Large doses of E can sometimes push up the blood pressure a little for the time being. If you have had an excessive flow you may need extra iron. The mineral oils used in skin care preparations rob the body of vitamins A, D, E and K, so avoid such cosmetics if you can.

Eat foods containing plenty of the B vitamins, calcium and iron – wholegrains, wheat germ, liver and brewer's yeast, yogurt and other dairy foods, some molasses. Kelp tablets are a good source of extra minerals, including the extra iodine which some women need now. Lecithin is often useful for a dry skin and pollen has been found effective in minimizing menopausal symptoms (SEE pages 121 and 127 for these two).

Read the *Whole Foods* section. Your practitioner will tell you that a good diet comes first and any supplements you may need come second.

Biochemists agree that vitamins can replace hormones in certain circumstances, and your practitioner may decide to give you vitamin A to substitute for oestrogen and vitamin C to act for progesterone. The body can change one vital substance into another with the help of the pituitary gland, and this process is helped by vitamin E. Many practitioners believe that the adrenal glands – if healthy – partly take over the secretory role of the ovaries following the menopause[2] and this is confirmed by health authority Dr Hans Selye.

The herbal remedy, Vitex Agnus Castus, is a specific for the menopause. It does not contain any hormones, but by working on the pituitary gland it enables the body to regulate its own hormones naturally, and in this way helps the woman to go through her menopause more smoothly (SEE *Additional therapies* at the end of this section).

To conclude, it is clear that there are several ways to prevent or alleviate unpleasant symptoms associated with the menopause. Diet, with the supplements and herbal medicines mentioned above, is of major importance in this.

But the way you cope with the change of life depends a lot on your attitude. Now is the time to find the courage and energy for new interests and challenges. Now you can pamper your health and looks, too, to an extent never possible when you were a hard-working younger woman. A few lines on your face don't alter the fact that sexual response is a fundamental part of human physiology and does not die out as you get older unless you let it. Your need, and your partner's need, for love and its physical expression are still the same.

Additional therapies
Herbalism: Vitex Agnus Castus is produced by Inter-Medics Limited, of 52 Walsworth Road, Hitchin, Hertfordshire and is obtainable by prescription through a naturopath, medical herbalist or other qualified natural therapeutics practitioner: SEE *Herbalism* in the appendix (page 405) if you wish to consult a medical herbalist.
Homoeopathy: SEE appendix, page 405.
Osteopathy (to normalize trigger points associated with the menopause): SEE appendix, page 405.
Relaxation: SEE appendix, page 405.
Yoga: SEE appendix, page 405.

Books mentioned in this section
Life Change by Barbara Evans (Pan 1979).

Nails and Food

The nails comprise three layers of a dead, horny substance (mostly protein) called keratin. Contrary to popular belief, they contain relatively little calcium.

Poor nails can be caused by inadequate circulation, bad nutrition or cold weather (they grow more slowly in the winter months). Like every other part of the body, they are dependent on what we eat.

Nails need in particular the vitamins A and D, the minerals calcium and iodine, and protein. Marked longitudinal ridges and brittle nails can reflect a lack of iron; a copper deficiency, with allied deficiencies of zinc and vitamin B6, can cause white spots on the nails.

The best food for your nails is the best food for you. So keep off refined and junk foods. Your bread should be wholemeal and your other cereals – rice for instance – should be wholegrain. Eat plenty of fresh vegetables, in salads or short cooked, raw fresh fruit, and sufficient protein.

Kelp is good for the nails (SEE *Kelp* page 120) and a food which is claimed to prevent brittle nails is the seaweed, Nori. Evening primrose oil is a proven remedy for brittle nails (SEE *Evening primrose oil* page 111). A traditional treatment for the nails is flavourless gelatin; this must be added to milk or bouillon before it is taken for it to be effective. Dietary treatment for the slow-growing nails takes at least six months to show results.

A good treatment for your nails is to soak them in warm wheat germ oil for three to four minutes, massaging the oil in afterwards. Store the oil in your fridge to keep it fresh.

Additional therapy
Biochemic tissue salts are recommended for nails: SEE pages 107–8. Combination K for brittle nails; combination D for diseased nails.

Older People and Food

'I can't say which, come eventide,
More tedious I find;
Competing with the juvenile stride,
Or meeting the juvenile mind.
So I think it rorty, yes, and nifty,
To be with people over fifty.'

OGDEN NASH, *You can be a Republican,*
I'm a Gerontocrat

Old age is the time when all the policemen are young lads, and everybody whispers. The world is going to the dogs, and someone has fixed the pavement so you can't run for the bus any more.

In our youth-obsessed society, old age is a nuisance. But – with the blessing of good health – the years bring with them many benefits; improved judgement, serenity, a sense of having seen it all and knowing most of the answers. Many of our politicians could claim the old age pension, and people who are enthusiastic about life go on until they drop, ignoring little things like greying hair and creaking joints. We are, in fact, old when we feel it.

People in England and Wales now can expect to live about thirty years longer than people born in the middle of the last century. This improvement in the expectation of life began between about 1850 and the 1930s, rising more quickly up to the 1950s. It was due mainly to better nutrition, sanitation and housing, with cleaner water and better general hygiene. Now, over half the male population of Britain reaches the age of 70 and about half the women 75. But during the past fifty years the incidence of several chronic degenerative diseases – heart disease, bronchitis, high blood pressure, cancer – has increased rapidly and more and more people are kept alive, or half alive, by surgery and drugs. This is survival – but is it living?

The rate at which we turn into shuffling oldsters is influenced by heredity, the support we get from family, friends, religious beliefs, activities we love – and of course our health. Our attitudes can sustain us or they can poison us. The hate and fear we carry around, or the love and confidence, have a profound effect on our vitality and rate of ageing.

The ageing process

We are not built like Oliver Wendell Holmes' Wonderful One-Hoss Shay, which retained all its faculties unimpaired until it suddenly fell apart. We get old little by little, almost imperceptibly, unless this gradual decline is accelerated by an added stress such as bereavement or illness. Many older people are taking drugs for chronic degenerative illnesses now and there is no doubt that an ageing system can have difficulty in coping with these toxins. Drug side-effects can damage the tissues and hasten the onset of degenerative changes.

As the body ages, activity lessens. Muscles lose bulk and strength and body fat may increase. Ligaments shorten, bones become porous and brittle and we tend to stoop. Skin dries and becomes less elastic and sensitive, hair loses its colour, teeth deteriorate and the senses of taste, smell and touch, sight and hearing are often impaired. The metabolic rate (speed of the body's internal workings) drops. Lung capacity decreases, and the heart valves and arteries can harden (one explanation for the increased blood pressure often found in the old). As we get older, the body is often less able to deal effectively with sugar, too.

Due partly to hardened arteries and constricted smaller blood vessels, circulation slows down. This decreased circulation is one reason why the brain and nervous system are so profoundly influenced by ageing. The bloodstream is less efficient at bringing nutrients to the cells and taking away wastes, and this inefficiency creates a lack of oxygen and encourages cellular degeneration. We have myriads of brain cells and they are dying every day and not being replaced; as we get older these cells die in greater numbers. Memory fails; senility, says Robert Downs, is 'loss of recent memory, . . . in all probability it is a direct effect of cellular ageing due to poor circulation'.[1]

It is obvious, therefore, that the process of ageing is strongly affected, and perhaps largely dependent on, the quality of the blood and its capacity to reach and nourish the cells and carry away waste. We are as old as our circulation. People who flourish – rather than just survive – to a ripe old age do so partly because their body cells are getting what they need.

In view of their deteriorating circulation, it is not surprising that many old people feel the cold acutely. Some of them have a normal temperature of about 95°F or 35°C; hypothermia is the medical term for a body temperature below normal (this condition is made worse by drugs such as barbiturates and other sedatives). They fail to shiver naturally and are therefore extremely vulnerable to cold.

It has been found that, in old tissues, large protein molecules lying close together for long periods become welded to each other so that the whole structure is rigid, and this prevents the molecules from working properly. Protein repair and maintenance probably become more difficult with age, so that eventually vital functions are affected. Another factor believed to exacerbate ageing is the presence of 'free radicals' – substances formed by oxygen acting with fats – which clog the metabolic machinery. Natural radioactivity is believed to encourage cellular decay to some extent.

We have seen how closely the onset of old age depends on the state of the blood and its circulation round the body. There is a current theory which attributes *all* the symptoms of ageing to that arch-clogger of the bloodstream, cholesterol. This substance is partly found in our food and partly produced by the liver, and, since the more food we eat the more cholesterol we produce we are advised to cut down by eating less, as well as avoiding high-cholesterol foods.

It is a well-established fact that laboratory animals – and people, too – eating good quality food but less of it do better and live longer than their overfed counterparts. Less, and better quality, food has long been recommended by naturopaths. But excess cholesterol, whether ingested in food or produced by our bodies, is only one factor among many others in the ageing process. The situation is far more complex than the 'cholesterol and age' theorists would have us believe.

Cholesterol, of course, is a fat. And it's interesting to note that, as we get past forty or so, the time taken for the body to clear fats from the blood gets longer. This is a powerful argument for cutting down on *all* fats as we get older.

Nutritional deficiencies

Older people are less active, so they need fewer calories (a very few make poor use of their calorie intake so they need more calories and not fewer). They often have a reduced ability to absorb *nutrients*. In general, then, older people need food with fewer calories than before, but with more essential nutrients. There is current interest in the possibility that as the body ages it becomes less efficient at converting the essential fatty acid linoleic acid, into the valuable group of substances known as prostaglandins (SEE *Evening Primrose Oil* pages 111–14).

Many older people are taking drugs for various illnesses and this may upset, for instance, the potassium balance in the body, or destroy an already meagre intake of vitamin C. Iron deficiency anaemia can develop from internal bleeding caused by taking a lot of aspirin. Old people who do not go out in the sunshine much may lack vitamin D, which can be formed by sunlight on the skin, and lack of D can interfere with calcium absorption and thus cause a deficiency of calcium. The commonest deficiencies in the old are vitamins C, D, B1 and folic acid, iron, calcium, phosphorus and protein.

Dr Gaston Pawan, senior lecturer in metabolism at the Middlesex Hospital Medical School, has made a special study of the ageing process. He visited Los Viejos – a tribe in Southern Ecuador who live very long and active lives, sometimes up to 120 years. Dr Pawan found that these people work hard, get up early and go to bed early; their stresses are few. They eat very little meat, with plenty of fresh vegetables and fruit, some bland white cheese and wine – about 1200 calories a day. They eat no refined or processed foods.

This study echoes earlier work done in the 1920s, when Robert McCarrison lived among the Hunzas, poor peasants living 8000 feet up in the Himalayas. Like Los Viejos, these people live long and active lives, have an excellent physique and enjoy remarkable freedom from disease. When McCarrison did his research the Hunzas were, like Los Viejos, frugal eaters. They were living on a diet of wholemeal chapatti, yogurt, cheese, plenty of vegetables often eaten raw, and lots of apricots; they ate meat on feast days. They drank glacial water, rich in minerals. Their life-style called for a lot of strenuous exercise. Unhappily, since those days the Hunzas have started to enjoy the questionable benefits of Western influences including refined foods, and their health record now is less outstanding. Even so, a more recent examination[2] of 25 Hunzas aged between 90 and 100 found *no* cardiovascular symptoms, and their blood pressure and cholesterol levels were well below the Western average. These results, in such old people, are astonishing.

It is clear, therefore, that not only the *quality* of nutrition, but the *quantity*, has a decisive effect on health. Another study over two years of 4000 people aged 20 and over, carried out by Dr A.B. Nicholls at the University of Montreal, showed that over-eating can be as dangerous to the heart and arteries as the much-condemned high fat diet.

Protein should form about 10% of your diet. Remember that meat is not essential for health, but if you prefer to eat it then organ meats, particularly liver and kidneys, are best. Eat a little fish and cheese (try to cut down on very fatty cheeses such as camembert) and include pulses, soya, wheat germ and brewer's yeast. Whole grains, nuts and seeds are good sources of both natural fats and unrefined carbohydrates; try to reduce your fat consumption to about 10% of your total diet. Eat plenty of fresh raw salads and fruit and short-cooked vegetables, where practicable leaving them in their skins. Naturopath Alan Moyle recommends garlic every day for older people (this can be taken as a supplement if you prefer). Use honey and molasses for sweetening, and drink plenty of unsweetened fruit and vegetable juices, home-made if possible.

If you are constipated, try bran (SEE *Constipation* page 282). If you cannot tolerate it after a fair trial, take sunflower oil and seeds, prunes, figs, beetroot, mushrooms, black molasses, honey and a *little* spinach in your diet – within reason; these foods are gentle natural laxatives. Molasses can be taken once a day. Start with one dessertspoonful in water and adjust the quantity to suit yourself.

Avoid refined flour products and foods containing white sugar; avoid fried and other very fatty foods, and convenience foods in general. Cut down on salt, tea, coffee, synthetic squashes and cola drinks; the occasional glass of wine won't hurt you however.

Readers are invited to look at *Bonus Foods and Supplements* pages 107–38 in particular the pages on *Sprouting Seeds and Grains* and *Raw Juices* (juices recommended for the elderly are apple, grape, orange, carrot and beetroot); many older people find chewing fibrous fruits and vegetables difficult and raw juices are ideal for them. Eat less food, at more frequent intervals, and start a meal whenever possible with some salad or fruit. The very old should eat spinach, lettuce, tomatoes, plums and prunes very sparingly.

Grow your own vegetables without artificial chemicals if you can. Retirement is often a welcome opportunity to concentrate on gardening. 'The weight of evidence for maintaining health, preventing disease and delaying the degenerative effects of life, is that a balanced diet of organically-grown foods (or food as little contaminated or denatured as possible) is absolutely vital.'[3] (Please also SEE *Whole Foods* pages 101–6.)

The most difficult age for people to change their eating habits for the better is the mid-fifties. This is the time when diseases start to appear which will make life difficult later on. It is never too late, however, to change. Illnesses can be arrested, cured, and best of all *prevented* by good nutrition and sensible living.

Supplements

It is better to get all the vitamins and minerals we need from the food we eat. But this is not always possible nowadays. Crops are often grown in mineral-deficient soil; many vitamins decay during storage, particularly vitamin C, and both vitamins and minerals are reduced when food is cooked.

Additionally, older people often fail to metabolize the nutrients they take in, and suffer from deficiencies accordingly. Many naturopaths consider that supplements are necessary for older people. This does not mean, of course, that a sensible diet can be dispensed with. All nutrients work together, so supplements on their own are much less effective.

Pollen has been found valuable for the mental exhaustion and confusion sometimes accompanying age (SEE *Pollen*, pages 127–8). Lecithin granules (SEE pages 121–3) can also be very effective for this. Lecithin helps to clear from the blood the fats which remain there longer with advancing age, and it contains the B vitamins choline and inositol, for good circulation and brain function. Pumpkin seeds have been successfully used by a German doctor for prostate troubles (SEE *Sprouting Seeds and Grains* pages 133–5).

Vitamin D with calcium has proved effective for the brittle bones (osteoporosis) which often appear in the elderly.[4] Because vitamin D can be toxic in large quantities, follow the recommended dose or consult your practitioner. Vitamin D can be made from sunlight too and is easily absorbed this way. Calcium on its own is often very useful for older people; other minerals they tend to lack are magnesium, zinc, potassium and selenium. Like vitamins E and C, selenium is an anti-oxidant, protecting against cellular degeneration. Ask your practitioner about dosage.

Vitamin E is recommended by naturopaths for a healthy circulation and is thought to be an important factor against ageing. A deficiency can lead to cell damage. Do not go above 100 I.U. a day of E without consulting your practitioner; it can sometimes raise the blood pressure a little.

Royal jelly (SEE page 131) contains large quantities of the B vitamin pantothenic acid, and American biochemist Roger J. Williams found that mice given royal jelly lived longer than those without. Another B vitamin, PABA (para-aminobenzoic acid) has been used by Dr Anna Aslan in Rumania to slow down premature ageing. It appears to enhance glandular function. B6 is known to help protect the arteries and help control blood fats, and some researchers associate B12 with mental alertness. Folic acid is often deficient in older people, who sometimes also lack vitamin K.

Substances about which relatively little is known yet are the bioflavonoids, also known as vitamin P. They have been found to correct disorders related to poor capillary function and work best when combined with vitamin C. It would seem a good idea therefore to use them for poor circulation as well as vitamin E.

Garlic has long been known for its reduction of high blood fat levels and high blood pressure and its protective effect against infections makes it a very valuable supplement.

Perhaps the single most important vitamin for older people is C. Vitamin C has been linked to the rate of mortality in the old and 'an ingestion of less than 50mg vitamin C a day has been correlated with an increase in mortality of 48% above average'.[5] This vitamin is a vital factor in preventing infections and is currently being used to treat cancer. With B12 and hormones, vitamin C helps to keep the cell membranes healthy and can relieve fatigue. It is necessary also to build collagen (the main part of connective tissue) and this is probably linked with the flexibility or stiffness of the joints. Vitamin C tends to decrease artery disease by altering the blood composition slightly and it is clear, therefore, that plenty of C is essential for older people. Unfortunately, they are often deficient in this vitamin, which has to be ingested every day. It cannot either be made or stored by the body. It is found in fresh fruits and raw vegetables and older people may find these hard to chew or cannot be bothered to eat them. As we have seen, too, if a person is taking drugs, vitamin C is often destroyed. For further advice on diet and supplements, please consult a naturopath (SEE page 405) or a nutritionally aware doctor.

There is, therefore, a lot we can do simply by intelligent eating to see that old age does not overtake us before its due time. Moderate exercise, relaxation, friends and above all an interest in life and a loving family; all these combine with good nutrition to make old age a happy and fruitful time.

Additional therapies
Exercise: SEE appendix, page 405.
Relaxation: SEE appendix, page 405.
Yoga: SEE appendix, page 405.

Recommended reading
The Time of Your Life, published by Help the Aged and The Health Education Countil at £1.95. Write to the Health Education Council, 78 New Oxford Street, London, WC1A 1AH or telephone 01 637 1881.
The Pritikin Program for Diet and Exercise by Nathan Pritikin (Bantam 1981).

The Pill

The contraceptive Pill contains hormones which prevent natural menstruation, and therefore conception. Some types of Pill have only progestogen (synthesized progesterone), but most have a mixture of oestrogen and progestogen.

Taking progestogen reduces the level of progesterone in the blood, and taking oestrogen raises the level of oestrogen. This prevents the pituitary gland from releasing hormones which encourage the egg cell in the ovary to ripen and as a result you cannot become fertile. (Some authorities consider the Pill to have its main effect on cervical mucus and not always on ovulation itself.) When you stop taking the Pill for a few days, the change in hormone levels causes the womb lining to disintegrate, and the bleeding which results is very like normal menstruation.

There are almost 30 different varieties of oral contraceptive on the British market and it is assumed, although not yet proved, that the latest ultra-low-dose pills are safer.

Side-effects

The Pill alters liver function, which has far-reaching effects throughout the body since the liver is involved in so many processes.

Blood changes occur, and these are:
    alterations in blood fats, including a rise in blood cholesterol.
    alteration in blood sugar levels.
    alteration in blood clotting factors.
Hormonal changes.
Mineral and vitamin changes; release of stored vitamin A and a fall in B6: the Pill puts up the body's need for C, B12, B2, folic acid, other B vitamins and vitamin E; a fall in zinc and selenium; a rise in copper, iron (since loss of blood with the Pill is less, iron is conserved).
Changes in the levels of binding globulins, which carry hormones and minerals round the blood.
Changes in the factors affecting blood pressure.
Fluid retention.
Alterations in the immunity/allergy system.

With these widespread changes it is not surprising that many other risks have been noted. For instance Dr Barbara Evans in her book *Life Change* says that several authoritative studies 'have all established that during the reproductive years of a woman's life oral contraceptives increase the likelihood of her developing deep vein thrombosis and pulmonary embolism [clot in the lung] at least five times.' *The Lancet* reported in October 1977 that among long-term users of the Pill the extra death rate due to circulatory diseases each year is 20 per 100 000 women – four to five times the rate for those women who have never taken the Pill. This extra death rate rises with age. Changes in blood clotting factors, together with artery walls already damaged by other causes, may result in a heart attack and stroke.

That this blood clotting (thrombosis) only happens in the deep veins is given by some authorities as a reason why moderate varicose veins need not stop you taking the Pill. These surface varicosities, however, may stand out and your legs may ache if you go on the Pill, so something must be happening to these veins as well as to the deeper ones.

Reporting on the higher blood sugar levels often occurring in Pill-takers, *The Lancet* dated 6 March 1971 states that in a group of 66 women who used it, systolic blood pressure (one of the two ways of measuring it) had increased after one year in 50 cases.

A chilling report in *The General Practitioner* dated 1 August 1980 warns that women who take the Pill in the three months before conception are two to three times more likely to have babies with spina bifida than women who do not use oral contraceptives during this time. I am told by a consulting medical herbalist that this may be due to the Pill's effect on mucus, damaging it so that it allows through sub-standard sperm.

Among the Pill's other possible side-effects is an increased tendency to cystitis. It is interesting to note that in his book *The Pill*, Dr John Guillebaud quite rightly says 'it is a general principle of medicine that if a drug is really to be blamed for a side-effect, it is better to stop the drug than to use yet another drug to treat the side-effect', following this a little later with the bland statement that, if you suffer from cystitis, 'your doctor may sometimes advise taking a couple of antibiotic tablets shortly before intercourse as a *regular preventive routine*' (my italics).

Depression is commonly helped by the Pill, but a few women complain that it makes them feel worse. Migraine sufferers usually find that the Pill makes their headaches more frequent, or causes them for the first time, only a very few saying that it seems to prevent them. Other kinds of headache are often blamed on the Pill. Some contact lens wearers find that their eyes get sore when they start taking the Pill, and a few women complain of a dry vagina. Cervical erosion is twice as common in Pill-users, but this is harmless.

For smokers, the risks are much greater. The risk of subarachnoid haemorrhage (a kind of stroke) in cigarette smokers on the Pill is 22 times that of women who neither smoke nor take oral contraceptives.[1]

For most women, however, actual menstrual troubles are greatly improved by the Pill. The blood that appears once a month is not true menstruation, and when the Pill's hormones are removed for one week out of every four a thin lining comes away from the uterus with less bleeding than happens naturally.

Guillebaud warns that a link between the Pill and some forms of cancer might be traced some time during the next few years, commenting that this is very likely, in view of the Pill's widespread effects upon the body. Because some cancers do not develop until some twenty years or so after exposure to the carcinogen, *'most of the news, good or bad, is yet to come'* (Guillebaud's italics).

Finally, an article in *The Practitioner* (February 1980) makes the point that drug interactions may result in a reduction in the effectiveness of the Pill or a change in the effects or side-effects of any other drug being taken. So, as well as its effects when taken on its own, the Pill may alter the actions of other drugs.

Although these alterations of your body chemistry are very worrying, statistically your chances of developing an illness from them are very small. As we shall see, too, there are ways of helping your body nutritionally so that it can cope better with oral contraceptives. Neither of these statements means that I am recommending you to take the Pill. If you are – justifiably – worried about taking it, then you can add to your possible side-effects another one: anxiety.

When not to take the Pill
Women with any of the following conditions should not take oral contraceptives:

Circulatory disease, including thrombosis or conditions predisposing to it.
Naturally high blood-fat levels.
Hormone-dependent tumours of the breast or uterus.
Impaired liver function.
Impaired pituitary function.
Abnormal genital bleeding.
Lactation (and of course pregnancy!).
Severe diabetes.
Gross obesity.
'Crescendo' type migraines.

Angina pectoris and some other types of heart disease.
Drug regimes with potential inter-action.

Women with the following conditions should avoid the Pill if possible:

Some breast diseases.
High blood pressure.
Migraine headaches.
Epilepsy.
Fibroids.
Idiopathic cholestatic jaundice in previous pregnancy.
Sickle-cell anaemia.
Gall-bladder disease.
Heavy smoking – 20 a day, especially at 35 years and over.

Whether you are at risk also depends on your age and how long you have been taking the Pill.

Should you decide to give up taking the Pill, you should supplement your diet for a few months with vitamin A at the recommended dosage. Tests on animals have proved that the Pill depletes body stores of A and therefore women who give up taking it may experience a temporary deficiency which will cause them to menstruate heavily for the time being.

Coping with the Pill

Obviously, because of the vitamin and mineral deficiencies sustained by women taking oral contraceptives, it is wise to include plenty of foods which will supply these essential substances. The vitamins C, B2, B6, B12, folic acid, the other B vitamins and vitamin E, and the minerals zinc and selenium are found in wholegrains, wheat germ, brewer's yeast, fresh raw fruits and vegetables and liver (SEE *Whole Foods* and *Vitamins and Minerals* sections pages 68–106). You may like to boost your intake of B vitamins by taking lecithin which also lowers blood fats, helps the body to use B6, and is claimed to act as a mild diuretic for excess fluid retention. It is wise to cut down on, or cut out, refined sugar, which can put up blood fats and disturb blood sugar mechanism and which destroys B vitamins.

In the case of vitamin B6, it has been established that women taking the Pill may need as much as 20 to 25mg a day to normalize their B6 level. This is a lot – much more than could be supplied in food. B6 has many tasks in the body, including helping to keep the blood sugar levels normal (Pill-takers sometimes have mild diabetes), helping to use protein and to produce the red, oxygen-carrying part of the blood called haemoglobin. B6 is essential for healthy arteries. Another key function of this vitamin is helping to make a substance necessary for brain function called serotonin, without which depression and sleep disturbances may result. B6 is also needed to make GABA (Gamma Aminobutyric Acid); this substance has a calming effect and so, here again, a deficiency of B6 can have a detrimental effect on the brain.

A sound diet comes first and supplements come second. If you are on the Pill and you decide to counteract its effects by using supplements, please consult a naturopath (SEE appendix page 405) or a nutritionally aware doctor for advice.

Books mentioned in this section
Life Change by Barbara Evans (Pan 1979)
The Pill by John Guillebaud (Oxford University Press 1980).

Pregnancy, Lactation and Food

Healthy children?
Britain has the highest perinatal mortality rate of any comparable Western country.[1] During 1979, 5125 babies were stillborn in England and Wales. 8064 were born alive but died within their first year.[2] More than 7% of our babies arrive dead or clearly malformed. These tragedies are obvious. We do not know how many babies are damaged in other, more subtle ways. For instance, brain development reaches its maximum at about 40 weeks' gestation, declining over the first two years or so after the child is born. Children whose brains do not grow properly before birth may have impaired mental development with a low IQ. (Brain development after birth depends to a large extent upon the amount of sensory stimulation, including cuddling and attention, that the baby gets.)

Birth defects are to some extent hereditary. But the bulk of the evidence points to environmental factors – diet, drugs and other toxins, the mother's activities during her pregnancy (perhaps she tries to overwork), the home circumstances, and so on. Foetal ecology is the study of these factors.

Substances causing birth defects are called teratogens, and among the substances capable of doing damage in a mild or terrible form are certain drugs. 'The simple fact is', writes Dr Vernon Coleman in Foresight's *Guidelines for Future Parents* (SEE *Information* at end), 'that if a drug is powerful enough to have a useful effect on the body it is powerful enough to have a dangerous effect as well.' Doctors have to be doubly cautious in prescribing drugs for a pregnant woman.

The benzodiazepines have been promoted as a safe alternative to the barbiturates. They include Valium, Librium, Mogadon and Norbrium. Some of these drugs may, if taken during the last three months of pregnancy, cause the baby to be deformed. Some of them get into the breast milk, tranquillizing the baby as well.

The oedema (water retention) which about one-third of British or American women suffer from when they are pregnant is believed to be due to too much salt in the diet. Many doctors therefore restrict salt and prescribe diuretic drugs to get rid of the water. The need for extra salt in the body during pregnancy was however recognized by the 1969 White House Conference on Food, Nutrition and Health, which stated that sodium retention is a normal physiological adjustment during pregnancy and condemned the 'promiscuous use' of diuretics. (The vitamin B6 treatment for water retention is described later.) Diuretics cause the body to excrete nutrients as well as fluid; potassium and magnesium are among the vital substances lost. In her book *Let's Have Healthy Children* Adelle Davis says that although all nutrients have not yet been studied individually, diuretics can produce deficiencies of about 35. This is too much at any time – and much too much when the woman is carrying a growing baby.

The Pill leads to several nutritional deficiencies, notably a lack of B6, and also alters liver function. These effects are worse if the woman also smokes, drinks or takes a tranquillizer such as Valium, when the risks of a damaged baby will be greater. Smoking increases the amounts of most nutrients needed by the baby, especially vitamin C. Please do not smoke while you are planning, carrying or nursing a baby.

The American Food and Drug Administration, investigating a possible link between high caffeine consumption and birth defects, suggests that both pregnant women and those who hope to conceive should limit the amount of coffee and tea they drink. In the UK women are usually given this advice in any case. The American March of Dimes Birth Defects Foundation suggests that coffee should be limited to six cups and tea or cola drinks to fourteen cups. This of course is just a guess, since coffee differs in the amount of caffeine it contains. Six cups of coffee is a lot, and fourteen cups of tea is about enough to take a bath in.

The Foetal Alcohol Syndrome (FAS) describes abnormalities found in babies whose mothers drank a lot of alcohol during and possibly before pregnancy. Dr David Woollam of Emmanuel College, Cambridge, advises that *no* alcohol during pregnancy is the only really safe rule.

There may be a connection between birth defects and the poisonous metals lead and cadmium. Professor Derek Bryce-Smith, the academic leader of the UK anti-lead campaign, found in a small pilot study that the cadmium and lead levels in stillborn, malformed babies were generally about 5 to 10 times higher than in normal babies. Calcium and zinc levels on the other hand tended to be very low.

'It seems amazing that anybody should regard it as unorthodox . . . to pay special attention to the bodily health and nutritional status of parents before the child is conceived. It seems so blindingly obvious . . .' PROFESSOR DEREK BRYCE-SMITH, interviewed in the American magazine *Bestways*, January 1981.

Child care begins with the parents, *before conception*. Writing in the British Nutrition Foundation Bulletin,[1] nutritionist Jane E. Morgan states that the mother's diet before conception has an important influence on her capacity to bear a healthy baby, and emphasizes that her diet at this time is even more crucial than during her pregnancy. According to F. E. Hytten, the health of the father is equally important.[3]

After conception, foetal development is especially rapid between the second week and second month of pregnancy. So this earlier part of the pregnancy is particularly important from a nutrition point of view. But from well before conception until the end of breast-feeding, the food the mother eats strongly influences the health of her child.

Pregnancy puts stress on the woman, and her food has to nourish the unborn child as well as herself. This is probably the time when the deficiencies and additions in our Western refined foods can do the most damage. According to Weston A. Price in his book, *Nutrition and Physical Degeneration*, our refined denatured Western diet is directly related to the deformities in our children. There may be several other factors involved, some of which perhaps are out of our control. But we can – and must – control our diet.

Nutritional research for healthy babies

'If all the prospective human mothers could be fed as expertly as prospective animal mothers in the laboratory, most sterility, spontaneous abortions, stillbirths, and premature births would disappear; the birth of deformed and mentally retarded babies would be largely a thing of the past.' From *Nutrition Against Disease* by ROGER J. WILLIAMS

A lot of research has been done into isolated vitamin and mineral deficiencies and their effects on pregnant laboratory animals. Fortunately for us, experiments of this kind have been limited to test animals. Without their forced co-operation, the importance of these nutrients would not have been illustrated with such overwhelming clarity. Only in the laboratory can foods be so stripped of the nutrient under study that it is virtually absent from the diet. A *deficiency* in our human diet can cause illness and damage. But a *total lack*, causing the appalling crippling seen in these experiments, must be very rare.

Some good breeding sows were fed a diet totally lacking in vitamin A during early pregnancy. In one litter of 11 pigs, every single piglet was born without eyeballs. There were no abnormalities in the young whose mothers had been given vitamin A.[4]

Severe deficiencies in the range of B vitamins gave rise to many foetal abnormalities in test animals, including brain disorders. Young rats deficient in B1 (thiamine) showed less intelligence in finding their way around mazes. A lack of riboflavin (B2) in laboratory animals caused deformed offspring.[5]

Every woman has in her body some of every amino acid, mineral and vitamin that a developing baby needs. Whether she has enough for a healthy baby is not so certain. She may be so poorly nourished that she produces a malformed baby, miscarries, or cannot become pregnant at all.

A woman's appetite increases when she is pregnant and during the first six months she accumulates about 30 000 extra calories, under the instructions of the hormone progesterone. During the last three months another hormone, lactogen, mobilizes this stored fat so that it can be used to feed the foetus which during the same time trebles its weight. Protein is also stored during early pregnancy and released later on.

Some doctors think that restricting weight gain during pregnancy helps to reduce the risk of convulsions and obesity. This is untrue. Eating less cuts down the birth-weight of the infant, which is an important part of his complete development, and a low maternal weight gain can result in failure to breast-feed.[6] The underweight woman should regain her normal weight before she conceives. (Cravings for certain foods are not harmful – unless you eat nothing else!)

The importance of a good general diet is underlined by some research at the Harvard School of Public Health.[7] 216 babies were individually rated in terms of their mothers' eating habits. 33 were born dead, deformed or premature, died soon after birth or were poorly physically developed. Of these failures, 26 came from mothers with poor diets, 6 from mothers with fair diets, and only 1 from a mother whose diet was rated as good. None of the diets studied was rated excellent. 33 small tragedies seems a lot out of only 216 babies.

A sound diet consisting of eggs, meat including liver, salad vegetables and fruit has been shown to prevent toxaemia.[8]

Before we go through the complete list of nutrients essential for a healthy baby, it is interesting to know about some work that has been done using a range of vitamin and mineral supplements. Professor R.W. Smithells at Leeds University gave vitamin and mineral supplements to women who had previously had malformed babies. These women had a higher than average chance of producing more defective offspring. Supplements were given for at least 28 days *before conception* and up until the date of the second missed menstrual period.

The incidence of defective babies born was 6 in every 1000, compared to 50 in every 1000 born to mothers who had not received the supplement.[9]

Researchers at Columbia University gave supplements of the B vitamins thiamine, riboflavin and niacin, with iron, to pregnant women. Although this study was not as strictly monitored as it could have been with experimental animals, nevertheless the IQ of the children whose mothers had received supplementation was significantly higher than those without.[10]

The high blood pressure of toxaemia has been corrected by the little-known B vitamin, choline, but toxaemia itself is associated with many deficiencies, including shortages of folic acid and vitamin E. Biotin, another little-researched B vitamin, has been given with liver[11] to nursing mothers and has cleared up seborrhoeic dermatitis in the baby.

Vitamin B6 is being widely used to help pregnant women. Many of the disorders associated with pregnancy yield to it, including piles, leg cramps, swollen, painful hands and feet, or hands and arms that 'go to sleep'. The need for B6 seems to grow as pregnancy advances and its shortage can cause nervousness and insomnia.

At least one-third of British and American women have oedema when they are pregnant. It may presage toxaemia, which affects both mother and child and can lead to convulsions (eclampsia). Dr John Ellis, in his book *Vitamin B6; the Doctor's Report,* writes that B6 can be used to prevent and treat both toxaemia and eclampsia in pregnancy. He controlled oedema in 225 of his pregnant patients quite safely with vitamin B6. Treating leg cramps with the same vitamin, he sometimes added magnesium and potassium. (Calcium has been used with B6 for leg cramps too.)

B6 has been used for several years against morning sickness (SEE *Information* at end of this section). In *Vitamins and Hormones,* volume 22, 1964, Dr W.H. Sebrell recommends it for the nausea and vomiting so common during the first three months of pregnancy.

Probably the most important B vitamin during pregnancy is folic acid. A deficiency of this vitamin can cause anaemia and, according to the British Nutrition Foundation Bulletin No. 8, unless dietary supplements are given, about 25% of pregnant women will develop folic acid anaemia. The Bulletin estimates that 50% to 60% of pregnant women may not be getting enough folic acid in their food. There seems to be more danger of a deficiency during the winter and early spring. In the UK, tablets of combined folic acid and iron are given routinely now to pregnant women. In his book *Vitamins in your Life and the Micronutrients* Dr E. DiCyab states that the foetus drains its mother of her folic acid to such an extent that she needs supplementation daily.

Folic acid deficiencies can cause miscarriages, megaloblastic anaemia, birth defects, toxaemia, premature birth, afterbirth haemorrhage and the premature separation of the placenta from the uterus wall before the baby is born. Children born to mothers deficient in folic acid can show delayed or abnormal development[12] and an early shortage can interfere with the body's ability to fight off diseases later on.[13] Laboratory rats completely deprived of folic acid either re-absorbed their offspring or produced babies with multiple abnormalities, including damage to the skeleton, heart, kidney, lungs, heart and blood vessels. Some of the animals were actually born without heads and some had their brains outside the skull.[14]

Pregnancy puts up the baby's demands for vitamin B12, and vegans in particular should take care to get enough of this vitamin. Women who have been taking the Pill will need even more B12 when they are pregnant.[15] It stimulates growth and improves health in human children.[16]

Human muscle contains about twice as much pantothenic acid as that of other animals. So, since laboratory animals need a lot of this vitamin during reproduction, we probably need a lot too; human milk contains plenty of pantothenic acid. Roger J. Williams, the biochemist who discovered this B vitamin, believes that providing pregnant women with 50mg per day would substantially decrease the number and severity of reproductive failures. It seems that the need for pantothenic acid goes up sharply just before birth. Laboratory rats completely deprived of it re-absorb their foetuses or the litters are born deformed.[17]

In the *Journal of Applied Nutrition* for winter 1971, Dr Fred R. Klenner reports that he gave vitamin C to 300 of his patients who were pregnant. Leg cramps were much reduced, the labour was shorter and less painful and there were no haemorrhages after the birth. Because C in large doses has a diruetic effect, none of his patients needed a catheter to drain off fluid (or diuretic drug either, presumably). Blood iron levels were easier to maintain, stretch marks lessened, skin elasticity improved, and there were no toxic manifestations during any of the pregnancies. Dr Klenner estimates that pregnant women need 4g a day during the first three months of pregnancy, 6g during the second and 10g during the third. (Vitamin C is also necessary for foetal brain development.)

Varicose veins and piles often develop during pregnancy and vitamin E can help (SEE *Varicose Veins and Piles* pages 382–7). Phlebitis in pregnant women can be triggered off when the expanding womb constricts the blood flow to the limbs. Vitamin E, with calcium, acts to improve circulation and, unlike drug anti-coagulants, it is safe.[18] In *The Complete Book of Vitamins* Dr Wilfrid E. Shute states that he and his brother have treated rheumatic heart disease in pregnant women with large doses of vitamin E. When iron supplements have failed, doctors have used vitamin E for premature babies born with a shortage of the vitamin and accompanying anaemia. The anaemia would not respond until vitamin E was added.[19] Vitamin E is also thought to help in preventing miscarriages. A deficiency increases the brain's need for oxygen and could therefore result in lowered intelligence. Dr R. Bayer, a German doctor who has made a special study of vitamin E, states that in thousands of deliveries he has never known a mentally retarded child to be born provided the *father* has taken vitamin E before the child was conceived. When dietary E is adequate, certain hormones are produced towards the end of the pregnancy which increase the elasticity of the vaginal tissues, and in her book *Let's Have Healthy Children* Adelle Davis states that vitamin E is probably more important than any other nutrient for an easy delivery.

Pregnant women should include foods containing vitamin K in their diet in order to protect themselves against excessive bleeding during childbirth. It is found in spinach, cabbage, pork liver, and other meats and vegetables, and is also manufactured in the intestine. It should not be taken as a supplement, as it may cause excessive clotting and coagulation in that form. There have been no reported cases of harm from vitamin K naturally present in food.

The bioflavonoids (or vitamin P) are among the nutrients used to treat piles in pregnant women. Dr T. Muller of the Hospices Civils in Strasbourg also gave bioflavonoids to expectant mothers with varicose veins; they were good for the pain and discomfort of the veins but did little for their appearance.

Calcium, the universal pain-killer, is valuable for an easy delivery. Calcium needs in later pregnancy are probably at their highest, but pregnant women may be able to adapt to some extent by increasing their absorption of the calcium they get in their foods. To be used by the body, calcium needs vitamin D.

Iron deficiency in pregnancy is probably widespread. An article in the British Nutrition Foundation Bulletin No. 30 states that the optimum level of dietary iron during pregnancy is unknown. But the requirement is high, and the authors advise the giving of supplements. There is more iron-deficiency anaemia in pregnant than in non-pregnant women, and women in later pregnancy need even more extra iron. Low birth-weight babies are more likely to be short of iron during infancy. On the other hand, if the diet lacks magnesium, B6 or choline, as it often does during pregnancy, excess iron from supplements can be absorbed and stored in the tissues, and this is damaging. Iron supplements can also destroy vitamin E to some extent if they are taken at the same time as an E supplement. The iron in food does not have this effect.

Totally zinc-deficient diets given to laboratory rats during the last third of their pregnancies produced appetite loss to such an extent that by the end of gestation some rats had stopped eating altogether. Growth of the foetuses was retarded.[20] Other studies showed that in these extreme dietary conditions some rats re-absorbed their foetuses, and that 90% of the babies born were deformed. A combined deficiency of zinc and manganese reduced the maternal instincts of laboratory animals without affecting the birthweights of the litters.[21] (Women who are pregnant, or who are on the Pill, have lower than normal blood levels of zinc.[22])

There are more minerals in hard water and there is a link between areas of the country with the highest infant mortality rates and birth defects, and places where the water supply is soft and acid.[23]

Protein is vital to a healthy pregnancy. One of the amino acids which make up protein, tryptophan, was withheld from pregnant rats. They re-absorbed their foetuses, while those rats getting tryptophan gave birth to healthy young.[24]

Linoleic acid is an essential fatty acid, abundant in

unrefined oils, especially sunflower oil. Dr Norman F. Gant, of the Southwestern Medical School in Dallas, believes that linoleic acid may prevent some pregnancy complications, including pregnancy-induced high blood pressure. He used sunflower oil in his research.

Nutrition for breast-feeding
Breast-feeding is best for your baby and its advantages are fully discussed in the section *Breast-Feeding* (pages 141–5). If you are worried about your ability to breast-feed, the information at the end of that section and the dietary advice given here will help you.

Lactation, like pregnancy, is a time to make sure that you are eating the best possible diet. Your baby cannot get anything in your breast milk which you have not first eaten.

The exceptions to this rule are the minerals calcium and phosphorus. Dozens of studies have shown that these minerals can be taken from the mother's bones and used for her breast milk. If this happens – in addition to some calcium being excreted as well – then she is said to be in 'negative calcium balance'. It is therefore even more important to watch your calcium intake when breast-feeding – probably adding calcium supplements to your diet – than it is during pregnancy.

Eating refined starches and white sugars increases the content of saturated fats in breast milk; this also happens of course if you eat a lot of solid, saturated fats.[25] A wholefood diet is low in all kinds of fat but contains the essential fatty acids.

The liquid need for a nursing mother is about three quarts a day; drinking any more does not increase the milk. Unless you are allergic to cow's milk, you should drink between one and two pints a day.

One of the B vitamins, inositol, stimulated milk production in rats to such an extent that it was dubbed the lactation vitamin. This vitamin, together with the other B vitamins, is found in liver, wheat germ and brewer's yeast, the foods recommended by American nutritionist Adelle Davis to help good breast-feeding. (Drinking beer used to stimulate the milk flow – if you didn't mind a tipsy baby.) These B vitamin foods also contain extra protein and the need for protein goes up while you are nursing your baby. A good way of adding more protein is to add an egg and some skimmed milk to your glass of ordinary milk, or you could try the energy drink described in the *Fatigue* section (pages 303-9) which is full of the protein and B vitamins you need.

Incidentally, baby oil may contain mineral oil, and should not be put on your nipples. When your baby swallows it, it could leach the vitamins A, D, E and K from his body – so if your nipples are sore use some vegetable oil on them instead.

How long should you nurse your baby? Breast-feeding for any length of time is good for him; nurse him as long as you wish (and for as long as the milk is there, of course). Adelle Davis recommends breast-feeding for up to six months;[26] some women breast-feed their babies for as long as eight months.

Whole foods for healthy babies

Whole foods come first and supplements, if they are needed, a resounding second. According to nutritional expert Dr James Lambert Mount, a good diet is just as successful as supplements in protecting your baby and is basically a sounder approach. Please, therefore, SEE the *Whole Foods* section (pages 101-6) if you are planning to conceive, or are carrying or feeding a baby. Whole foods are delicious and you will enjoy eating a healthier diet. If you have up until now eaten mostly refined and convenience foods, then go gently with the change over several weeks to give your digestive system a chance to adjust to the new way of eating. Wholemeal bread, for instance, and raw salads need a lot of chewing!

Put yourself in the hands of a naturopath or a nutritionally aware doctor for advice on diet and on any additional supplements you may need before and during pregnancy and while you are nursing your baby. This will extend the care you are already getting from your ante-natal clinic.

Information

Morning sickness affects over half of pregnant women. By the end of the third month this condition, probably due to hormonal changes, is usually past. Dr Barbara Pickard, a research biologist, offers guidance for women who wish to act before they are pregnant to prevent morning sickness. Her excellent advice is based on the minimizing of this condition with foods rich in vitamin B6. Dr Pickard has written a booklet on this subject. Please sent 50p and a stamped and addressed envelope to: The Department of Animal Physiology

and Nutrition, Leeds University, Leeds LS2 9JT, or Lane End Farm, Denton, Ilkley, West Yorkshire, LS29 0HP.

Raspberry leaf tea: An infusion of raspberry leaves has been used for many years to allay labour pains in the Midlands and West Country. J.H. Burn, then Professor of Pharmacology at the University of Oxford, tested it on animals and found that it had a definite action on the uterus.[27] Raspberry leaf tea is obtainable from a health food store; please ask a qualified medical herbalist (SEE appendix page 405) about dosage.

Foresight: Formed by a group of women, this charity is setting up a number of clinics where prospective parents can get a thorough overhaul a few months in advance of the intended pregnancy. Screening for food and other allergies is given and couples tested for mineral levels, including poisonous minerals such as lead.

Information on nutrition, breast-feeding and other aspects of child care is provided. These clinics are under the supervision of Profession John Dickerson, Professor of Human Nutrition and Consultant Adviser in Clinical Nutrition to the South West Thames Regional Health Authority. Foresight has published *Guidelines for Future Parents* – a booklet costing £1 plus 20p for postage. If you wish to know more, please write to: Mrs Peter Barnes, Foresight, Woodhurst, Hydestile, Godalming, Surrey, GU8 4AY.

Relaxation for pregnancy: please SEE *Relaxation* in the appendix (page 405).

Recommended reading
Let's Have Healthy Children by Adelle Davis (Unwin 1975).

Books mentioned in this section
Nutrition and Physical Degeneration by Weston A. Price (Price-Pottinger, USA, 1977).

Vitamin B6: The Doctor's Report by John Ellis (Harper and Row, USA, 1973).

Vitamins in Your Life and the Micronutrients by E. DiCyan (Fireside, USA, 1975).

The Complete Book of Vitamins by Wilfrid E. Shute (Rodale Press 1977).

Skin and Food

The skin is a waterproof protective layer of marvellous complexity: supple, self-renewing and tough. It is an active, adaptable organ and a good shield against infection.

The skin acts as a barrier to bacteria, and a relay station for the messages of touch. It reacts to strong feelings and other stimuli by going pale, blushing and sweating. It can absorb certain substances and uses sunlight on its surface to make vitamin D, which is then absorbed into the body.

The sweat glands work with the blood vessels to regulate body temperature and they wash out toxins from the body, using the minerals potassium and sodium; a major organ of elimination, the skin is sometimes called the third kidney. Sebaceous glands near the surface produce sebum for lubrication.

The skin has two main layers. The top layer is the epidermis, without blood vessels, constantly shedding old cells as new cells move up to take their place. The next layer is the jelly-like dermis, with a network of blood vessels and nerves supported by collagen. Nails, hair and sweat glands grow from the dermis.

Sunlight is good for the skin – in moderation. Too much sun is damaging and can even result in skin cancer. Heavy tanning impairs the manufacture of vitamin D on the skin surface and ages the skin.

Some drugs, for instance the Pill, can cause a change in skin colour, as can menstruation, pregnancy and the menopause.

'Scarcely a deficiency exists which does not manifest itself by pathological changes in the skin,' says biochemist Roger J. Williams.[1] Vitamin A has an important effect on the skin, which reacts early to a mild deficiency. The resulting rough, bumpy skin used to be called 'toad skin' and looks like goose pimples. A lack of riboflavin (vitamin B2) shows as inflamed areas at the corners of the mouth, and a lack of thyroid can produce rough, unhealthy skin. A shortage of the B vitamin niacin can cause a rash like prickly heat; the skin becomes oily and scaly, with fine wrinkles and a coarse texture. Williams lists vitamins A, C, D, E, all the B vitamins except B12 and the unsaturated fatty acids to maintain skin health and to this list

must be added protein and the minerals magnesium and zinc. It is clear that a good skin, at any age, depends on good nutrition and good health.

Exaggerated claims are made for vitamin E, but it does help burns and scars to heal. American dermatologist Dr Irwin I. Lubowe reports that the use of highly-concentrated vitamin E on the skin has improved roughness and lines. It has a more profound effect as well. When polyunsaturated fats are deprived of their natural anti-oxidant, vitamin E, these fats will react with oxygen and form 'free radicals' – unpleasant substances which damage the cells and cause premature ageing of the skin. Vitamin E will work against this.

Vitamin A has been used to treat acne with some success and B6 can be effective against the kind of acne that flares up just before menstruation.[2] Tests at the University of Miami School of Medicine prove that the baffling skin condition, psoriasis, will often respond to vitamin A. Zinc promotes rapid healing of burns and other wounds, and a lack of magnesium has been related to skin ulcerations.[3]

Vital for the skin are the essential fatty acids, or EFAs, found in polyunsaturated fats and unrefined oils. Work on laboratory animals shows that EFA deficiencies cause thick, dry and scaly skin. Dr George Burr, working at the University of Minnesota, induced eczema in himself and a long-suffering colleague by cutting out EFAs. American nutritionist Adelle Davis describes a striking case of a small boy covered in eczema and very lethargic who was almost miraculously cured by the EFAs in soybean oil.

As the skin gets older, the sebaceous glands produce less sebum. The skin secretes less water, becomes less elastic and thinner. Older skins do not shed the top cells as easily as they did before, and this can make them look muddy. The supporting collagen becomes less flexible.

All this is an argument in favour of nutrients which can delay these processes. Vitamin E is often recommended at middle-age and we have seen that it helps prevent premature skin ageing. Collagen depends heavily on vitamin C which is, like E, an anti-oxidant, helping to delay cellular damage and consequent skin ageing. Another valuable substance is lecithin. Lecithin contains the EFAs which the skin needs and also helps the body to cope properly with fats. Slow or faulty fat metabolism can give rise to many skin diseases and lecithin has been used for eczema, some forms of acne and psoriasis, with some success.

These are specific nutrients, but the skin, like any other part of the body, needs good all-round nutrition to function well and look good. Eat whole cereals, including wholemeal bread, plenty of fresh raw fruits and salads and drink fruit and vegetable juices (SEE *Whole Foods* section pages 101–6). Refined foods containing white flour and white sugar, fried foods, convenience foods . . . none of these helps your skin. The delicate surface capillaries can be injured and thread veins caused by lots of tea and coffee, alcohol and spicy foods (and also by extremes of temperature). There is some evidence that sugar changes the sebum content of the skin, implying that it may be involved in seborrhoeic dermatitis. Smoking encourages premature wrinkles and a poor complexion.

Poor digestion and elimination are reflected in the skin, as are tension and negative feelings. Deep breathing and plenty of exercise give a glow to your skin and any inverted yoga pose is especially good, bringing the blood to the head. Learn to relax and get enough sleep. Your skin is a mirror of your wellbeing, and if all this advice sounds like a prescription for better health all over – it is.

Additional therapies
Deep breathing: SEE appendix page 405.
Exercise: SEE appendix page 405.
Relaxation: SEE appendix page 405.
Yoga: SEE appendix page 405.

Teeth and Food

Film star David Niven was out East when he caught sight of a ravishing, mysterious Oriental beauty. She turned her perfect oval face to him and smiled, revealing a complete set of stainless steel false teeth.

There are those among us, however, who may prefer to retain the assets that nature has given us . . .

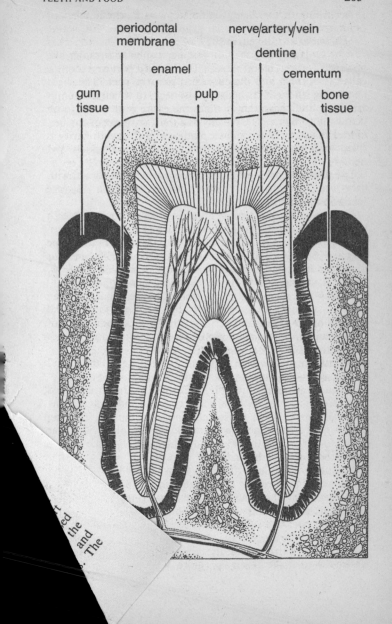

gum tissue · periodontal membrane · enamel · pulp · nerve/artery/vein · dentine · cementum · bone tissue

According to the Dental Estimates Board, the number of estimates for full and partial synthetic dentures for *young people under 21* totalled, in 1979, 42 070.[1]

A tooth is a strong shell of dentine, a substance rather like bone but without blood vessels. The exposed part of a tooth is called the crown and the concealed part the root. The slight narrowing where the two meet is the neck, to which the gum is attached, and cementum outlines the entire root of the tooth below the gum line. The crown has a thick covering of enamel, harder than any other animal matter, and the tooth cavity is filled with pulp and well supplied with blood vessels and nerves.

The two categories of dental trouble we are concerned with here are tooth decay (dental caries) and gum disease (periodontal disease).

It appears that our remote ancestors had rather better teeth than we have. Professor H.L. Hardwick examined 1014 teeth in Anglo-Saxon skulls and compared them with the same number belonging to his contemporaries. 9.5% of our ancestors had dental caries, compared with 48.6% of us. Indeed dental caries now has reached epidemic proportions.

Because the enamel of young teeth is less resistant, children have a lot of tooth decay. In adults, the caries rate falls off and diseases of the gum take over. (In spite of this, about 75% of schoolchildren now have gum disease.[2]) Most people do not even realize that they have unhealthy gums.

The two enemies which attack our teeth – dental decay and gum disease – are caused primarily by plaque.

Plaque is an almost invisible, sticky white substance formed by a combination of food particles, enzymes and bacteria. The minerals in the saliva cause the plaque to harden, forming calculus, or tartar. Bacteria in the plaque combine with sugar in the food particles to make acid, which dissolves the enamel of the tooth and produces decay.

Plaque and calculus irritate the gums, so the body reacts by dilating the blood vessels in the gums and sending more white blood cells. Calculus forces the gum away from the root of the tooth, allowing the entry of more food debris. This is the sta of gum disease. The gums swell to accommodate the increas number of white blood cells, and as the disease progresses bony socket surrounding the tooth is also attacked destroyed to make room for more white blood cell protective gum tissues, meanwhile, recede down the root of the tooth and pus starts to form where the bone has been lost. Eventually the condition develops from bleeding gums – gingivitis – to bleeding and swollen gums with the infection draining into the rest of the body. When the disease has spread deeply, forming pockets, it is called periodontal disease; it finally degenerates into pyorrhoea. Dentists may find it necessary to extract teeth if the gum tissue round them is diseased, and The British Dental Association states that more teeth are lost through pyorrhoea than any other cause.

Healthy gums, therefore, anchoring each tooth firmly to the jawbone, are the foundation of a healthy mouth. But although the teeth are protected with tough enamel, the gums are vulnerable. The plaque in the crevices between the necks of the teeth is a dense concentration of bacteria which can cause gum disease. And gum disease, if left untreated, can lead to the loss of every tooth in your mouth.

Healthy gums are firm and pinkish and fill in all the spaces between the teeth; they have little dot-like indentations on them closest to the teeth and there should be a slight collar round the gum where it meets the tooth. Unhealthy gums may look smooth and puffy and have signs of inflammation; they will probably bleed easily – hence 'pink toothbrush'. Pale gums can be a sign of iron-deficiency anaemia. Pregnancy, the Pill and certain other drugs can affect them, causing swelling and bleeding. Heavy smokers often have discoloured gums.

The blame for most plaque can be firmly laid on refined sugars and refined flour. (Please note that any kind of sugar eaten separate from its natural source – that is, sugar refined out of sugar cane and sugar beet – will cause plaque. Even black molasses will damage the teeth if they are not cleaned afterwards.)

Returning here to the skulls of our ancient ancestors, it has been established that the slow rise in the incidence of caries from the Bronze Age onwards was chiefly due to the refining of flour, but the much faster rise in recent times is caused by the refining of sugar. Although the starch in flour can be changed by bacteria into sugar fairly quickly, any refined sugar will find it still easier to ferment into the acids which do our teeth so much harm. Sugar in its various forms, therefore, causes tooth decay to increase, and this has been conclusively proved. Caramels and toffees are worse than, say, milk chocolate because, like sugar and flour, they are sticky and adhere to the teeth.

Sugar can even cause pain in the teeth. The cementum which outlines the tooth root below the gum line has nerve endings and is therefore sensitive. As the gum recedes with age the cementum gradually becomes less sensitive. But with a high sugar intake the gum recedes too quickly for the cementum to lose its sensitivity naturally and the result is pain.

Snacks of sweets and biscuits given to children between meals are a major cause of tooth decay. Babies given a dummy to suck containing sweet syrup have teeth which literally rot as they erupt, causing rampant caries. At the age of two or three, these children can have mouths full of blackened stumps. 'If nothing else were achieved in the nutritional sphere over the next 50 years but the control of sweet eating and confectionery advertising,' says doctor and writer James Lambert Mount, 'this would be worth-while.' And he goes on to ask, 'what is more sacred, vested financial interests, or children's health?'[3]

On the other hand, sugars taken in their natural form will do the teeth nothing but good. Fruit, for instance, containing fruit sugar, only benefits both teeth and gums as the fibre in the fruit acts as an abrasive, helping to clear food debris from the teeth as it is chewed. A two-year study between 1955 and 1957[4] proved that schoolchildren given slices of apple after meals not only had less caries, but less gum disease than the others. In another study, improvement in the condition of the gums was noticed after only four days in a group of volunteers who were fed on fruit, fresh raw vegetables and good quality protein.[5]

Chewing hard, fibrous food also encourages optimum growth of facial, skull and jaw bones. It helps to avoid malocclusion, where the palate is not wide enough to hold the teeth and they cannot be spaced out properly.

Care and nutrition of the teeth

This starts with your toothbrush. For leaflets on the care of the teeth SEE the *Information* section at the end of this chapter; for professional advice consult your dentist or dental hygienist.

I am not going to discuss in detail the fluoride question which provokes so much heat. But I would like to say that, even if fluoridation of the water prevents decay – and evidence strongly suggests that in fact it only delays it – not enough research has been done into its effect *on the whole body*. Fluoride is added to the water where it is not naturally present and where the minerals usually accompanying it – calcium and magnesium – are not found. What is the effect of this? Further, fluoridation *increases* the incidence of gum disease, which is widespread in children and even commoner among adults, and it is strongly suspected of linking up with cancer. [6]

Teeth begin early. The permanent teeth begin their existence five months before a child is born. Experiments prove that diet is closely linked with both the development and the maintenance of healthy teeth and gums, so we should distinguish between foods we should steer clear of in order to protect our teeth, like white sugar and refined sticky flour, and the foods which help our teeth – fresh, chewy fruits, vegetables and wholegrains. [7] These foods not only supply us with the nutrients we need for a healthy body, including strong teeth and gums but they demand thorough mastication – equally important.

Minerals essential for the teeth include calcium, phosphorus, molybdenum (which helps prevent caries), zinc, vanadium, boron, lithium, strontium, fluorine. Calcium needs to combine with phosphorus in building the teeth, in a natural ratio of about one to one. In many of our foods, this ratio is unbalanced and too much phosphorus is eaten, so a deficiency of phosphorus is unlikely.

It has been found that changes in the hormonal systems of pregnant women lower their resistance to plaque, and that women often need more calcium in the later months of pregnancy.

The hard enamel and dentine covering a tooth appear unchanging and inert. But these structures have been built by living cells, and there is some evidence that mineral loss from the teeth can be replaced and the cavity 'remineralized'. Some researchers believe that, if decay starts, healthy teeth can throw up a wall of hardened dentine to stop it. (This can work the other way around, too; if a person is deficient in calcium the bones and teeth can release some for the rest of the body to use.) Dr Sheiham of the London Hospital Medical College Dental School states that 'remineralization occurs quite often. In one study more than half the early lesions were diagnosed as sound at later examination.' The teeth, therefore, are far from lifeless, and calcium supplementation might well prove useful to protect them.

The jawbone shrinkage which often occurs with age is uncomfortable for denture wearers as it causes ill-fitting teeth. Many dentists accept this as normal, and dental adhesive manufacturers make money out of it. But extra calcium can slow down this process. One study showed that denture wearers given 750mg of calcium and 375 units of vitamin D a day (the two need each other to work properly) lost about 36% less bone from their jaws than an unsupplemented group; further work at the University of Gothenburg in Sweden showed that calcium supplementation can actually reverse jawbone loss. There is also some evidence that vitamin C may inhibit jawbone shrinkage.

Vitamin A is also needed to build tooth enamel. Where there is a serious deficiency, both bone growth and the sloughing off of old bone cells are retarded.

Vitamin B6 may reduce tooth decay by as much as 50%. Two studies showed that Cuban children who chewed whole, fibrous sugarcane (which contains quite a lot of B6) had fewer caries and, not surprisingly, a higher amount of the vitamin in their blood than another group tested from New York City.

The cells lining the gum crevice have one of the highest turnover rates in the body – they completely renew themselves every three to seven days. Bad nutrition may impair this renewal and prevent the gums from going their job. 'It cannot be too strongly emphasised that all living cells associated in any way with the teeth, those in the gums, in the pulp of the teeth, in the periodontal membrane which lies between the teeth and the bone of the jaw, and those in the salivary glands, all require complete nutrition.'[8] Nutrients for these cells include iron, copper and pantothenic acid.

A vitamin C deficiency almost doubles the ease with which bacterial toxins can penetrate mouth tissues and the addition of a modest 100mg a day to the diet of volunteers caused dramatic improvements in bleeding, sore, infected gums.[9]

American dentist Dr Vogel is currently using 4mg a day of folic acid to protect women on the Pill from gum disease, and calcium supplementation also appears to work well.

Many illnesses and toxic conditions are made worse by bad teeth and diseased gums. Teeth and gums, like any other part of the body, exert an influence on the whole and cannot be thought about in isolation.

Please SEE the *Whole Foods* section (pages 101–6) for the best way of eating for healthy teeth and gums. Any supplements which may be necessary must be *in addition* to a sound diet – please consult a naturopath (SEE appendix) or a nutritionally aware dentist.

Information

Leaflets on care of the teeth and gums are obtainable from:
Your local Health Education Officer (address in phone book; free of charge).
The Health Education Council, 78 New Oxford Street, London WC1A 1AH (free of charge).

Vegetarian and Vegan Eating

'Vegetarian' was taken by the English vegetarians – who were trying to make a point – from the Latin *vegetus*, meaning 'whole, sound, fresh or lively'. It does not mean that they live solely on vegetables. Those who coined this word defined a vegetarian as 'one who abstains from flesh, fish and fowl, and who may or may not use milk, eggs and cheese.'

People eating no animal flesh, or foods of animal origin either (dairy foods), are vegans.

Vegetarianism is not just a Western minority fad. Many people throughout man's history have lived largely on a vegetarian diet, reserving meat for feast days and other treats. Many Buddhists and Hindus are vegetarians and Taoist writings say that a meatless diet is required for spiritual development. In the East, it was often the priestly class who chose to be vegetarians and the lower classes who ate meat.

Many people are vegetarians for ethical reasons, too. George Bernard Shaw, Alexander Pope and Hitler are famous vegetarians, the last provoking a comment from Jay Dinshah, founder of the American Vegetarian Society: 'no one has ever claimed that vegetarianism is a sure cure for insanity.'

'All the while
I pray to Buddha,
I keep on killing
Mosquitoes'
Japanese poet Issa

I am not going to discuss the ethical arguments in favour of giving up meat. There is no doubt that animals in factory-farming are cruelly reared and slaughtered to meet our huge demands for this expensive protein. Raising these animals needs a lot of land, and to get 1lb of edible meat you need several times this amount of feed for the animals. In any world this is pretty bad economics and in today's world it is absurd.

What about our fish supplies? Many marine scientists believe that we have now fished the oceans to the limit. Fish harvests have been declining for several years, due partly to pollution and partly to over-fishing, and the impact of fish-farming on the world food crisis can only be slight.

The fatted calf
We in the West take meat for granted and often eat it several times a day. True, it is a complete protein and contains vitamins, minerals and saturated fats. But some carcases of animals intensively reared for meat contain far more fat than do wild or free-range animals (about 30% compared with about 4%).

Medication in the form of antibiotics and hormones put into the food and bodies of farm animals causes a real risk of residues in their meat. Because of these vast quantities of antibiotics, resistant strains of bacteria are created in the meat which fail to respond, in the meat-eating human being, to antibiotics prescribed for him. A short tour round the chemicals now being poured down the throats of animals, injected into them or otherwise inflicted upon them in the name of farm efficiency makes the head spin. There are of course pesticides and other chemicals in fruits and vegetables but a recent American test found that these are about one-tenth of the residues in flesh foods.

When animals are slaughtered, there is 'a definite incentive not to comply with personal hygiene regulations if this means slowing down the kill-rate.'[1] Hardly any British or EEC slaughterhouses have the means for bacterial examination of the meat. Another hazard from flesh foods arises from the fact that meat, fish and poultry are liable to disturb the benevolent micro-organisms which normally inhabit the human intestine, leading to gastric disturbances.

Fish are not exempt from our present policy of industriously polluting everything in sight. An unfortunate herring caught in Lake Ontario was found to contain 28 known or suspected carcinogens.[2] Little research has yet been done on salt-water fish and one hopes that the seas are cleaner than the lakes . . .

Let's compare ourselves with true carnivores.

We have front incisor teeth, with small canines on either side, and molars along the jaw lines. Our incisors are useful for shredding fruit, vegetables and nuts which are further ground up by the molars, and we have a mobile jaw for chewing our food to a paste before swallowing it. The true flesh-eaters have large canines and rip their foods to pieces before gulping it down in lumps. Life is fast for the predator.

Our intestinal tract is longer than our torso and, although this is fine for vegetable matter, it is not so good for flesh foods, which quickly decompose and become toxic. The carnivore's tract is relatively shorter so that the meat can pass quickly through. The form of its gut and its flora and secretions are different; its alimentary canal secretes enough hydrochloric acid to dissolve bones, and chewed hunks of flesh and gristle are quickly broken down and the toxins excreted.

Our saliva contains amylase, an enzyme which predigests starch from plants. A carnivore's saliva does not.

Although we sometimes call ourselves omnivores, we have very little in common physiologically with other animals who also eat just about everything, such as the fox and rat; there is in fact no order Omnivora. Our immediate relatives are the great apes, the chimpanzee, gorilla, orang-utang and gibbon; humans and African apes are 'biologically so close as to be nearly inseparable in many essentials,' says physical anthropologist S.L. Washburn. So if we look at the way these animals feed, we might learn something about our own past eating habits and from that the feeding we are best adapted to.

Researcher Dr Jane Goodall has seen wild chimpanzees in Tanzania eat fruits, seeds, leaves, insects, honey, birds' eggs and small birds and mammals. Meat-eating seems to occur in cycles. So it's likely that we were not vegetarians all the time. Since meat on four legs must have been difficult to run down on two legs, it has been argued that we only ate meat when we could get it. This theory takes both our anatomy, and animal research, into account.

It is concluded, therefore, that early man was a hunter-gatherer and then, as now, a general feeder and able to survive without animal foods. We will eat anything that won't kill us if we like the taste of it.

But there is still room for doubt about what we ate early in our history. 'How can we speak authoritatively about what we ate, when who we were is still largely unknown?' asks Vic Sussman in his book *The Vegetarian Alternative*.

Meatless eating: the advantages

It has been shown by several investigations that vegetarian diets lower blood cholesterol[3] and vegan diets lower it still more. This could be due to the lower amounts of saturated fats in a meatless diet or to the higher amounts of pectin in many fruits and vegetables (pectin lowers blood cholesterol). It might link up with the high content of dietary fibre or roughage. Although it is true that a vegetarian who eats dairy foods will be getting some saturated fat, the rest of his diet will be low in fat and a vegan will get very little. Lower levels of blood cholesterol are believed to help protect against heart and artery disease (SEE *Fats* pages 23–35).

An Australian study has found that the blood pressure of vegetarians is 'significantly less' than that of meat-eaters.[4] This research was carried out on Seventh Day Adventists, a strict religious group about half of whom are vegetarians. They do not take coffee, tea, alcohol, spices or refined foods either. Their rates of 'nutrition-related' cancer – which includes colonic, rectal and intestinal cancer – are 50% to 70% lower than those for the general population. These figures strongly suggest that a vegetarian diet may also protect against some kinds of cancer. Their risks of dying from heart disease, too, are lower than average.

A good vegetarian or vegan diet has about two to four times more dietary fibre than is found in meat-based diets. Fibre, plus the large quantities of fruit and vegetables also typical of this way of eating, gives plenty of bulk without too many calories and this also helps to control a person's weight. Additionally, 'recent studies have shown that the increase in cereal fibre in the vegetarian diet has given vegetarians about one-third the risk of diverticular disease of non-vegetarians. I think a lot can be said for a vegetarian diet.'[5]

Briefly, fibre prevents constipation and many allied illnesses, including the diverticular disease mentioned above, by providing the soft mass the colon needs in order to get rid of body wastes quickly and efficiently. (SEE *Fibre* pages 35–42).

There is a correlation between eating animal proteins and the formation of kidney stones. This is discussed in an article with the arresting title 'Should Recurrent Oxalate Stone-formers Become Vegetarians?'[6] It's also possible that high-meat diets, by over-stimulating the system, add to the risk of diabetes. A high-fibre diet has the opposite effect by slowing down absorption of sugar into the blood and therefore helping to stabilize the diabetic's blood sugar level. A vegetarian diet has been shown to increase the manufacture in the gut of certain B vitamins.[7]

Two British researchers successfully treated four cases of severe angina pectoris with a vegan diet. All four patients were symptomless and free of pain and able to 'engage in strenuous activities' by the fifth or sixth month of treatment.[8]

A long-term prospective research project has now been started by the University of Oxford in collaboration with the Vegetarian Society to study the health of vegetarians.

Possible deficiencies

Because vegetarians and vegans don't eat meat, and meat contains iron, do they get anaemic?

Iron deficiency is common even among meat-eaters. So vegetarians and vegans should take care to get enough, even though numerous studies have shown that the intake of iron in a good vegetarian diet is within acceptable limits. Although iron from flesh foods is more easily absorbed than that from plants, vegetarians' high intake of fresh raw fruits and vegetables, with plenty of vitamin C, is probably a factor in helping them to make the most of their dietary iron (vitamin C helps iron assimilation).

Non-meat foods containing iron are: soybeans (plenty of easily assimilable iron), molasses, brewer's yeast, wheat germ and wheat bran, wholewheat cereals including wholewheat bread, pulses and legumes; green leaves especially spinach, turnip and beet tops, dandelion greens; dried fruits, mushrooms, potatoes, sunflower and pumpkin seeds, sprouting seeds and grains. White bread and other white flour products are enriched with iron, but it is often not absorbed properly. (Red kidney beans should always be soaked for at least 18 hours and boiled for at least 15 minutes before being eaten. They contain toxic factors which must be destroyed.)

Although there is plenty of protein in their diets, vegetarians and vegans can occasionally become protein-deficient. Readers may like to turn to the *Protein* section (pages 51–7), which explains this in more detail.

Vitamin B12 is an essential vitamin. It is needed by every cell in the body and its deficiency can lead to megaloblastic anaemia, damage to the nervous system and mental symptoms. Since it is found in foods of animal origin (including dairy foods) and in some fermented foods, it will be lacking in the vegan diet and perhaps deficient in the vegetarian diet as well. Cereals, nuts, pulses, fruits and vegetables do not contain vitamin B12 unless contaminated by the micro-organisms that produce it, and its deficiency can be masked by the presence of folic acid. It has been identified in seaweed growing near sewage, and is said to be in certain other plants in minute amounts.

The incidence in vegans of any symptoms of vitamin B12 deficiency, however, is very small,[9] and there is some evidence that many people who do not eat foods containing this vitamin can make it for themselves in the gut, since when tested they are not deficient. This cannot be relied upon for everybody, however, and you can buy vegan foods with B12 added at health food stores or you can take a supplement; very little is needed. Spirulina contains plenty of this vitamin (SEE page 132).

A report on the health of pre-school vegan children from 19 families were given at a Nutrition Society meeting in May 1980. The mothers had all followed a vegan diet during pregnancy and lactation and 25 children were studied, with an average age of about 30 months. All the children appeared to be healthy. Their growth was normal, although they tended to be shorter and lighter than other children. The report concludes that 'although energy and calcium intakes were below those recommended, their diets were generally satis- factory. However, a few children had low intakes of riboflavin (vitamin B2), and vitamin B12. There is obviously a need for vegan mothers to ensure that their children receive an adequate supply of these vitamins.' In an article in the British Nutrition Foundation Bulletin (27) Dr Sanders advises the vegan mother to eat a properly balanced vegan diet during pregnancy and lactation and supplement it with B12, vitamin D and calcium gluconate (especially if she lives in a soft water area). He emphasises that considerable care and some nutritional knowledge are required to provide a good vegan diet for young children, but states that properly balanced vegan and vegetarian diets do not endanger health.

To summarize the *possible* disadvantages of meatless eating, these are:

1 Deficiency of vitamin B12 (particularly in vegans).
2 Too many starchy foods.
3 Too few proteins.
4 Lack of calcium, riboflavin (B2), vitamin D, iodine (vegans).

Please note I am assuming that a vegetarian knows enough about nutrition to avoid refined, sugary and convenience foods. A vegetarian – and more especially a vegan – needs to be well-informed.

But what IS a vegetarian?

Vegetarians often have other beliefs and habits which are so closely bound up with their vegetarianism that it is difficult to disentangle them. For example, a vegetarian may enjoy open air sports and take lots of exercise; it would be difficult to say then how much his good health is due to his diet, and how much to his physical fitness. The presence of other factors is illustrated most clearly by the Seventh Day Adventists, who have been widely studied because many of them are vegetarians and they enjoy above-average health. But their way of life – which includes their way of eating, of course – involves regular exercise, and a high value is set on family stability, education and religious observance. It is therefore impossible to disentangle their food from their lifestyle and it is obvious that *all* these factors have a bearing on their health.

There is another important distinction.

You can compare a vegetarian with the average 'omnivorous' eater. But what does this really mean? There are two comparisons to be made – one between the well-informed vegetarian (or vegan) and the equally well-informed person who follows a wholefood diet including meat; the other between the same vegetarian and the person living mostly on refined and convenience foods.

We can list the advantages of a good, intelligent vegetarian or vegan diet:

1   Low fat (particularly for the vegan).
2   High fibre.
3   Enough, and not too much, protein.
4   Low calories.
5   High vitamins and minerals (in fresh raw fruits and vegetables).
6   A wide range of high quality foods, as little tampered with as possible.
7   No convenience foods, few additives, little sugar and salt.
8   Low cost.

We can see that many of the benefits listed here apply also to the non-vegetarian, but wholefood, way of eating too. But if we compare these same advantages with the characteristics of the mountains of junk eaten by so many people, *this* distinction is strikingly obvious.

It is probably true that a wholefood way of eating, with occasional meat, would suit many of us very well. Some people who decide in favour of whole foods find themselves becoming part-time vegetarians in this way; there is no doubt that complete vegetarianism does not suit everybody.

Information
The Vegetarian Society, 53 Marloes Road, Kensington, London W8 6LA (telephone 01 937 7739) will answer all your queries and offers countless books, holds courses and sponsors scientific research.

The International Vegetarian Health Food Handbook, obtainable from the Society at £1.75 plus postage of 35p includes among much useful information a list of vegetarian hotels, restaurants and health food stores. The Vegan Society, at 47 Highlands Road, Leatherhead, Surrey answers all vegan enquiries.

Recommended reading
Readers might like to obtain a copy of the excellent *The Vegetarian Alternative* by Vic Sussman, published by the Rodale Press. Their address is Potten End, Berkhamsted, Hertfordshire HP4.2BR (telephone Berkhamsted 71313).

PART THREE

Illnesses –
The Nutritional Approach

Allergies to Food

What is an allergy?

If you are allergic, you are trigger-happy. Your body is firing from the hip in an empty street. Quick on the draw – but all the villains are out of town. Something in you is over-reacting to a substance that leaves most people cold.

' "Allergy", by definition,' writes naturopath Leon Chaitow, 'is an altered or changed reaction on the part of the body to a specific substance, which causes no symptoms to the non-sensitive individual. Quite literally, one man's meat is another man's poison.'[1]

What happens when we are allergic? And – still more important – why are some people allergic and not others?

We are all blessed with an immune system which defends us against infection. In the allergic person it is believed that this system makes a mistake and labels a harmless substance 'enemy'. Antibodies and chemicals are released to deal with the 'enemy', and spare antibodies rampage round the body, causing inflammation. One of the chemicals released is histamine which, carried round by the bloodstream, causes body tissues to be over-sensitive to the invaders and makes capillary walls more permeable, causing swelling and mucus.

Some people cannot control their production of antibodies, and some allergies may be due to the lack of an enzyme. Both these defects may be inherited.

Allergic reactions show up most often as skin or respiratory problems such as asthma or hay fever, and allergies to foods often show up as stomach upsets, but they can produce almost any other allergic symptom as well. A single irritant substance, or allergen, can cause reactions at several different sites in the body. Allergens have to get on to or into the body to cause any trouble so they must be breathed in, swallowed, touched or injected. Allergic reactions vary from trivial discomfort to anaphylactic shock, which can kill. These reactions may be sudden and temporary (sneezing), or they may last for years (eczema). The first exposure to the offending allergen makes the body sensitive to it, and the second or third exposures to the same substance will bring about an allergic reaction.

Allergy runs in families. If both parents have an allergy, the child has a 75% chance of being allergic too. If only one parent is allergic, the chance drops to about 50%. It is thought that as many as 30% of all people attending their GP have an allergy of one sort or another.

To describe the range of allergic reactions is a pretty depressing activity. A growing body of medical opinion believes that arthritis, depression and mental illness, alcoholism, obesity, stomach ulcers, bedwetting and possibly some cancers should join asthma, hay fever and nettle-rash as the signs of an individual's intolerance of certain substances, including foods, in his environment.

As well as these definite illnesses, an allergic reaction carries with it other unpleasant symptoms as the affected part of the body rebels. Symptoms include:

persistent fatigue, depression, irritability
joint pains, back and neck pains
fluctuations in weight
puffiness of hands, face, stomach, ankles
swollen glands
palpitations, especially after eating
excessive sweating unrelated to exercise
red eyes, running or blocked nose.

These symptoms may accompany an actual illness, or they may exist alone.

Every allergic person has a target area, the part of his body which is sensitive to the allergen, but an allergic reaction is also universal, affecting every cell in the victim's body.

Body allergies

Stepping back a few paces, we can see that allergy belongs in a wider picture, that of ecology. Ecology deals with the relationships of living things to their environment and to each other. The longer a living creature has been exposed to a substance, the better its adaptation to it.

And this is where allergy comes in. The clinical ecologist studies individual susceptibility and adaptation to the air, water, drugs, clothes, living places and above all the *food* which we all use now. These parts of our environment have a far-reaching influence on us, and they are changing rapidly – changing more quickly, in many instances, than we are able to adapt to them.

Intolerance to certain foods was familiar even to Hippocrates. But the ancient Greeks did not have to live in a world increasingly polluted with chemicals in the air, the water, even in our clothes and our homes. They did not have our impressive, and depressing, array of drugs. They did not eat the mind-boggling range of additives and other chemicals that we add to our refined, processed foods. Discussing the reasons for allergies in his book *Not All in the Mind* Dr Richard Mackarness blames our adulterated, refined food for many allergies. His researches indicate that it is often not the foods themselves to which his patients are allergic, *but the chemicals which have been added to them* (please SEE the section on the *Modern Food Industry*, pages 42–51).

It is true that food additives have been extensively tested, but only for a narrow range of conditions. They have been used on animals to discover if they can cause cancer or cell damage, and they are only tested singly. But we take them in *together* – and they may not have been tested for the other diseases, including allergy, that they may cause. We would be wise to view all additives with caution – a large question mark still hangs over many of them.

Allergic reactions

There are two kinds of allergic reactions. The first one is the obvious kind – the sufferer instantly reacts when he eats a strawberry, for instance, or even walks past a fish-shop. This allergy is easy to see and there is no waiting for symptoms to appear, as an allergic patient will tell you. You simply eat the offending food and put up with what happens afterwards.

It is also possible to become addicted over a long period of time to the food to which we are allergic, as an alcoholic is addicted to his drink. Here's what happens in this 'masked allergy'.

1 As a result of several exposures to, or doses of, the offending substance, the person becomes sensitive to it.

2 As his exposures continue, the person notices an unpleasant reaction each time.

3 His reaction goes through a change now, and he feels good after each exposure.

4 He may go without his allergen for a while now, and he will experience unpleasant withdrawal symptoms – a hangover. He resumes his allergic food again and feels better, and he then

tends to eat the offending food more and more often so that he does not go through any more hangovers, but keeps on feeling good. Regular intake of his allergen will seem to keep him well for years, and the length of this stage will depend on how well his body can adapt to the allergen each time he takes it in. This is addiction.

5   Eventually his powers of adaptation to the allergen run out and he gets to the stage where his body is exhausted. He needs more and more of his allergen, at shorter and shorter intervals, to keep from feeling lousy.

This pattern of addiction is clearly illustrated by the alcoholic, but some people are addicted to sweet, starchy foods, and will raid the larder to stave off a carbohydrate hangover. Addiction is linked with the later stages of the slow-acting, less obvious allergies.

We tend to get masked allergies to the foods we eat most often. The more familiar the food is to us, the more severe the allergic reaction, and the more difficult it is to pinpoint the cause.

A rash from eating shellfish or strawberries is easy to recognize. But it is much harder to see that the bread or eggs we eat every day may be causing our bouts of catarrh, headache and depression. Wheat, eaten in bread every day by almost everybody, is one of the commonest producers of allergic reactions.

Pinpointing an allergy

Allergy symptoms are superb mimics. Therefore, before you assume that you are allergic to some substance, you must make absolutely sure that your illness, or discomfort, is not due to some other cause. Your practitioner should be able to help you with this. Migraine, for example, can sometimes be due to low blood sugar or several other causes. Because allergies can result in such a wide range of symptoms, they are frequently blamed where they do not exist. (Dr Peter Nixon of the Charing Cross Hospital has found that several of his Total Allergy Syndrome patients were in fact only suffering from hyperventilation, or over-breathing.)

One method of allergy testing is to place the patient on a four- to five-day fast, during which he takes nothing but water. During this period of no food, and therefore of no food allergen, his symptoms will go down if he is allergic. Then he is given a test feeding of a single food, and watched for his reaction. Because he has been without the allergen food for several days, his reaction is usually sharp and unmistakeable. (This test must be carried out in a hospital under supervision. If you are allergic to a common food which we eat every day, such as milk, wheat or beef, you will be dealing with a serious illness.)

Another way is cutting out a group of foods for several days – for instance, all cereals, or all dairy foods – and then re-introducing it and seeing what happens.

The term 'allergy' was restricted in the past to those substances which provoked a reaction on the skin and led to asthma, hay fever, and so on. By giving carefully graded injections, it was often found possible to desensitize the patient so that he no longer reacted to his allergen (pollen, house dust, etc.). But skin tests were found to be misleading when used for food allergy testing, perhaps because a food may cause a reaction in a person only when he is below par or emotionally upset, or perhaps because the injected food is in a different state from the food actually eaten.

Sometimes small quantities of the allergen are put under the tongue for sublingual tests and this is a useful method. Some American food allergists use intradermal tests, in which food extracts are injected into the skin. The value of this method is still being debated.

If you want to test yourself for food allergies at home, you can try the pulse test, invented by a Dr Coca, although this is not entirely reliable. For this, take your pulse and keep a record of it for at least a week. Test your pulse:

on waking
just before each meal
half an hour after each meal
just before going to bed

If the pulse remains below 84 a minute, then there is probably no allergy present. If there is a swing of more than 6 beats a minute up or down, then you are probably allergic (allow for a rapid pulse after violent exercise, of course). By noting down everything you eat and drink, and comparing this with your changes in pulse rate, you may be able to pinpoint any possible allergens in your food.

If the pulse test is positive, miss a meal one night, and test your pulse the next morning on waking. Then eat or drink a small quantity of the suspected food on its own, re-testing your pulse over the next hour or so. If there is a rapid rise of 6 or more beats a minute, or the onset of allergic symptoms, then the test is positive (this can however be complicated by a delayed reaction). Symptoms to watch for are sneezing, sniffling, a runny or blocked-up nose, itching, coughing, a tight chest and wheezing, bloat, gas, heartburn, palpitations, nausea and vomiting, cramps, diarrhoea, chilling or flushing, sweating, fatigue, headache (including migraine), aches and pains.

After several months during which you strictly avoid your allergen food, you may gain a tolerance to it if you take it in small, spaced doses. Some food allergies, however, are resistant and no tolerance can be gained in this way. Many people are allergic to more than one food, and food allergy usually accompanies allergies to other substances, e.g. house dust, tobacco, paint, etc.

Drug treatments
There are various drugs for the treatment of allergies.

Antihistamines work against the effects produced by histamine, thus reducing the intensity of the allergic reaction. They always produce side-effects, of varying intensities. They can depress the brain, leading to drowsiness and sleep, and other side-effects include dizziness, noises in the ears, lack of co-ordination, blurred vision, mood changes, nervousness, delusions, insomnia, tremors and tingling, appetite loss, nausea and vomiting, diarrhoea or constipation, dry mouth, coughing, frequency and difficulty in passing urine, palpitations, headache, tightness in the chest, weak, heavy-feeling hands. Very rarely, they can cause serious blood disorders, and you can even become allergic to them. A healthy liver can destroy histamine, but a damaged liver cannot. Antihistamine drugs can easily harm the liver and their toxicity puts a strain on the adrenal glands, whipping a tired horse, and eventually worsening the patient's health.

The corticosteroids will put a stop to almost any allergic symptoms and stop inflammation. Continuous doses can produce hairiness, moon face, muscle weakness, nervous disorders, and can encourage the adrenal glands to leave off producing natural hormones. When the drug is stopped the patient can suffer a horrible rebound of symptoms.

Disodium (or sodium) cromoglycate (marketed as Intal, Nalcrom, Rynacrom and, in the USA, Cromolyn) appears to block certain allergic reactions and is often used for asthma and a running nose due to an allergy. It may cause irritation of the throat and bronchii, especially during an infective illness, and it should not be taken in the early stages of pregnancy. Its sudden withdrawal may trigger off an attack of asthma.

Some allergic people find that aspirin helps their asthma if it is due to pollen, and in his book *Eating and Allergy* Robert Eagle suggests that people with an acute food allergy can protect themselves by taking a hefty dose of aspirin before a meal. Presumably nobody has considered the effects that this 'hefty dose' can have on the allergic person's poor unsuspecting stomach.

It is of course possible to be allergic to any drug, for instance, penicillin or aspirin, occasionally an anti-allergy drug or even vitamin pills which are coloured or which contain preservatives.

But it's not as simple as that . . .

To avoid allergen foods, or to have to take anti-allergy drugs with their potentially damaging side-effects, is not good enough. Avoidance is not a cure. Knocking the symptoms – and often the hapless patient too – on the head is not a cure either. More questions need to be asked.

Why is there so much allergic illness around? If we look at what happens to the body when a person is allergic, perhaps we can get closer to ways to prevent and cure this disabling and sometimes very dangerous array of symptoms.

Allergy is a reaction to our environment. Is it possible that, in our chemically polluted world, our powers of adaptation have broken down so that those of us who tend to be allergic are the first casualties? Does our food, for instance, have so many additives put into it and so many nutrients taken out that it is no longer able to nourish our immune system, which protects us against allergy?

For allergy means stress. Any allergic reaction puts a strain on the body. The allergy itself is often a result of physical or emotional stress, a decision factor which can tip the balance and push the body into illness.

The relationship between health and food is the subject of

this book. Let's look at the way we can attack allergy, and its attendant stress, through nutrition. Not simply by leaving out the offending food, although this of course can be an essential beginning to the treatment. But by strengthening the patient's powers of resistance to the *allergic state itself* with good nutrition and possibly the use of supplements, so that his immune system no longer flies into a panic at the approach of the humble ear of wheat, or piece of cheese, or cup of coffee.

Food allergy is a condition that is either inherited or acquired. If it is acquired, then a combination of stress and a diet of refined carbohydrates is almost always involved. Allergies vary widely, and many are only transitory. A food or any other substance which causes an allergic reaction can be harmless when the patient is feeling calmer and better. The substances giving most trouble to the food allergy victim, whether his illness is inherited or acquired, are mostly within the range of foods that man has added to his diet along the centuries: cereal products, dairy produce and – in very recent times – the whole gamut of refined foods, low in essential nutrients and high in synthetic colourings, flavourings and preservatives.

Although in general an allergy victim is more likely to be allergic to cereals, dairy produce and junk foods, he can, in his lowered state of health, be allergic to *any* food.

It has been found by some doctors that adherence to a strictly limited diet, although removing the allergic symptoms for the time being, only results in the long run in more allergic symptoms showing up. 'The limitations of the clinical ecologists' approach', writes naturopath Leon Chaitow, 'are that they do not take the logical further step of reforming patients' diets so that not only are irritant foods avoided, but a positive state of health is built up to help prevent further sensitivities or allergies from developing. An allergy is, after all, only a symptom of an underlying imbalance in the system. Correction of this is the fundamental task, and it requires nutritional reform together with supplements to enable organ systems and functions to normalize.'[1]

Allergy is rapidly becoming a fashionable complaint. But its effective treatment can demand changes from the sufferer requiring real effort. Unless he overhauls his diet his body will be unable to throw off the tendency to be allergic. His allergic symptoms may simply shift from one allergen to another, until in the end he is forced to sit in a plastic bubble eating mashed potatoes.

Elimination diets, although useful to pinpoint the allergy, are usually nutritionally inadequate. They should be used for detective work only and the long-term emphasis must be placed on building health as well as on avoiding the offending substance. Indeed, some inadequate diets prescribed for allergic people, by exhausting the adrenals, causing indigestion, impairing liver function, and increasing cell permeability to foreign substances, may only make matters worse. People on a very pure (i.e. allergen-free) diet, can in this way get more sensitive and more allergic than ever.

The nutritional approach needs dietary advice (as well as avoidance of the trigger foods) which will built up the patient's health. It will probably also need vitamin and mineral supplements, and other therapies (SEE end of this section) may also be useful.

American nutritionist Adelle Davis recommends a health-building diet for perhaps a month, together with the avoidance of the offending food. Then the allergen can be tried in small amounts, and gradually increased when the body is able to cope with it.

Several nutritionally aware doctors in this country believe that the avoidance of incompatible foods – basically, the avoidance of starch and protein mixtures at the same meal – can prevent an allergy. (For a full description of this approach please SEE *Compatible Eating* pages 151–5.) Dr Daniel Munro tested his allergic patients for the toxic proteins which can be produced when incompatible foods are eaten and describes this in his book *Man Alive You're Half Dead*. He found that a meal of mixed, incompatible foods produced more histamine. Through this work he was able to advise his allergic patients to eat a compatible diet, and many of them lost their allergic symptoms. Complete, easy digestion of food is of prime importance in treating all allergies, and food allergies cannot occur when foods are completely digested. (Yogurt has been found to inhibit the production of histamine, if taken regularly.)

The body's first line of defence against the stress of allergic reactions is the adrenal glands. The nutrients involved in producing hormones from the adrenals to supply this protection are protein, vitamin C, pantothenic acid and vitamin B6.

Vitamin C is notably vital for these hormones and is therefore equally vital in the diet of an allergic person.

The second line of defence is strong, less permeable capillary walls. By strengthening the collagen, or intercellular cement, vitamin C helps to achieve this. Vitamins E and A also normalize cell permeability. Vitamin A and E have been given together for four months before the pollen season starts to prevent hay fever, with success. C also has a natural antihistamine effect, as do the B vitamins pantothenic acid and B6.

Vitamin C has been used on its own both to prevent and treat allergic reactions. The dose recommended for allergic people is half a gram a day, increasing if necessary by no more than one gram a week until the dose reaches five grams a day. If you have any adverse reactions such as loose bowels, reduce the dose. You should in any case take high doses of any supplements only under the guidance of a naturopath or nutritionally informed doctor.

The B vitamin pantothenic acid is widely dubbed the anti-stress vitamin. Tests on volunteers have shown that allergic symptoms and those produced by pantothenic acid deficiencies are strikingly similar. Often the simple addition of this vitamin brings relief to allergy sufferers. Because of their rapid growth, infants and children need a lot of pantothenic acid; this may partly explain why children are so often allergic, and why they so often grow out of it eventually when their need for this vitamin goes down. A reason why babies so often develop allergies is that they cannot tolerate cow's milk.

A study of 32 children with bronchial asthma and allergic eczema showed that, when the children were given an excellent diet, together with supplements of vitamins C, E, A and the B range, most recovered in a single month. All recovered within two months.[2] This is crucial evidence that a superior diet and supplements, rather than simply the avoidance of trigger foods, can result in the cure of allergic conditions.

This view is further confirmed by biochemist Roger J. Williams, who states that allergies cause stress and that the body needs a good supply of the dietary essentials to cope with that stress. He recommends the possible use of supplements for allergic conditions.[3]

Minerals come into the picture too. In a letter from Dr Dorothy West to me she states 'it has been found that people with allergies usually have a grossly distorted mineral pattern, being short of some, loaded with others and especially tending to have accumulations of toxic metals. A good diet goes a long way towards correcting this.'

Low blood sugar, or hypoglycaemia, encourages the body to react in an allergic way, and the person with low blood sugar is more likely to suffer an allergic reaction when his blood sugar is at its lowest. By discouraging sudden swings in blood sugar levels, the unrefined carbohydrates in a wholefood diet (wholegrains, wholemeal bread, fruits and vegetables) help to make an allergic reaction less likely. (Please SEE the *Whole Foods* and *low Blood Sugar* sections, pages 101 and 340.)

If you are allergic, you are strongly advised to put yourself in the hands of a qualified naturopath (SEE appendix page 405) or a nutritionally aware doctor (SEE *Information* section below).

Additional therapies and information
Acupuncture: SEE appendix (page 405).
Herbalism: SEE appendix (page 405).
Homoeopathy: SEE appendix (page 405).

For a list of doctors interested in treating allergies, write to: Action Against Allergy, 43 The Downs, London SW20 8HG (telephone 01 947 5082).

The organization Sanity supports enquiry into the nutritional and biochemical factors in mental illness and this includes work on allergy. Write to Sanity, Chairman Mrs M. Hall, 77 Moss Lane, Pinner, Middlesex HA5 3AZ.

Recommended reading
Not All in the Mind by Richard Mackarness, (Pan 1976).
Food Allergy: a Practical Easy Guide by Rita Greer and Robert Woodward, (Roberts Publications for Bunterbird Limited, 225 Putney Bridge Road, London SW15 2PY, 1981)
The First Clinical Ecology Cookbook by Rita Greer. Cooking without some common allergens. You can obtain a copy from Ms Greer, 44 Wallisdean Avenue, Portsmouth, Hampshire. Price £3 including postage.

Books mentioned in this section
Eating and Allergy by Robert Eagle (Futura 1979).
Man Alive You're Half Dead by Daniel Munro (Bartholomew House, USA, 1956).

Arthritis and Rheumatism

In 1936 Dr D.C. Hare of London's Royal Free Hospital took an unprecedented step. She put a group of patients severely crippled with arthritis on a diet recommended to her by the Swiss Bircher-Benner Clinic. This consisted of milk, raw fruit and raw vegetables together with Bircher-Benner muesli (see index) and cream. No drugs were used.

After a few weeks she noted remarkable improvement and relief of pain in her patients and the final result was seven complete recoveries of mobility and three partial recoveries. All twelve patients were considerably better by the end of the treatment. This trial was later repeated with similar excellent results and the patients filmed so that their new mobility could be recorded.

All the patients concerned in this work had been classified as incurable. [1]

Extract from a letter to me from the Arthritis and Rheumatism Council dated 9 June 1980:
'Although a number of writers have recommended various diets for the treatment of arthritis and rheumatism, in general the medical profession *does not feel that diet plays a great part in the treatment of these diseases* (my italics) . . . our research is mainly concerned with finding the cause and, once this problem has been solved, the question of the best form of treatment will surely be shown.'

'The cause is staring them in the face' (Dr I.P. Drysdale, Vice-Dean of the British College of Naturopathy and Osteopathy, talking to me).

The Arthritis and Rheumatism Council states that rheumatism is Britain's most widespread disease and that only 1 person in 50 will escape some form of rheumatic disease by the time they reach the age of 70. About 37 million working days are lost annually through rheumatism and arthritis – and this figure is conservative.

Arthritis
Arthritis is the inflammation of a joint, giving pain and

restricting movement. The two main categories of this disease are osteoarthritis, with possible bone erosion at weight-bearing points, and rheumatoid arthritis. Other types are spondylitis (and its later condition, spondylosis); cervical spondylitis and ankylosing spondylitis where the spinal joints eventually lock; sacroilitis and gout. Traumatic arthritis follows an injury or severe strain.

In all arthritic conditions it is almost certain that rheumatic changes are also present, particularly with joint injuries. Long-standing rheumatic conditions are likewise usually found with arthritic disease in the underlying joints.

Do you really have arthritis?

A recent statement by the General Council and Register of Osteopaths blames doctors for using the general term 'arthritis' when spinal X-rays merely reveal an ageing process; in one study 85% of people over 50 were told that they had spinal arthritis – an unlikely percentage. 'Every day', says the Council, 'hundreds of people who have been told "you must learn to live with it" are obtaining relief at the hands of registered osteopaths' and they deplore the thought of people suffering unnecessarily simply because of a wrong diagnosis. Readers who also like to know that back pain often responds to one gram of vitamin C a day, or to calcium and vitamin D supplementation (ask a naturopath or a nutritionally aware doctor about dosage).

Rheumatism

All rheumatic conditions are inflammatory and they eventually produce degenerative changes in the affected places. The inflammation affects the soft tissues; muscles, ligaments, tendons, sheaths, etc.

Types of rheumatism are fibrositis (previously muscular rheumatism) of which panniculitis is a form; neuritis, affecting nerves and their sheaths (neuritis of the sciatic nerve is called sciatica), synovitis (or captulitis) which is characterized by the increased secretion of synovial fluid as well as inflammation; tenosynovitis, bursitis. Lumbago is a vague term covering pain in the lumbar region and usually indicates an early rheumatic condition, and frozen shoulder and tennis elbow are basically rheumatic disorders as well.

In acute rheumatism, or rheumatic fever, the heart is likely to be affected; the very acute form of this disease is now uncommon and subacute rheumatism, with the same risks, is more usual.

Drug treatments

Drugs for these conditions are among the most dangerous. Virtually every drug used in the treatment of rheumatoid arthritis is potentially toxic.[2]

Cortisone, for instance, is naturally present in the body but when given artificially it can produce oedema, excessive hair growth, high blood pressure, ulcers, pancreatitis, diabetes-like symptoms, demineralized bones and severe infections – even mental disturbances and bone fractures. It also causes the tissues to retain salt and water, thus creating a deficiency of the salt-balancing mineral, potassium. ACTH (corticotrophin) can damage the adrenal glands. In some circumstances cortico-steroid drugs can be fatal.

Butazolidin (or phenylbutazone) can cause oedema, nausea and rash. Indocid (indomethacin) can cause dizziness, headache and gastro-intestinal upsets. Even aspirin destroys vitamin C, and this loss will of course be more significant when the drug is taken a lot. Pain-killing drugs encourage the over-use of damaged joints and muscles – until the effects wear off - and this can cause further harm.

As for gold injections, it is difficult to understand why this treatment has persisted; it has resulted in the death of many patients.[3] So has Opren.

Joint replacement, although a miracle to the grateful patient, does not eradicate the disease, but removes the main site of it. More pain and crippling may result. A hip replacement operation can cost about £400.

Causes

Impairment of kidney function is a major cause of the modern degenerative diseases, and this is often associated with arthritis and rheumatism. Seldom, if ever, is there a single cause.

Deficient nutrition will affect the whole body, including the joints and soft tissues. The defective use of calcium by the body will mean that too much is deposited, distorting and thickening the joints, or too little, depleting the bones of this essential mineral. The synovial fluid which lubricates the joints is a viscous solution of various minerals with about 1% of protein. These constituents must be provided in our food. If one of the required minerals is deficient, or if the cells are poisoned with toxins, poor lubrication will be the result.

Gout is on the increase and it was found by Professor John Yudkin that people with gout take more sugar than others. Further, gout is characterized by needles made of uric acid crystals combined with sodium. Kidneys injured by drugs may not be able to dispose of the uric acid in the form of urea, so that it collects and makes the gout worse. In order to excrete uric acid the body needs the B vitamin, pantothenic acid. Sufferers from gout may therefore be short of pantothenic acid and this theory is strengthened by the fact that gout usually follows some kind of stress and that during stress pantothenic acid is used up rapidly by the body. Some cases of rheumatoid arthritis may be linked to low blood sugar (SEE *Low Blood Sugar* pages 340–5).

No germ for arthritis or rheumatism has ever been identified. There are in fact thousands of germs with us, both on the skin surface and inside the body, which are self-regulating; many of them are beneficial. The streptococcus bacterium, once thought to be the cause of rheumatism, is a normal part of intestinal flora. It appears elsewhere in the body during rheumatic fever, but it also does this in a number of other septic and feverish conditions and it is not alleged to be the cause of those. There are many viruses present in the body too, but none of these has ever been identified as the specific cause of rheumatism or arthritis.

Concerning climate – there is almost as much arthritis in Jamaica as there is here. So for arthritis, at least, we cannot blame the weather.

Naturopathic treatment is based on the fact that we can make ourselves ill by living in the wrong way and principally by eating unbalanced denatured food. The form the illness takes depends on the strengths and weaknesses of the individual body and its ability to fight back, and when we treat our bodies with less care than we would give to a car or a row of lettuces in the back garden we must expect a protest sooner or later. We can damage ourselves in two ways – by poisoning our cells with the wrong food and other pollutants, and by depriving those cells of the nutrients they need.

Nutritional treatments

Rheumatic and arthritic diseases invariably involve the whole body, with changes in the vital tissues, including the blood. They do not begin in a healthy body; in all cases, even in those of injury, disturbances of health will have started beforehand. These disorders are characterized by inflammation, which doctors will try to suppress. This is treating the symptom and not the cause. Additionally, any treatment which does not rest upon the principle of treating the whole body instead of isolated bits of it will fail. Care must be given both to detoxifying the poisoned tissues and to providing the cells with the best possible nourishment so that they can fight the disease effectively themselves.

It has been frequently said that it is impossible to regain movement in joints which are completely fused (ankylosed), or complete healing where the tissues involved are damaged beyond repair. In her book *Let's Get Well* nutritionist Adelle Davis describes some nutritional cures and writes, 'Persons frequently believe that when arthritic spurs have formed or joints are cemented together, as are the vertebrae in spondylitis, nothing can be done. Because I have worked with many who had results similar to the ones cited, I wholeheartedly disagree.'

Drugless treatments
Several doctors have used individual vitamins in large doses to treat arthritis, with some success. Dr William Kaufman used the B vitamin, niacin, to treat his arthritis patients. He found that it improved the movement in their joints, but results varied widely. He also used B6 and riboflavin and these proved effective for relieving pain and locking of joints, numbness, cramps and night paralysis. Biochemist E.C. Barton-Wright and Dr W.A. Eliott made extensive studies of the role of pantothenic acid in treating arthritis, with some good results. They found that sufferers had less of the vitamin in their blood than healthy people. More recent work confirms that pantothenic acid reduces arthritic symptoms significantly, but further improvement is not obtained by stepping up the dose, and progress does not continue. The biochemist who discovered pantothenic acid, Dr Roger J. Williams, observes that this vitamin is no doubt only one of the nutrients required and that the whole nutritional chain of life is needed by deficient cells.[4]

Adelle Davis believes that arthritis is a disease of adrenal exhaustion – in other words, due to one kind of stress of another. She also states that the need for pantothenic acid is paramount, and uses a lot of other supplements too; vitamin A, the B vitamins, C, D, E and brewer's yeast.[5] Her diet and supplements are designed to stimulate natural adrenal production. She has known several patients whose arthritis was linked to their feelings of hostility and rage, and world authority on stress, Dr Hans Selye, confirms that stress can induce arthritis in laboratory animals.

American doctor John M. Ellis has successfully treated arthritis with vitamin B6. Large doses of vitamin C – 4g a day – have been shown to reduce arthritic pain. Patients who take large doses of aspirin should also take vitamin C, to lessen some of the side-effects of the drug. Vitamin C is drained from the body by prolonged stress.

It is believed that some forms of arthritis are associated with a food allergy. The Dong diet, devised by Dr Colin Dong, is based on this idea. The main ingredients of the Dong diet are fish, vegetables and rice. Cereals, dairy produce and red meat are avoided, as are all foods containing artificial additives. This treatment is fully described in *New Hope for the Arthritic* (SEE *Recommended Reading* at the end of this section).

Many patients suffering from rheumatic and arthritic diseases have improved considerably after cutting out all foods to which they are allergic. Nearly all the people who respond to this form of treatment have previously suffered from some other common allergic complaint (SEE *Allergies and Food* pages 219–29).

English doctor Hugh Trowell agrees that arthritis is an auto-immunity disease (an allergy), but adds that it is also a disease associated with eating too many refined carbohydrates.

It is in *nutrition* that we must look for the cure of arthritis and rheumatism. A programme of whole nutrition is more likely to work than a fragmented approach using supplements, although these methods may work well together.

A plan of nutritional therapy based on whole, natural foods is essential, firstly for relief and ultimately for cure. Improvement depends partly on the degree of damage already inflicted on the body. For much of the dietary information here, I am indebted to the excellent *Why Endure Rheumatism and Arthritis?* by Clifford Quick.

First stage – fruit fast For two days, eat nothing but fresh, ripe raw grapes and melon, about four or five ounces of each at the usual meal times. Wash the grapes well but do not skin them. No drinks should be taken; there is enough fluid in the fruits.

You may find that you pass a lot of urine during this fruit fast. These foods have a natural diuretic action and this is entirely beneficial.

Second stage Continue the following diet for the next seven days:

On rising Small glass of half-and-half carrot juice and fruit juice (selected from apple, grape, or pineapple). Avoid citrus fruit juices (oranges, grapefruit, satsuma, lemon), and rhubarb and plum juices. You can make carrot juice yourself by grating some carrot into three or four thicknesses of muslin, twisting the muslin round, and squeezing out the juice.

Breakfast Choose two kinds of fruit only from apples, pears, grapes, melon, peach, pineapple.

Mid-morning A yeast and vegetable extract drink such as Barmene or Tastex (from your health food store) hot or cold as you wish.

Lunch A raw salad, from three only of the following cut, grated or shredded ingredients; Dutch white cabbage, lettuce, Chinese lettuce, watercress, raw red cabbage, celery, raw carrot, grated raw beetroot, grated raw swede or parsnip, onion or leek, ripe tomato, cucumber (with skin on), parsley, endive, chicory, sliced green or red peppers. A salad dressing can if desired be made from unrefined oil and lemon juice or cider vinegar; or some natural yogurt with chopped chives, mint or parsley, with a little honey added if liked. With the salad, take a portion of cottage cheese.

To follow Fruit, as for breakfast.

Tea As mid-morning break, or some weak china tea, without sugar.

Supper Fruit, as for breakfast. Follow with about half a pint of natural yogurt, with a small dessertspoonful of molasses added.

This first part of the nutritional plan will provide an alkaline residue in the body which helps to reduce the relative acidosis common in rheumatic sufferers, while also providing vital minerals and vitamins. If this first part of the treatment is followed strictly it should soon be possible to begin to cut down the dosage of any drug being taken.

Third stage Follow the Food Therapy plan outlined on

pages 396–401, with the following modification:

On rising Continue your half-and-half fruit and vegetable juice as before. You may now vary your vegetable juices; there will probably be a range in your health food store. Keep to vegetarian proteins, and avoid all citrus fruits, rhubarb, plums and their juices.

At your meals containing protein, avoid concentrated starches (bread and potatoes) and vice versa. This 'compatible' way of eating is sometimes beneficial for arthritis (please see the section on *Compatible Eating*). It is very simple to give this added boost to your dietary treatment.

Before you undertake your Food Therapy, it will be necessary for you to know how and why it works. Please, therefore, read the *Nature Cure* section first (pages 391–6).

Please note that the dietary treatment is on general lines only, and that you may also need additional vitamins and minerals. For individual guidance on both your Food Therapy plan and any supplementation, please consult a naturopath (SEE appendix) or a nutritionally aware doctor.

Additional therapies

Acupuncture: SEE appendix (page 405).

Devil's claw: Professor Zorn of the Physiological and Chemical Institute of the University of Jena has found from his trials of this root that it is helpful in the treatment of arthritis. It is available from health food stores.

Evening primrose oil: Writing in *The Lancet* (2:508,1977) J.N. McCormick et al state that this oil was effective for a substantial number of patients with rheumatoid arthritis (SEE *Evening Primrose Oil* pages 111–14).

Herbalism: SEE appendix (page 405).

Homoeopathy: Homoeopathic treatment of 23 patients with rheumatoid arthritis was described by Dr R.G. Gibson et al in the *Brit. J. Clin. Pharmac.* (9, 453-459 1980). Significant improvements, without side-effects, were reported. (SEE appendix page 405).

New Zealand green lipped mussel extract: Clinical trials carried out by Dr R.G. Gibson et al and reported in *The Practitioner* for September 1980 resulted in improvement for 76% of the rheumatoid and 45% of the osteoarthritic patients. This extract, obtainable from health food stores, should not be taken by people who are allergic to fish or shellfish.

Osteopathy: SEE appendix page 405.
Water treatment: please consult a naturopath.

Recommended reading
Why Endure Rheumatism and Arthritis? by Clifford Quick (Allen and Unwin 1980).

Readers with easy access to a swimming pool will find *Pain-Free Arthritis* by Dvera Berson (New English Library 1980) of interest. It contains exercises to be practised in water.
New Hope for the Arthritic published by Diefmart, Unit 112, Shepherd's Bush Centre, London W12.

Books mentioned in this section
Let's Get Well by Adelle Davis (Unwin 1975).

Asthma and Hay Fever

Definitions
Asthma and hay fever are respiratory diseases. There are about 2 million asthmatics in the UK,[1] and about 3 million sufferers from hay fever.[2]

Asthma is heavy, difficult breathing. While the asthmatic can, with effort, breathe in during an attack, it is extremely hard for him to breathe out. This causes a lack of oxygen and too much carbon dioxide, producing a frightening sense of suffocation. One reason for the asthmatic's difficult breathing is the spasmodic contraction of the small bronchii, or breathing tubes, leading to and from the lungs. The mucous membrane lining and bronchii get congested and swollen like the lining of the nose when you have a heavy cold and this also makes the air passages narrower. The asthmatic cough is an attempt to expel the mucus collected in the air passages. Breathing in partly counters this narrowing effect, because expanding the chest creates a partial vacuum which tends to widen the tubes, but breathing out raises the pressure around them, increasing the constriction.

Asthma is often associated with bronchitis, nervous disorders, and hay fever. Cardiac asthma is an attack of difficult breathing with a rapid heartbeat, and renal asthma is difficult breathing in kidney disease. Neither of these two is a true asthmatic condition.

Although there may be depression and irritability first, an asthmatic attack is usually sudden. The patient often wakes up in the early hours of the morning feeling anxious and afraid. His chest feels tight and heavy and he is unable to expand it properly. He may sneeze or cough, and his distress gets worse as he tries to breathe. Pulse is rapid and weak, hands and feet are cold, his face is wet with sweat and either pale or livid. The attack may last for minutes or several hours and its easing is often marked by the coughing up of mucus.

Frequent asthmatic attacks are liable to produce emphysema (SEE *Bronchitis and Emphysema* pages 247–56). This is over-distension of the air spaces in the lungs, with tissue destruction and the formation of large sacs.

Hay fever is an inflammation of the mucous membranes lining the eyes, nose and air passages. It usually arises during the months of May to July when haymaking is in progress, and strictly speaking it is a seasonal complaint due to grass pollens, but the term can be stretched to include any allergic reaction happening in the nose. Anything in the air, in fact, to which a person is allergic can set off an attack at any time. Catarrh of the nose (rhinitis) makes some people more prone to attacks of hay fever.

In hay fever you get the symptoms of a very bad running cold, with a streaming, itchy nose and eyes, and perhaps a dry cough with violent sneezing. An asthmatic attack can also arise. The immediate cause of all this is histamine produced by the body.

Drugs

There are many drugs for the treatment of asthma. Broncho-dilators open up the airways and make breathing easier. There are two groups of bronchodilators; the sympathomimetic drugs which mimic chemicals produced by the body, and the theophylline derivatives. The sympathomimetics include salbutamol (Ventolin), ephedrine (in various preparations) and isoprenaline (Medihaler Iso, Saventrine, isoprenaline hydro-chloride, isoprenaline sulphate, isoproterenol hydrochloride). In spite of the evidence linking the increase in recent deaths with the inappropriate use of isoprenaline, *it is still being prescribed.*

Salbutamol is safer than isoprenaline. Its main effects are on the bronchial tubes and not on the heart. It may, however, cause dizziness, nervousness, trembling and weakness. Some patients cannot tolerate ephedrine; if it is given in large doses it can cause nausea and vomiting, giddiness, trembling and muscular weakness, insomnia, headache, sweating, thirst, palpitations and anxiety. It should be given with caution to patients with heart disease.

The second group of bronchodilators, the theophylline derivatives, includes Choledyl (choline theophyllinate) and Nuelin (theophylline). They may cause stomach irritation, nausea and vomiting.

Sodium cromoglycate (Intal) is used to prevent attacks of allergic asthma and in the form of Lomusol and Rynacrom for an allergic runny nose, or rhinitis. It can cause irritation of the throat and bronchial tubes, particularly if the sufferer already has an infection, and its sudden withdrawal may trigger off an asthmatic attack.

The corticosteroid drugs are used in the treatment of a number of chest diseases, especially asthma. The term corticosteroid is broad, embracing the wide variety of these drugs.

Short courses of prednisolone, a corticosteroid, are given for bronchial asthma. This drug appears under prednisolone pivalate (Ultracortenol) and prednisolone sodium phosphate (Codelsol, Prednosol and Predsol). A maintenance daily dose of above 7.5mg of prednisolone or its equivalent may produce serious adverse side-effects.

The side-effects of the corticosteroid, or steroid, group of drugs vary widely. But according to Peter Parish, author of *Medicines: a Guide for Everybody*, every patient using them should carry a warning card; if these drugs are used for longer than a few weeks the body will fail to react to stress in the normal way, with the result that the patient may collapse and even die. Their use should be tapered off very gradually over several weeks. Corticosteroids in general have profound effects on the body. They affect its salt and water balance, inducing salt and water retention and potassium loss, and they put up the blood pressure. They affect the protein metabolism, producing weakened bones which can fracture and retarded bone growth in children; they affect the fat metabolism.

resulting in fat being laid down on the face ('moon-face'), shoulders ('buffalo-hump') and stomach. They increase the risk of kidney stone, cause skin wasting with a stripey appearance and the delayed healing of wounds, and reduce resistance to infection. They can cause mood changes and disorders of the nervous system and, as we have seen, if they are suddenly stopped the patient may collapse.

An attack of hay fever triggers off the production of histamine by the body, and it is this substance which causes the symptoms. Anti-histamine drugs for hay fever act, not by preventing the release of histamine, but by occupying its sites of action. The main side-effect of these drugs is that they make you drowsy; other side-effects include dizziness, noises in the ears, lack of co-ordination, blurred and double vision, mood changes and nervousness, delusions, insomnia, appetite loss, nausea and vomiting, diarrhoea or constipation, a dry mouth, coughing, frequency of problems in passing urine, palpitations and tightness in the chest, tremors, tingling, heaviness and weakness of the hands. You can even become allergic to these drugs and, very rarely, they can cause serious blood disorders. An overdoese, which can cause excitement and convulsions, is serious and difficult to treat. They can produce alarming reactions in some children – over-stimulation, fever and convulsions. Because they irritate the stomach, they should always be taken with a little food. Peter Parish advises his readers who are just starting a course to 'try taking the first dose on a Friday and then you have the weekend to overcome or become accustomed to the adverse effects'.

Sodium cromoglycate (Intal), already described among the drugs for asthma, is also used to treat hay fever.

It may be seen from this brief description that the drugs used to treat hay fever and especially asthma are very dangerous. They are useful in relieving the symptoms, but may leave the unhappy patient with another set of symptoms to cope with. They burden the system with their toxicity and do nothing to tackle the *root cause* of either illness. They can indeed do a lot of damage – perhaps permanent damage – to the body.

Causes

Allergy plays a big part in asthma and hay fever. A person in lowered health is more prone to allergies. If an allergen can be identified in either asthma or hay fever, it is sometimes possible to desensitize the patient. The allergen is injected in gradually increasing doses until the patient is immune to its effects. If you are found to be sensitive to grass pollen, for instance, and this is giving you hay fever, you can have a series of injections of the offending substances, usually in increasing strengths over a period of time, to desensitize you. The courses are usually given in winter and may have to be repeated for several years. This method is laborious and unpredictable, because there are so many species of grass and other plants which could carry the allergen pollen.

Although desensitization is said to work quite well for a number of people this approach, like drug treatments, ignores the lowered state of health of the patient, in particular the poorly functioning immune system and lack of resistance to disease which accompany asthma and hay fever. In a letter to me, naturopath Terry Moule writes, 'As far as desensitization injections are concerned I personally do not believe in them since it is not really a natural means to tackle the problem, and certainly from my own experience in many cases they are not really effective.' It is quite possible for the person to escape as far as possible from the substances, including food, to which he is allergic, and still suffer allergic reactions.

There are several factors which predispose to asthma and hay fever. One is bad breathing. The inefficient exchange of oxygen and carbon dioxide through shallow breathing deprives the body of oxygen and allows the blood level of carbon dioxide to rise. An oxygen deficiency permits waste products to accumulate which interfere with the health of the bloodstream and can contribute to an allergic attack; it also has a direct effect upon the nervous system – an important consideration in these illnesses. Poor posture stops the lungs from working properly and encourages muscular tensions, particularly in the head, neck, shoulders, ribs and spine. Smoking is an irritant and will make any respiratory condition worse.

Constipation is an important factor too. And, as well as the bowels and kidneys, the skin is an organ of elimination – toxins are effectively discharged through a healthy skin. If elimination in general is inadequate the body will make catarrh in an attempt to throw off the toxins and this heavy mucous, not only in the chest but in the stomach and the whole alimentary tract, is often a forerunner of asthma and hay fever.

There can also be a connection between asthma and low blood sugar (SEE *Low Blood Sugar* pages 340–5).

The vagus nerve is a main link between the heart, lungs, stomach and brain, linking up the nervous pathways. Over-eating and over-drinking can therefore have a direct influence on both asthma and hay fever. Industrial fumes and irritants from aerosol sprays can make matters worse and trigger an attack and several drugs, including aspirin, some laxatives, bromides and sulphonamide, can cause asthma.

Nervous exhaustion and psychological factors – anxiety, fear and other negative emotions – are of major importance in these two psychosomatic illnesses. An asthmatic attack is very frightening and a person's dread of it happening again may make the whole thing worse. Hay fever can be part of an unconscious desire to cry, and breathing problems can have their roots in chronic emotional tension reflected in a tight, unmoving diaphragm.

The wholeness or otherwise of what we eat – the nutrients left out and the chemicals put in – is an integral part of health. This is as true of asthma and hay fever as it is of any other chronic degenerative condition. In his book *Nature Cure for Asthma and Hay Fever*, naturopath Alan Moyle states that the diet factor is chiefly responsible for the incidence of asthma and hay fever.

The nutritional approach

The sufferer from asthma or hay fever will be routinely advised to avoid any foods which trigger off an attack. In naturopathic treatment, however, this is not the whole story; nutritional therapy is designed both to help him throw off accumulated poisons and strengthen his immune system so that he is no longer allergic.

We have seen that both asthma and hay fever involve catarrh. This heavy mucous is formed more readily when starchy, refined foods are eaten; it can even arise when too many whole, unrefined starches are taken in the diet. Milk and the harder cheeses are catarrh-forming, and so are junk foods which load the body with wastes which it will try to get rid of by forming mucous and discharging it.

Please turn to the *Food Therapy* section (pages 396–401) and follow the dietary plan given there. Cut out cow's milk, using soya milk as a substitute, and cut down on starches. You could

take just a little whole cereal for your breakfast, topping up
with plenty of fresh fruit, or you could have the fruit breakfast
on its own. Please note that rhubarb should not be eaten by
the asthmatic; you may find that the acid citrus fruits disagree
with you as well.

You will gather from reading the *Food Therapy* section that
alkali foods – fruits and vegetables – are better for you than
acid foods. This is particularly true of the asthmatic and hay
fever sufferer. The Food Therapy diet is designed to cut down
on acid foods. Meat is acid-forming and pork should be
avoided by the asthmatic. Lamb's liver is good and, if you
really feel you need some other meat occasionally, chicken is
better for you than bacon or beef. Better still, have some fish.

It may also help to add some carrageen moss to your fruit
drinks; this moss is very useful in the treatment of respiratory
conditions and can be bought at a health food store. Yogurt is
thought to inhibit the production of histamine, which produces
the symptoms of allergy, so eat about one-third of a pint of
natural yogurt every day.

Since asthma and hay fever are often due to allergies, it may
also be helpful for you to avoid combining high-protein and
high-starch foods at the same meal. This is further explained in
Compatible Eating (pages 151–5), and has proved valuable for
many sufferers from allergy.

Fasting is especially useful for these two conditions, because
it gives the body a chance to discharge its toxins through the
catarrh, which will eventually dry up. You should try to fast
on fruit juices one day a week (please read the *Fasting* section).
If this is really impossible for you, then you could arrange one
day a week to eat nothing but fruit. This is still a cleansing
process, although not so radical. If you have been taking drugs
for your illness the fasting will give your body a chance to get
rid of these toxins too, which have a deleterious effect on your
general health.

Several isolated nutrients have been found valuable in the
treatment of asthma and hay fever. The most important is
vitamin C, which has an antihistamine action. When 300mg of
C were given every 15 minutes to a group of asthmatics during
attacks, some got relief almost immediately and the rest within
an hour. Further attacks were prevented when 1½g of the
vitamin were taken every day.[3] Similarly, hay fever sufferers
showed a marked improvement when given between 200 and

500mg a day. In *Let's Get Well* Adelle Davis writes, 'on several occasions I have seen persons with severe hay fever whose stream of tears ceased flowing within minutes after 2–3g of vitamin C were given them.' So, for that matter, have I. A hay fever sufferer who knows he has to go into the country or to any other place which will trigger off an attack should take 2–3g of vitamin C before setting out. When given together with vitamin E daily for four months before the hay-fever season, C has kept many people free of symptoms during high summer. Working on mild bronchial asthma, Dr A. Houhuys found that a single dose of 500mg of vitamin C can prevent asthmatic breathing. The benefits last for up to six hours, and relatively small maintenance doses of 250mg throughout the day will give protection against an asthmatic attack.[4] Another study showed that vitamin C supplementation helps people in dust-laden environments to breathe better than any drugs.[5] The bioflavonoids (vitamin P) may help the vitamin C to work effectively.

A Californian doctor, Granville F. Knight, treats his hay fever patients with a wholefood diet, excluding all refined starches and sugars, and a supplement of B-complex. The B vitamin pantothenic acid can moderate allergic reactions by reducing histamine production.[6] It is also useful for the nasal stuffiness accompanying hay fever and one 100mg tablet has been found to relieve this quickly.[7]

Dr Robert Downs of Albuquerque's Southwest Center of the Healing Arts treats asthma with a diet high in protein and iron with supplements of A, C, pantothenic acid and dessicated liver. He also recommends vitamin B15 to stop asthmatic attacks from airborne allergies and to help correct the lack of oxygen and high levels of carbon dioxide commonly found in asthmatics. He states that some of his asthmatic patients have attacks when their blood sugar is low (SEE *Low Blood Sugar* pages 340–5); this can be avoided by replacing refined starches with whole, unrefined carbo-hydrates and eating small meals and snacks, rather than 'bingeing' once or twice a day.[8]

In the *Journal of Vitaminology*, 18, 1972, Dr M. Kanimura described his work on vitamin E and allergies. He injected human volunteers with histamine, and their allergic reactions were reduced by about a third after they had been given 300 I.U. of vitamin E for several days.

Finally, pollen (SEE pages 127–8) is effective against hay fever if taken continuously starting well before the hay fever season. Garlic (SEE pages 114–15) is useful for respiratory disorders. Both are obtainable from your health food store.

Please note that Food Therapy comes first and any supplements which may be useful come a resounding second. Before you undertake your Food Therapy, it will be necessary for you to know how and why it works. Please, therefore, read the *Nature Cure* section first.

This dietary treatment is on general lines only, and you may also need additional vitamins and minerals. For individual guidance on both your Food Therapy plan and any supplementation, please consult a naturopath (SEE appendix page 405) or a nutritionally aware doctor.

Breathing

In both asthma and hay fever there is often rigidity of the chest, upper spine and shoulders. Contraction of the ribs and the intercostal muscles which swing the ribs in and out arises in all asthmatic conditions. Asthmatics are notoriously bad breathers. Good breathing is helpful for hay fever sufferers but *no treatment of asthma is complete without breathing exercises.*

The Knowles method of breath training has helped many hundreds of asthmatics. Please write to Miss M. Knowles, 46 Fleetwood Close, Chalfont St Giles, Buckinghamshire HP8 4DR, for more information. I can recommend this system myself. The Asthma Research Council, 12 Pembridge Square, London W2 4EH, were in the process of revising their booklet on breathing exercises when this book was being completed.

Additional therapies

Acupuncture: SEE appendix, page 405.

Herbalism: SEE appendix, page 405.

Homoeopathy: SEE appendix, page 405.

Relaxation: because of the link between asthma and hay fever and tension, relaxation will help. Your breathing will help you to relax, but you are advised to use a specific technique as well: SEE appendix, page 405.

Water treatment

Hip bath (useful during fast): Stay in a hot bath, sitting with the knees drawn up or the feet on the end of the bath, for 10 to

15 minutes, topping up with hot water when necessary. The water should come up to the navel. Finish by sponging the hips and lower back with cold water.

Cold friction rub (daily): Dip a coarse towel into cold water and lightly wring it out. Starting from the feet and working upwards, scrub every part of the body with the wet towel. The first few times, you may like to stand with your feet in a bowl of warm water during your rub. If your skin does not glow afterwards, leave the rub for a few weeks and then try again, when you will probably have enough vitality to react to it.

Steam inhalation: You can inhale steam over a bowl of hot water, but this will cramp your chest a little. It is better to sit in front of (but not too near!) an ordinary kettle with the jet of steam playing on the nose, throat and chest, for about 10 minutes. Conclude with cold water applications to the same parts. You can add a little pine oil to the water.

Natural unimpeded sunlight and *fresh air* are good for all respiratory conditions.

Recommended reading
Nature Cure for Asthma and Hay Fever by Alan Moyle (Thorsons 1978).

Books mentioned in this section
Medicines: A guide for Everybody by Peter Parish (Penguin 1980).
Let's Get Well by Adelle Davis (Unwin 1975).

Bronchitis and Emphysema

Figures and definitions
Bronchitis is known as the 'English disease'. The death rate from chronic bronchitis in the UK is higher than the rate for all related diseases anywhere else. It accounts for over 20 000 deaths per year and is one of the principal killer diseases in the very young and in older people. It is among the diseases for which people go most often to their GP, ranking third after

the common cold and rheumatic/arthritic conditions.[1] It has been estimated that in middle age, one in four men will be bronchitic.[2] Among men between 45 and 64 it is the second most frequent reason for admission to hospital (heart trouble comes first); in hospital admissions for women it ranks fourth.[3] The percentage of hospital admissions for bronchitis has *doubled* in the period 1969–1979.[2]

Emphysema can follow bronchitis as the lungs deteriorate further, and its incidence, too, is increasing in the West.[4]

Understanding bronchitis and emphysema

It is necessary for the victim of either or both of these diseases, if he is to undertake naturopathic treatment, to understand the way his lungs work.

The lungs occupy most of the chest. When we breathe in, the expansion of the chest lowers the air pressure in the lungs, creating 'negative pressure' and drawing the air through the nose or mouth and into the lungs. When we breathe out, the air is expelled from the lungs by the contracting volume of the chest cavity. Breathing in, if we are breathing well, causes the chest to expand in all directions.

The diaphragm is a dome-shaped muscle dividing the chest from the abdomen and stretched across the body just above the waist. As the chest enlarges to take in air, the intercostal muscles attached to the ribs raise them upwards and outwards and the diaphragm flattens to make more room. Chest expansion is most marked with the lower ribs; these, like the rest, are attached to the spine at the back, but at the front they are not similarly attached to the breastbone and are free, 'floating' ribs. Because of this the greatest movement takes place in the lower and not in the upper chest. When we breathe in properly the muscles of the abdominal walls are also called into play to influence the floating ribs and the diaphragm and, during exertion or when breathing is difficult, certain neck and shoulder muscles may also be used.

The lungs are not just large bags which fill up with air. The system of breathing tubes, or bronchi, leading from the nose and mouth to form the body of the lungs looks rather like an inverted tree (SEE diagram). The trunk is divided into more bronchi and each of these subdivides again into many smaller branches down to the smallest, called the bronchioles, with a diameter of only about 1mm. These finally terminate in tiny

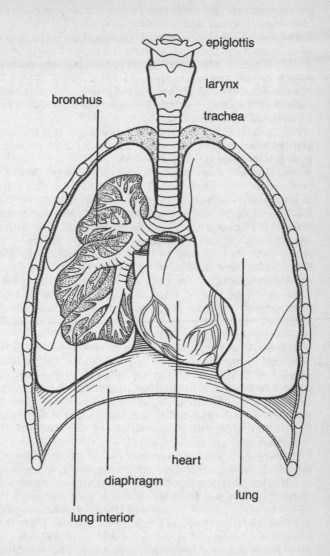

air sacs with very thin walls called alveoli. Our lungs probably contain about 750 million of these alveoli.

The lungs have two circulatory systems. One carries blood to the lungs themselves and the other is a network along which the bloodstream collects oxygen from the lungs and unloads carbon dioxide and other unwanted gases. In the process of breathing the lungs take in oxygen and breathe out these other gases, a vital exchange which, if stopped for more than a few minutes, will result in death.

Bronchitis is an inflammation of the air passages in the lungs and can be acute or chronic. Most acute cases are precipitated by a virus infection and a bacterial infection follows. There is a severe, long cold or a cough, dry with clear phlegm. Mucus is produced in the inflamed breathing tubes and the cough tries to get rid of this mucus by expelling it. Tiny hairs called cilia line the windpipe and bronchi and these carry the mucus towards the throat where it can be expectorated. The patient feels feverish and unwell; he may have a heavy feeling in the chest, with pain or a sense of irritation between the shoulder blades, and there is often a high temperature. The illness usually only lasts a few days. If inflammation continues however it may lead to broncho-pneumonia or even lobar pneumonia. It may leave the person with a catarrhal tendency which will encourage another attack and this can eventually bring about chronic bronchitis.

Chronic, long-term bronchitis is a serious illness and is the type most commonly found in England. There is a persistent cough with sputum which can be yellowish or greenish and thick; breathing is difficult, fast and noisy due to mucus obstructing the breathing tubes and cilia which help to expel this mucus are smoothed over and cannot work. It may lead to bronchiectasis (degeneration of the walls of the bronchial tubes) and emphysema.

Emphysema is most often seen as part of advanced chronic bronchitis, although it may also complicate other long-standing lung diseases. It concerns the tiny air sacs, the alveoli. These tiny cells get distended and lose their elasticity; the network of capillaries supplying them degenerates too, reducing the blood flow and making things worse. When they break down, groups of alveoli leave scar tissue and large air sacs, which are very inefficient substitutes. The ventilating surface of the lungs is therefore very much reduced. The strain of constant coughing and of trying to breathe with mucus-blocked air passages and bacterial damage to lung tissue all contribute to this condition. Eventually, the chest can become fixed at the position of full inspiration and breathing is very difficult. The cartilages joining the ribs to the breast bone can become rigid, causing a 'barrel chest' and the diaphragm is permanently flat. To try and help with breathing, the shoulders heave up and the neck muscles get very tense.

Causes
The Clean Air Act swept away a lot of soot, but left sulphur dioxide still in the atmosphere. This chemical is equally irritating to the lungs. Cold damp air is also an irritant, as are extremes of air temperature – sitting hunched in front of a roaring fire and then going into a freezing bedroom.

Bad posture, lack of exercise and nervous tension result in poor use of the lungs and this is a contributory factor. The onset of fibrositis in the chest walls and arthritis in the chest joints reduces the flexibility of the chest, impairing breathing capacity. Tobacco smoke is dangerous and harmful to the lungs, quite apart from its detrimental effect on the rest of the body. Poisonous industrial fumes can damage the lungs and encourage bronchitis.

Bad eating is another important factor. The person becomes deficient in the nutrients his body needs in order to defend itself against illness, and he overloads his system with refined, manipulated foods which leave a toxic residue. Mucus can be the body's attempt to discharge some of these toxins.

Acute bronchitis often starts with a bacterial infection, coming on top of all these contributory factors. But the body is constantly throwing off the germs it does not want. It is only the unhealthy body which is vulnerable.

Germs exist all over us and inside us. There are teeming colonies of germs on the skin, in the colon and in the respiratory passages. The mucous secretion in the respiratory passages contains a natural antibiotic, lysozyme, assisted by lactic fermentation, which allows beneficial bacteria to grow and dissolves unwanted bacteria or renders it harmless; the germs of various well-known diseases, the pneumonia germ for instance, are normally present in a healthy person's mouth and throat. Viruses are also subject to control by the body's own defences.

The high temperature and fever often associated with bronchitis and many other illnesses are simply the body's attempt to heal itself. 'Give me a fever,' said Hippocrates, the father of medicine, 'and I will cure the patient.' The fever speeds up all the body's biochemical processes. This includes the disposal of toxins and the action of its defence mechanisms, which will produce an antibody designed with exquisite accuracy to knock out or disarm that particular infection.

Nature cure is not concerned therefore with using a drug to suppress the body's efforts to heal itself and to destroy the bacterial infection which is one of the factors causing acute bronchitis. It is concerned with helping the body to destroy the infection in its own way and throw off the toxins which are adding to the illness.

The causes of emphysema are the same.

The orthodox treatment

In an acute attack of bronchitis, an orthodox doctor will try to suppress both the chest inflammation and the cough. The inflammation and accompanying fever serve to eliminate the bacteria which have got out of hand and are causing the illness. The cough is the body's attempt to clear itself of unwanted mucus. By suppressing these actions with drugs he is paving the way for a more chronic form of the disease.

Antibiotics are used for the infection in bronchitis. They kill or inhibit the growth of bacteria, destroying beneficial bacteria as well. The latter, most of which colonize the intestinal tract, are essential for normal digestion and the manufacture of certain vitamins. Their destruction gives the unwanted bacteria a chance to multiply still further and this is why the infection, if not knocked out by the drugs, often recurs soon after the course of antibiotics has been finished. This disturbance of the healthy bacterial ratio can be hard to treat. It is commoner with 'broad spectrum' antibiotics, and occurs more often in children and in elderly and debilitated patients.

Adverse effects from antibiotics are on the increase. They often cause diarrhoea and nausea and, because they must be broken down by the liver, they can cause problems for those with liver weaknesses. The broad spectrum antibiotic tetracycline, for instance, can affect human cells and cause liver, kidney and eye damage. It can deposit itself in teeth and bones, causing permanently discoloured teeth in children and even in some adults. Allergic reactions to antibiotics include skin rashes, swollen face, fever, painful joints, bone-marrow damage and jaundice.

If an antibiotic knocks out the infection, it still does nothing to strengthen the immune system and improve health. The body then has to cope with its lowered state of vitality, plus the harmful effects of the antibiotic itself.

Some cough mixtures suppress the act of coughing so that the body cannot rid itself of mucus. Some – the expectorants – can stimulate an over-secretion of mucus, which will block up the air spaces still more.

None of these drugs does anything about the causes of bronchitis. The mortality figures alone on bronchitis must cast doubts on the effectiveness of orthodox medical treatment.

There are no drugs to treat emphysema.

The nutritional approach

We have seen that bronchitis does not flourish in a strong healthy body, nourished on the right food. If you will turn to the *Food Therapy* section (pages 396–401) you will see that the diet cuts out all refined and junk foods and contains some whole starches and a preponderance of fruits and vegetables.

All starches and sugars are mucus-forming, whether refined or not. So follow the Food Therapy plan, but cut down on the breads, cereals and potatoes. Take, for instance, an all-fruit breakfast if you can. Cow's milk and hard cheeses are very catarrh-forming, so stick to the soft cheeses such as cottage cheese and use soya milk as a substitute for cow's milk.

Fit in a regular fast on fruit juices and water – please read the *Fasting* section (pages 159–163). You could follow the Food Therapy plan for two or three weeks and then fast for two or three days, or you could fast for one day once a week and follow the plan the rest of the time. If it is really impossible for you to fast completely, then take fruit and fruit juices only for the periods suggested for your fast. The important thing is to decide on your dietary programme and stick to it. (During your all-fruit days, avoid the very acid fruits – citrus fruits and plums – and do not eat rhubarb.)

If you have an acute attack, go to bed and fast, taking a little fruit juice diluted with bottled mineral water every three hours. You can also have some hot diluted lemon or apple juice. Expectorate as much as you can. Tepid sponging is good at this time, and hot flannels, either dry or wrung out in hot water, can be applied to the chest (rub in a little vegetable oil first to protect the skin). When the attack is over and your temperature, if it was high, is normal again, break your fast with a little ripe, raw, sub-acid fruit and continue with your Food Therapy plan.

In bronchitis and all other conditions involving catarrh or mucus the body may use the discharge to expel accumulated wastes. You may occasionally find during your treatment, therefore, that you are coughing up more phlegm than before, but there is no need to feel discouraged. This 'healing crisis' is fully explained in the *Nature Cure* section (pages 391–6) and it is important for you to understand it. 'A bout of acute bronchitis, if properly managed, may actually serve towards curing a condition of previously established chronic bronchitis.'[5] You will feel better if you realize that a healing crisis can be the first major step back to vitality and health. You will also find the *Nature Cure* section useful in explaining how and why your dietary treatment works, too.

Little research has been done into the effects of isolated nutrients on bronchitis and emphysema.

In 1952, however, a London doctor, Max Odens, set up long-term trials with 17 of his patients aged 48 to 67 who were chronic bronchitics. In addition to their usual therapy, they took supplements of vitamin A. He reported this work much later in the German publication *Vitalstoffe* for December 1967, stating that even in the severe winter of 1952/53, his patients continued to improve. A lack of vitamin A in babies is related to increased susceptibility to infections, including bronchitis. Russian researchers have used vitamin B15 for emphysema.

Vitamin E has been used to treat bronchitis (Dr Carl Pfeiffer in the magazine *Prevention* for July 1981) and the emphysema associated with cystic fibrosis improves after vitamin E is given.[6] Generous amounts of this vitamin can often relieve breathing difficulties, and the alveoli cannot be strong and healthy without[7] enough of the vitamins A, C and folic acid, together with protein.

Garlic is a traditional remedy for all respiratory illnesses. Garlic pearles, which are odourless until they dissolve in the stomach, are obtainable from your health food store.

If the diet itself is not improved, however, the illness can be expected to get worse.

Breathing exercises and other exercise

No treatment for bronchitis or emphysema is complete without breathing exercises. Deep breathing, if practised regularly, will help the lungs to expel mucus and will improve the breathing capacity. The bronchitic, because of his clogged breathing tubes, is not getting enough air and this makes him breathless. Deep breathing will help him make the best use of his lungs. The sufferer from emphysema is even more restricted and again breathing exercises are essential for the same reason.

The Knowles method of breathing training is helpful for bronchitis and emphysema. Please write to: Miss M. Knowles, 46 Fleetwood Close, Chalfont St Giles, Buckinghamshire HP8 4DR, for more information. I can recommend this method myself.

The Chest, Heart and Stroke Association, of Tavistock House North, Tavistock Square, London WC1H 9JE, have published a booklet called *Breathing exercises for chronic bronchitis and emphysema.* Single copies are free on receipt of a stamped addressed envelope (9in × 6in).

Exercise is also valuable; it helps to lessen both breathlessness and the fear of breathlessness, keeps heart and muscles fit and improves your well-being. If you can take a brisk walk every day you will be helping your lungs to function more efficiently. The Chest, Heart and Stroke Association will also send you a copy of their free leaflet *Exercise can help your breathlessness* on receipt of a stamped addressed envelope (9in × 6in).

In both bronchitis and emphysema, the limit of a naturopathic cure is measured both by the determination of the patient and the extent of lung deterioration that has already taken place. You are strongly advised to put yourself in the hands of a qualified naturopath (SEE appendix page 405) or a nutritionally aware doctor before starting your treatment.

From the orthodox medical standpoint, emphysema is incurable. Emphysema is an illness involving actual structural damage to the lungs and this cannot be reversed. However, with the purifying and revitalizing diet outlined in the *Food Therapy* section (possibly with added supplements), together with breathing exerises and expert naturopathic help, a great deal can be done both to halt the progress of the disease and to make breathing easier and fuller. Nature cure treatment will often help the body to compensate and adapt, making good use of the lung capacity still remaining.

Additional therapies

Acupuncture (bronchitis; can also be helpful in emphysema): SEE appendix page 405.

Exercise (both bronchitis and emphysema): SEE appendix page 405 and consult your practitioner. Natural unimpeded sunlight and fresh air are good for all respiratory conditions.

Herbalism (both bronchitis and emphysema): SEE appendix page 405.

Homoeopathy (both bronchitis and emphysema): SEE appendix page 405.

Osteopathy (bronchitis only): SEE appendix page 405.

Relaxation (both bronchitis and emphysema): SEE appendix page 405.

Recommended reading

Nature Cure for Bronchitis and Emphysema by Clifford Quick (Thorsons 1979).

Cancer

In Britain and many other Western countries, one death in five is from cancer.

The average cancer rates for the years 1951 to 1955 in Britain were 2183 for males and 1848 for females. This is the number of cancer deaths per million people.

By 1978 these rates had risen to 2848 and 2328. This means that in 1978 23.1% of the men who died, and 20.2% of the women, died of cancer. [1]

In 1900, cancer was the eighth most common cause of death. In 1970, it was the second. [2]

Cancer rates are frighteningly high, and we have all had

experience of a relative or friend with the disease. Often – too often – the person does not recover.

Survival is an elastic term; for most types of cancer five years with no sign of the tumour means survival, but for some others 15 years is needed to satisfy the criterion.

What is cancer?

Cancer is a group name. There are over 200 kinds of cancer, each with its own characteristics.

This family of diseases has in common the uncontrolled growth of cells. A healthy cell has its job to do and its place in the body and it keeps to these, passing the good habits on to its offspring. A cancer cell, however, has escaped from the body's controlling mechanisms and this renegade cell will pass on its independent behaviour to succeeding generations. Rather like hooligans in a modern city, cancer cells ignore the rules – but they make sure they get plenty of nourishment from the body whose laws they refuse to obey. Cancers fall into three main groups:

1   *Carcinomas:* the most common kind. Malignant tumours in the coating or lining tissues of the body – cancer of the breast, mouth, stomach, lungs, prostate, gastro-intestinal tract, skin.

2   *Sarcomas:* less common. These cancers occur in connective tissue – muscle, bone, cartilage.

3   *Cancers of blood-forming tissues:* these are leukaemia, tumours in lymphoid tissue, and, the rarest kind, tumours in the bone marrow.

So long as it keeps to its parent organ, the disease is called a stage one cancer. A stage two cancer is one that is still confined to its original organ, but has managed to spread into the nearest lymph glands as well. Stage three is when the cancer has spread to the nearest organ or structure. Stage four is when the clumps of cancer cells get into the bloodstream and spread all over the body. This is called metastasis – another way of saying that secondary tumours establish themselves elsewhere.

Before the disease of cancer establishes itself, there exists in the body a pre-cancerous state. These pre-cancerous cells have not started growing fast or migrating yet, but can be seen to be abnormal under a microscope.

Orthodox treatments

Nobody can doubt the dedication and skill of those trying to find a cure for cancer. What must be questioned is the direction these efforts are taking.

Orthodox treatment attempts to destroy the cancer cells at their main site by X-rays or drugs, or remove the tumour by surgery. Hormone therapy and immunotherapy are more recent developments.

Radiotherapy This is treatment with ionizing radiation from radioactive substances or X-rays. Radiotherapy can be very effective for some skin cancers and bladder cancers. It is often used together with surgery.

Radiation makes use of the theory that many tumour cells divide more quickly than normal ones. By focussing the rays on the tumours, it is hoped to cripple the cancer. Radiation destroys the rapidly dividing cells and damages the ground substance of the part being treated, leaving a scarred and inhospitable environment for any remaining cancer cells. Not all tumours respond; the most malignant respond the best.

Tumours, however, unless they are interfering with a vital part, are seldom the direct cause of death. And a tumour has many normal cells, with connective tissue and blood vessels. Radiation usually does indeed reduce the size of the tumour, but it has been found that malignant cells are not, as was supposed, always the most sensitive. The tumour may shrink, but radiation can destroy healthy cells too and the proportion of malignant cells still thriving may actually increase.[3] During all this, the *actual cancer process* will go on.

Radiation can cause normal cells to become malignant.[4] An article in the *New York Times* of 21 July 1957 spoke of the repeated warnings of atomic officials and scientists that the medical use of radiation is far more dangerous than the radioactive fallout from atomic testings.

The body's immune system is fighting small cancers in us every day and throwing them off. So this system is our first line of defence. But radiation can damage the immune system, leaving the weakened body less able to help itself, and more vulnerable to other illnesses and infections too. If the irradiated area includes active bone marrow, radiotherapy can cause a marked drop in the white cells, with bleeding and again an increased susceptibility to infection.

Radiotherapy has a very depressing effect on the patient. There is lethargy, fatigue, nausea, lack of appetite and a general feeling of ill-health.

In a paper delivered to a National Cancer Conference in 1968, Dr Philip Rubin claimed that no increase in survival rates had been achieved by radiation. The effectiveness of this treatment has improved since then, but it is obviously still a questionable approach.

Surgery This is still the most common initial treatment. If the tumour is still at the stage where cancer cells have not spread and set up colonies elsewhere in the body, doctors often decide to remove it. Even if the tumour has spread, removal of the main growth may allow the body's immune system to mop up the rest. Some tumours cannot be removed, however, because of their position.

But post-surgery survival rates are disappointing. The overall survival rate after cancer surgery of all kinds is about 15 per cent.[5] This is with no metastases at the time of the operation. Patients often develop a further cancer a few months after surgery, grown from cells left in the body. Any cutting of the tumour, even by biopsy, tends to encourage the spread of malignant cells.

According to a Breast Cancer Symposium reported in the Breast Surgery Journal in 1969, 50% of women who have breast cancer surgery survive for five years. This is irrespective of the type of surgery used. Only 16% will survive for ten years or more and it has never been shown that these results are any better than no treatment at all.[5]

Hardin B. Jones, Professor of Medical Physics and Physiology at the University of California, spoke at a meeting of the American Cancer Society in 1969. He stated his researchers had shown that the apparent life expectation for people who had had *no* surgery seemed to be greater than for those who had!

Drugs There has been a boom in chemotherapy for cancer since the end of World War II. Drugs are very effective for fast-growing tumours. Because of them, we can now talk about cures for childhood leukaemia, Burkitt's lymphoma, Hodgkin's disease, and cancer developing from the tissues of the placenta in the womb – choriocarcinoma. This was impossible fifteen years ago. But these conditions form less than 5% of all malignant diseases.

Using the assumption that cancer cells divide faster than normal cells, it is argued that any chemical which would preferentially destroy these dividing cells would harm the cancer rather than the host. Almost every cancer drug acts like this. They are cell poisoners – cytotoxic.

Recent studies, however, show that for most human cancers the cell division rate is in fact *lower* than for a wide variety of normal tissues – the skin, lining of the gastrointestinal tract, parts of the bone marrow. These drugs, therefore, damage normal cells. It is clear now that the difference between a malignant growth and normal tissue is not the rate of cell division. The body cannot control the delinquent, malignant cells.

Cytotoxic drugs have some horrible side-effects. Continuous cytotoxic therapy will certainly reduce tumour growth. But it will also damage the bone marrow, the patient may bleed and get anaemic, and it may damage the immune system so that antibiotics have to be used as well to clear up the resulting infection. Other side-effects of cytotoxics include gastro-intestinal upsets, nausea, vomiting and diarrhoea, loss of hair, skin rashes, allergic reactions, peripheral nerve damage leading to muscular weakness, inflammation of the veins and skin ulcers, weight loss, bladder irritation, liver and kidney damage, loss of balance, visual disturbances, mental confusion, extreme depression, and occasionally death. It is known that these drugs can themselves cause malignancy as well as suppress it, and 'it is clear,' write Cameron and Pauling in their book *Cancer and Vitamin C,* [6] 'that if we go on like this, we shall kill the patient long before we can kill the tumour.'

A cytotoxic dose enough to kill cancer cells is only a shade lower than the fatal dose for normal cells. Because these drugs are so toxic, treatment has to be short or intermittent, to give the patient a chance to recover between each bout. He may die of an infection because these chemicals have damaged his body's ability to defend itself, and the cause of his death will be given as the infection not the cancer – which is strictly incorrect and produces misleading statistics.

This damage to the natural protection afforded by the immune system can be critical. Reduction of tumour size in the short term, or the stopping of cancer spread, is perhaps a questionable benefit when it accompanies such massive damage to the patient's immune system that he can no longer defend himself.

One group of cancer drugs, the anti-metabolites, is also being used after organ transplants, to suppress the immune system and stop the body rejecting the new tissue. The incidence of cancer amongst patients who have had immuno-suppressive drugs after an organ transplant is 2.5 to 4 times higher than the average.[7]

The benefits of chemotherapy do not appear very substantial. During the past 25 years, when cytotoxic drugs have become fashionable, survival rates for the majority of human cancers have shown no improvement.

This conclusion is echoed by Professor Hardin Jones, who stated in 1972 that his studies had proved conclusively that untreated cancer victims actually live up to four times longer than treated patients.[8]

Hormone therapy   The theory behind this is that by removing the source of, or suppressing, a particular hormone, doctors can induce regression of cancer in the target organ.

In 1897 a surgeon in Glasgow, Sir George Beatson, removed the ovaries from three of this patients with advanced breast cancer. In two of the women the disease underwent a significant remission. In Chicago in the 1930s Charles Huggins produced regression in patients suffering from cancer of the prostate gland by giving them female sex hormones and in this way suppressing the male hormone. In breast cancer, figures show that removal of the ovaries can induce remission of cancer in about 30% of patients. The opposite policy of giving oestrogens to breast cancer patients has also proved helpful in about 30% of cases. A longer life can be achieved in both cancer of the breast and prostate.

But any improvement is only temporary. It may last six months or longer, but anything over a year is unusual, and cancer almost invariably returns. Following removal of the ovaries to benefit breast cancer, the patient will almost certainly relapse after any remission. She may again respond to removal of the adrenal glands or destruction of the pituitary gland; these operations are performed because oestrogen, as well as being produced in the ovaries, is secreted by the adrenals and its production is controlled by the pituitary. These are major operations, to say the least.

Many types of tumour do not respond to this treatment. If hormone-producing glands are removed from a patient, he or she will obviously have to depend on hormone preparations to stay alive. Side-effects seem to be few, but naturopath Leon Chaitow warns that the use of hormones is potentially carcinogenic and comments, 'the future will no doubt produce a re-thinking of the indiscriminate use of hormones but that will be too late for many.'[5]

Research continues into this relatively new approach.

Immunotherapy   A search is always being made for a substance which will select and destroy only cancer cells. But we already have this mechanism inside ourselves; the immune system. The whole complex machinery, from the immediate recognition of an invader foreign to the body to the rapid manufacture of biochemical weapons designed for, and deadly to, their target, already exists in the immune system. A healthy immune system deals swiftly and effectively with the 100 000 or so cancer cells which develop in the normal human body every day.

These sophisticated defences weaken in old age and depend a great deal on the nutritional state of the body.

It has been found with some cancer patients that their cancers regressed after they had thrown off another infection and researchers believe that this is because the infection roused the immune system, encouraging it to beat off the cancer as well. Doctors Linus Pauling and Ewan Cameron suggest that an adequate intake of vitamin A, together with a stimulant such as a bacterial vaccine, may be enough to rouse the immune system to greater efforts. Several other methods are currently being tried.

The danger of side-effects in immunotherapy is extremely small, and research into it continues.

Some comments   Cancer is an illness which frightens us all, and death from it usually involves a lot of suffering. Although it is not the biggest killer, it is the most feared of all diseases and a major focus of world-wide research.

The cure rate for cancer, using orthodox treatments, is about one in three. This is not a good achievement, and even this success is usually short-lived, frequently no more than a matter of months. The results of treatments for the most common cancers have stayed the same for the past twenty years.

In cancer, as in all other illnesses treated with drugs, orthodox medicine balances one risk with another, weighing up the dangers of the treatment against the dangers of the disease. This is a frightening philosophy.

'To some it may seem hard to explain why cancer treatment

depends on widespread surgery, deliberate depletion of body energy, an attack on the defensive immune system and then dosage with cancer-producing rays and drugs to restore health . . . restoring health is not the object of treatment. It can't be, because everyone knows that it doesn't' (*Cancer – The Alternative Method of Treatment*, by Dr Isaac Bryant).

Cancer: the non-toxic approach

A discussion of the unorthodox approach to cancer must start with a look at causes. What are the factors – environmental, dietary, and psychological – which trigger off this disease? Why is there so much cancer around, and what can we do about it?

In 1808, a Dr J.L. Alibert took some cancerous material from a female breast tumour and made it into an emulsion which he injected into himself and, most irresponsibly, into three of his students. The only reaction was a severe feverish inflammation, lasting a few days. He repeated this experiment a few days afterwards on himself and a colleague, with the same result.

Doctors regard cancer as an invasive disease which has to be eliminated. But alternative medicine sees the tumour as growing only because a sick body permits it.

About 80% of our cancers are believed to be caused by our environment, which damages our health.[9] Connections have been traced between cancer and the following:

1 An unsatisfactory diet – nutrients left out and additives put in.
2 A shock such as bereavement, happening about two years before the cancer onset; constant stress; negative, suppressed feelings.
3 Bad housing.
4 Cigarette smoking.
5 The wrong job.
6 Genetic factors.

Other factors probably contributing are:

1 Radiation from X-rays and TV sets; atomic radiation from bomb tests.
2 Too much sunlight.
3 Chemicals in the environment, probably 5% of these are potentially carcinogenic; cancer-causing drugs.
4 Fluoridation in our water.[10]

Research has established that there is a 'cancer type' of person. The development of a serious illness such as cancer is a socially acceptable form of suicide. Some researchers think the disease may be started off by a virus, and others believe that any virus can invade a cell, causing it to become cancerous.

Nutrition and cancer Unhappily, the uprise in chemotherapy since World War II has thrown nutritional research into the shade. There are signs, however, that it is at last emerging.

We can discuss the nutritional angle in two different ways. We can look at the isolated, separate nutrients and additives which have been found to influence the development of cancer, and we can look at the nutritional picture as a whole. Let's start with the fragmented approach.

Whatever stops the normal cell from becoming cancerous must depend partly on nutrition. The immune system needs nutrients like any other part of the body, and this of course also applies to the cell.

Cancer often depresses the appetite and the cancer patient does not bother to eat. The proliferating cancer cells help themselves to the body's nutrients which makes matters worse. Some cancer patients actually starve to death.

Cancer therapy such as drugs and radiation may impair the absorption of nutrients. 'A better-fed patient is more likely to withstand the oppressive therapy we give today, but nutritional support is not being used very extensively,' says Dr Gio Gori of the National Cancer Institute.

Vitamin A A recent BUPA Medical Centre study has shown that men with the lowest vitamin A levels are more than twice as likely to develop cancer. 16 000 men were studied. All laboratory animals deficient in vitamin A develop cancer more easily, and both human and mouse epithelial (lining) cancers can be made to regress with vitamin A.[11] Most cancers are in the epithelial tissues; these tissues depend on vitamin A for health. Dr Sporn of the National Cancer Institute states that a shortage of vitamin A definitely means a greater susceptibility to cancer. This vitamin also appears to give some smokers a measure of protection against lung cancer.[12] This nutrient therefore is therapeutic in the treatment of precancerous cells and in prevention too, although probably less so in a fully developed spreading cancer. It is an anti-oxidant, helping to keep the harmful 'free radicals' in check.[13] These substances can damage cells and DNA molecules. Mutated cells are pre-cancerous, and mutation can be caused by damage to the cell membrane or by injury to the DNA molecules.

B vitamins   These have been less researched. In general, they help to increase appetite, prevent depression, detoxify drugs and other pollutants, maintain oxygen metabolism and stimulate immune response.

Normal cells use oxygen, cancer cells don't. Cancer cells thrive on glucose, but are killed by oxygen. So the B vitamins' role in promoting oxygen exchange is an important one. B15 in particular is thought to increase the efficiency of the cellular use of oxygen, and this nutrient may also help the liver to do its detoxifying job and stay healthy (liver activity is crucial in cancer). Laboratory animals made deficient in the B vitamins B1, B2, B3, pantothenic acid and choline get cancer more easily, and the B vitamin thiamine is found to be lacking in cancer patients. [14] In laboratory animals, PABA (Para-amino-benzoic acid) affords virtually complete protection against skin cancers.

Vitamin C   (The work done by Linus Pauling and Ewan Cameron using vitamin C in cancer treatment is described later in this section.)

Vitamin C boosts the immune system, the body's defence against cancer. It also stimulates the production of interferon, a natural substance produced by the body to deal with virus infections, helps to destroy carcinogenic chemicals, and reduces the ability of cancer cells to spread. A mixture of vitamins C and B2 has been shown to inhibit tumours and boost immunity levels in mice [15] and vitamin C recently added to test tube leukaemia cells reduced their number by 79% in 7 our of 28 cases. [16] Low levels of vitamin C have been found in women with breast cancer, [17] and the vitamin has been used – 1500mg a day – to prevent the recurrence of bladder cancer. [18] This vitamin is also a major anti-oxidant, acting to protect the cells against invasion by carcinogens.

Vitamin E   This is an anti-oxidant too. It improves resistance to bacterial infection, and stimulates the elimination of toxins. With vitamin E and the mineral selenium working together, the body's production of antibodies goes up. Some Australian research has found that mice fed extra E had only one-tenth as many bowel tumours (chemically induced) as other mice. [16] Vitamin E offers some protection against the side-effects of the very toxic anti-cancer drug Adriamycin and damage from radiation treatment.

Minerals The trace mineral *selenium* is the subject of much recent work. Geographical studies show that the local soil content of selenium is inversely related to cancer rates. Cancer incidence is reduced in laboratory animals given selenium. This mineral renders free radicals inactive; gives anti-oxidant protection to cell membranes; stimulates the immune system, and detoxifies. Selenium works with vitamin E.

Zinc seems to help prevent cancer in laboratory animals, and it is essential for the effective action of vitamin A. It is also intimately involved in immune function. [19]

An absence of *molybdenum* from the soil appears to increase the incidence of throat cancer. An *iodine* deficiency is believed to be related to breast cancer.

Although the relationship between *potassium, sodium* (salt) and cancer is unclear, most practitioners agree that potassium should be increased and sodium cut out as far as possible. Max Gerson gives potassium supplementation in his cancer therapy (SEE *Cancer, the Gerson Therapy* page 277, and also *Salt* page 57).

Fibre, fat and cancer Cancer of the bowel is the second commonest cancer in the West. It was rare before the 1920s.

This phenomenon is thought to be connected with our low-fibre diet. Fibre is not a nutrient; it is composed of the cell walls of plants. Its function in the body is to absorb water and help wastes through the bowel quickly; it prevents constipation, producing an easily evacuated, bulky, moist stool. Its lack in our food has been blamed for a host of Western diseases (SEE *Fibre* pages 35–42).

Without natural fibre, stools are smaller and much of the water is absorbed from them. They get hard and can stay in the body for several days. Waste does not just stream along like water in a pipe – some parts of it go faster than others and some of it can get stuck. Radio-opaque markers when swallowed show on X-ray that the points at which the bowel contents are often held up as they move along the colon are the cancer sites. [2] With fibre in the diet, the colonic wastes flow faster and more uniformly and these trouble spots don't occur.

There are carcinogens in our food. Because the bowel contents stay in one place longer than they should on a low-fibre diet, these harmful substances get plenty of time to act on the bowel lining. The speedy transit time of the bowel contents with fibre cuts down this delay and allows less time for the degradation of bile salts which occurs when bowel contents are static. When diluting the wastes by absorbing water, fibre may also dilute the carcinogens.

People who eat lots of fibre eat little fat, and the other way around. High-fibre eaters also excrete slightly more fat in their stools. Animal research at the Naylor Dana Institute for Disease Prevention has shown that high-fat diets increase the risk of breast cancer, and there is also a connection between a lot of fat and colon cancer. Some researchers believe that the huge quantities of fat we commonly eat in the West cause a type of bacterial flora which easily produces carcinogens. Laboratory rats bred without any bowel bacteria at all don't get the cancers that other rats get when exposed to the same carcinogens. This proves that bowel bacteria are essential for the production of bowel cancers.

A difference in dietary fat might be crucial in bowel cancer since a lot of fat and the absence of dietary fibre change the character of bowel bacteria – probably for the worse. People on a bulky, fibrous vegetarian diet have different stools from those eating other foods and this has a direct bearing on health.

There's no guarantee that if you eat fibre you will never get bowel cancer. But fibre seems to offer some protection.

The bacteria in yogurt, L. acidophilus, tend to inhibit enzymes that activate carcinogens in the bowel.[20]

Additives

'Will we continue to allow more than 90% of the tax dollars used for cancer research that tries to find cancer viruses and develops poisonous drugs as "therapy" when we already know that at least 90% of cancers are caused by environmental and food pollutants?' (*Cancer and its Nutritional Therapies* by RICHARD A. PASSWATER).

The additives put into our food are probably harmful in many cases, in spite of being tested. The food additive AF-2 was extensively tested before being released and this included a negative result, using animals, for cancer. But in the Ames test, invented by Dr Bruce Ames, this additive showed up positive and was later shown to cause cancer in laboratory animals.[9]

Still being argued over is the legal use of nitrates and nitrites as preservatives and flavouring agents in hot dogs, bacon, canned ham, most luncheon meats, smoked fish, etc. Under laboratory conditions, nitrites can combine in the stomach with partially digested proteins to create new compounds known as nitrosamines. These are powerful carcinogenic chemicals. (Tests at the Eppley Institute for Research in Cancer show that, when there is enough vitamin C, this transformation is almost completely blocked.[21])

Alcohol, cola drinks and coffee have all been identified as factors in bladder cancer in laboratory animals. Carcinogens are formed in rancid polyunsaturated fats when meat fat is heated to very high temperatures. Many pollutants produce free radicals.

Overeating and cancer It appears that too much food, as well as too many additives, can encourage cancer.

Dr Albert Tannenbaum carried out some research while he was director of the Department of Cancer Research, Michael Reese Hospital, Chicago. By limiting the intake of calories, fat and excessive protein in laboratory mice, he managed to reduce their cancer incidence.[22] (Too many high protein foods which need enzymes for digestion may mean that not enough of those enzymes are left over to attack malignant cells; this also applies to too much fat.)

Nutrition in general Vitamins and minerals work together in a team. Alternative practitioners, therefore, when advising their patients about the treatment of cancer, usually give advice on all-round nutrition first, and supplements second.

In 1961, a paper appeared in the *American Journal of Proctology* by American surgeon D.C. Collins. Collins had operated on five patients for cancer, and at the time of the operation had noticed spreading of the cancer beyond the operation site. The cancers were of the colon, part of the large intestine, and rectum. After the operation, Collins put his patients on organically grown whole food. They *all* experienced spontaneous disappearance of the remaining cancers.

The Seventh-day Adventists in America do not smoke, drink, or take tea or coffee, and many are vegetarians. Their incidence of cancer is astonishingly low – less than half of the rest of the population.[23]

It is found that a vegetarian diet may decrease the cancer

risk. But it must be emphasised that there are good and bad vegetarian diets (SEE *Vegetarian and Vegan Eating* pages 209–16). You could live on doughnuts and coffee and call it a vegetarian diet. But you would not stay healthy on it for long.

The Hunzas, living in northern India, were studied by Robert McCarrison earlier in this century. Since then, they have been intensively studied by other medical researchers, including a team from the World Health Organization. The Hunzas are largely vegetarians, eating a lot of fresh and dried apricots (with the pits), fresh vegetables, wholegrains and various beans, some white cheese, a little meat, some wine. Although adulterated, refined foods are gradually filtering into their community now, at the time McCarrison made his survey *cancer was unknown to the Hunzas.*

Diet, therefore, can protect against cancer – and diet can produce the devitalized and poisoned state which invites it.

The medical establishment is realizing more and more that this is so. Dr Donald German, Clinical Professor of Radiology at the University of Missouri School of Medicine, states that diet is a major factor in cancer. This conclusion is echoed now by many other authorities.

Alternative treatments for cancer are based on diet. The curative diet must:

1 Eliminate all toxins.
2 Provide the body with what it needs to fight the cancer.

Meat and fish are cut out. They produce toxic breakdown products which the sick body cannot cope with. No dairy foods are taken either. The diet comprises wholemeal bread, soya, unsalted and fat-free nuts, seeds, natural yogurt and sprouting seeds and grains, fresh raw vegetables and fruits (organically grown), freshly pressed fruit and vegetable juices. No junk, convenience or preserved foods are eaten and no salt or sugar added.

Note: some people have recovered from cancer by treating themselves. But if you have cancer, and are interested in using the non-toxic approach,it is better for you to have professional guidance. Please SEE *Information* at the end of this section.

Cancer and the mind In 1971 Carl Simonton, a radiation oncologist at Fort Worth, Texas, took on a 60-year old man with incurable throat cancer. According to the diagnosis, this condition would have been incurable by radiation therapy. Nevertheless, after three months of treatment with radiation therapy and a special relaxation technique, the man recovered completely. A year and a half later, he had no sign of throat cancer. [24]

Simonton used Autogenic Training on his patient (SEE *Relaxation* page 406). This is a system of deep relaxation which can be practised by anyone. When completely relaxed, the patient is asked to visualize his disease, and his body's resources mobilizing to deal with it. Autogenic training can be used to influence a person's attitudes at a very deep level and, through visualization, the patient's whole physical and psychological strength is brought to bear on his illness. Through deep relaxation, too, he learns to throw off an important factor in cancer – stress.

In a 1974–78 study of 159 cancer patients treated by this method the average increase in survival time was one and a half to two times over that expected from orthodox treatment. 63 patients survived beyond 18 months; 20 showed enlargement of tumour size, 17 showed no further growth, 12 showed tumour decrease and 14 had *no evidence of cancer after treatment.* [25]

Development of this work continues, and it is now being conducted in London (SEE *Information* section). Autogenic training illustrates the enormous power that the mind has over the body, and the paramount importance of mental attitude in illness as in everything else. Optimistic patients do better in recovering from cancer, [26] and it has been found, in fact, that positive feelings of assertion can increase white cell activity and improve immune system response. [27]

Conversely, it has been shown that psychological stress reduces the effectiveness of the immune system. In laboratory mice subjected to stress, tumour incidence could be increased by up to 90%. It remained at 7% in a protected environment. Stress plays a vital role in cancer, as in almost all illnesses (SEE *Stress*).

Relaxation and meditation are currently being used by unorthodox practitioners in the treatment of cancer, together with psychotherapy.

Summary: the non-toxic treatments   Here is a list of many of the unorthodox cancer treatments now being used in varying combinations.

Foods   Raw fresh vegetables and fruit, fresh fruit and vegetable juices, sprouting seeds and grains, raw liver juice and liver extract, bran, yogurt, lecithin, brewer's yeast, wheat germ, garlic.

Supplements Vitamins A, B complex, B13, B15, B17 (laetrile), C, E, P (rutin or bioflavonoids). Minerals iron, copper, iodine, potassium, calcium, phosphorus, zinc, selenium, magnesium.

Other physical treatments Homoeopathic (Iscador); herbs (red clover, green alfalfa, violet leaves, ginseng, chapparal); enzymes; insulin; heparin; hydrazine sulphate; oxygen and ozone, BCG vaccine; neoblastine; orgone therapy; heat, natural unfiltered daylight (not hot sunlight); ultra-violet light; colonic irrigation and enemas; deep breathing and mild exercise; elimination of focal infections such as diseased teeth and tonsils.

Psychological Meditation, biofeedback, relaxation, psychotherapy.

Spiritual healing

Avoidance of pollutants including naked fluorescent light, cigarette smoke, alcohol, white sugar and salt, cosmetics, TV especially colour, harsh sunlight.

Some conclusions It will be seen from the foregoing list that many different therapies are used in the alternative treatment of cancer.

Cancer is a disease of the whole person. We have seen how it can be related to diet, to other environmental factors and to a person's attitude to life, particularly how he reacts to stress. Unorthodox, non-toxic treatments treat the whole person. Orthodox treatment, on the other hand, 'is not so much to create a healthy human being, as to attack his bad bits. It's hard luck if the patient himself gets in the way' (Dr Isaac Bryant, in *Cancer: the Alternative Method of Treatment*).

Tumour shrinkage cannot be regarded as successful cancer management. Successful management is, first of all, the creation of an enhanced state of health. From this comes the body's vitality and ability to dissolve the cancer itself, using its own weapon – the immune system.

Many physicians have found that non-toxic, alternative therapies help the patient to withstand the side-effects of the orthodox approach which they may consider necessary. If there is a growth on a site which obstructs vital processes and endangers life, for instance, surgery will be essential and the alternative approach will help the patient's body to mop up any remaining malignant cells. It also allows him to tolerate drugs and radiotherapy better.

But drugs and radiotherapy damage the body's immune system and reduce its ability to deal with the cancer naturally. It seems that because of this it may not always be possible to back both horses in cancer treatment and successfully make use of both approaches. It is not possible to give a firm decision on this point since the necessary research has not yet been done. Each case has to be considered on its own merits at present and each case is unique.

Alternative treatments 'appear to produce complete remissions in a third of cases where orthodox treatment has failed and make no difference in a third, except for healing, which never fails to help in another way. In the remaining third there is a variable slowing of the growth, gains in energy and loss of pain' (from *Non-Toxic Cancer Treatment*, SEE *Information*).

There follows here a description of some specific non-toxic treatments.

Cancer and Vitamin C
Linus Pauling, twice a Nobel Prize winner, is world-famous for his research into vitamin C, and Ewan Cameron is a surgeon who has been treating cancer patients for over thirty years. They spent eight years researching possible links between cancer and vitamin C.

Vitamin C is known to enhance the efficiency of the immune system and it also stimulates normal cells to fight against the enzymes given off by a malignant tumour. It has a general anti-viral effect and helps the body to throw off pollutants; there is a strong possibility that it leads to more of the natural anti-viral substance, interferon, being produced. It is essential for cell activity and resistance to illness. It is needed to make collagen, the principal constituent of all connective tissue; this means that it is used whenever new connective tissue is made, both in the healing of wounds and the enclosing of a cancerous tumour in scar tissue. This encapsulation of a tumour is a complex process involving many factors and one of these is the formation of protective collagen. This vitamin, therefore, is intimately involved in many body processes, both in health and disease.

Human beings are almost unique in the animal kingdom in

being unable either to manufacture or store vitamin C in their bodies. When laboratory rats develop tumours, they start to produce enormous quantities of vitamin C. In fact they produce the equivalent, in a man weighing 11 stone, of 16 grams a day. (Normal human level corresponds to an intake of about 50mg a day – SEE chart.) We can't do this – but it might help our resistance to cancer if we could.

Cancer patients have been observed to have very low blood levels and intakes of vitamin C. Indeed the average vitamin C level of a cancer patient is nearly 50% lower than that of a healthy person. After surgery, there is a further drop in the already low levels of vitamin C in the blood. If the patient takes drugs, the level will drop even further, and the same thing happens with radiotherapy. A women with breast cancer will have vitamin C levels about one-third lower than the average healthy person. After treatment by surgery, radiotherapy and drugs, the level will have dropped to about one-tenth of that of a healthy person. Orthodox treatment, therefore, has *interfered with the body's levels of a vital substance needed to combat the illness being treated.* Because

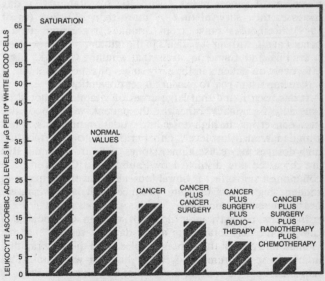

ASCORBIC ACID RESERVES IN HEALTH AND IN CANCER

vitamin C is needed for the functioning of so many essential processes, Pauling and Cameron feel that every doctor treating cancer should routinely correct the vitamin C deficiency caused both by the illness and its orthodox treatment.

Replacing the lost vitamin C, however, is a different matter from actually using this vitamin to treat cancer. This latter is what Pauling and Cameron have done.

In November 1971 Ewan Cameron began clinical trials at the Vale of Leven Hospital, Loch Lomondside, Scotland. In the eight years since they started, over 500 patients in the hospital with early and advanced cancer received vitamin C (together with routine nursing). Patients are usually given 10g a day, and almost without exception this is tolerated well without any side-effects.

Subjective evidence of positive change is usually apparent by the fifth to the tenth day of treatment. In many patients this response is very clear cut. The patient starts to feel better and there is general clinical improvement. During this time, objective evidence shows that the tumour growth has slowed down. Several trials with controls have established that the treatment of cancer patients with 10g of vitamin C a day increases their survival time by more than 330 days (as of 1979). Responses range from dramatic regressions to no benefit at all, with most patients in the middle.

Pauling and Cameron stress that vitamin C works most effectively on patients in the early stages of cancer, and that it has an important role to play in cancer prevention.

It has been found that large doses of vitamin C should be tapered off gradually, otherwise the patient, whose body has been converting the high doses into oxidation products, is left with dangerously low levels. Other criticisms to the effect that high dosages may cause kidney stones or destroy vitamin B12 are discussed and dismissed by Pauling and Cameron. The commonest side-effect is bowel looseness and flatulence, and sudden high dosages can produce diarrhoea, nausea, heartburn and intestinal gas.

In a few patients, large doses of vitamin C produced a catastrophic deterioration in a few days. It seemed that the vitamin had caused the tumour to bleed and die very rapidly, and because the tumours were so big this was fatal. This happened to 4 patients in a group of 50, and more work is obviously needed to control this effect.

American doctor Robert Downs believes that very high doses of vitamin C over a long period of time cause the body to lose essential minerals – calcium, magnesium, copper, iron, manganese and selenium which must be replaced.

In conclusion 'it is our opinion', say Pauling and Cameron in their book *Cancer and Vitamin C*, 'that supplemental vitamin C has value for the prevention of all forms of cancer in healthy human beings and also is of some benefit in the treatment of patients with cancer in every stage of the disease, and can be of great value to some patients. We believe that before long the use of this simple, safe, natural and inexpensive substance will become an accepted part of all regimes for the prevention and treatment of cancer.'

Laetrile

Laetrile is the name given to a naturally occurring substance found originally in the bitter almond plant by Dr Ernst Krebs. It is also known as amygdalin or vitamin B17 (its place in the B group of vitamins is still provisional).

Chemically, it can be thought of as benzaldehyde, hydrogen cyanide and glucuronic acid, all linked together. When the enzyme betaglucosidase reacts with laetrile, the release of cyanide occurs and many researchers believe that this cyanide kills the cancer cells. The releasing enzyme, betaglucosidase, is present only in large quantities in tumours. Laetrile's supporters believe that because of this appreciable quantities of cyanide from laetrile are released only in tumour cells; it is postulated that, because normal cells on the other hand have plenty of another enzyme, rhodanese, the cyanide is changed by this enzyme into thiocyanate, a harmless substance which is soon excreted.

German cancer specialist Dr Hans Nieper considers, however, that the constituent benzaldehyde is the active principle of amygdalin, and has treated his patients with it. His opinion is backed up by some Japanese research.[28]

Arguments still rage over laetrile and opinions are extreme. A trial was carried out by Dr Harold Manner of the University of Chicago over four years. 89% of his patients treated with laetrile underwent complete remission of their breast tumours and another 10% showed partial regression. In his control group, all the patients not receiving laetrile experienced tumour growth during this time. Another, apparently conflicting, example, is a trial in which dogs were treated with laetrile – and poisoned by it. But the dogs were given a vast overdose, and the substance was pre-digested, releasing dangerous cyanide, before it was administered to them.

Dr H. Moolenburgh, a Dutch physician with years of experience with laetrile, finds that many of his cancer patients feel better, have less pain and live longer than expected. Dr Kanematsu Sugiara of the Sloan-Kettering Institute in America believes however that laetrile is only a palliative and not a cure.

Laetrile must be used correctly. It is not advisable to take it on its own or without the guidance of an experienced practitioner. It must be part of a complete regime which includes first and foremost diet, with supplements and perhaps relaxation and psychotherapy. In his *An End to Cancer?* naturopath Leon Chaitow writes, 'any attempt simply to use laetrile as a treatment in its own right without these complementary adjuncts is certain to have little chance of success.'

This was taken into consideration by researchers in a recent clinical trial reported in the *New England Journal of Medicine* (1982: 306: 201–6). They tested laetrile on 178 patients, basing the work on current methods of treatment; whole foods and supplements were therefore included. The team state flatly that 'no substantive benefit was observed' in their patients, and that laetrile can be toxic.

This trial has been severely criticized by British laetrile experts on the grounds that the laetrile used was the wrong kind and that the wholefood diet was 'encouraged' only and not strictly adhered to. It is difficult to reconcile the negative results of this trial with the positive benefits noted by many other doctors.

Most patients seeking laetrile treatment have already been given surgery, drugs or radiotherapy and are terminal cases. At this stage of their illness, orthodox care does not expect more than one patient in a thousand to survive for five years.

Figures being supplied by physicians using laetrile as part of a total programme show that 15% of their patients survive for this time; there are signs that this figure could be higher. Less ill patients, with no spreading of the cancer, can probably anticipate an 80% survival rate for five years, according to these sources.[29] In the case of the stronger patients, this compares favourably with the 28% five-year survival figure for patients under orthodox treatment.

Readers can see for themselves, therefore, how controversial laetrile is. The discrepancy between the New England Journal of Medicine trial and other results needs to be explained.

Sources of Laetrile Widely distributed in nature, laetrile is found in the following:

Vegetables beetroot tops, cassava, spinach, sweet potatoes, yams, watercress.

Sprouting seeds and grains sprouting alfalfa, mung beans, lentils, buckwheat, wheat grass, bamboo shoots.

Pulses blackeye beans, lentils, lima beans, mung beans, green peas, chick peas, kidney beans, scarlet runner beans.

Cereals buckwheat, millet, oat groats, barley, brown rice, rye, vetch, wheat seeds.

Nuts almond, cashew, macadamia.

Seeds, kernels, pits apple, cherry, pear, peach, plum or prune, nectarine, linseed, apricot, bitter almond, sesame.

Fruit blackberries, cranberries, red and blackcurrents, elderberries, gooseberries, guavas, mulberries, raspberries, strawberries.

Please SEE *Information* at the end of this section if you wish to contact a practitioner who uses non-toxic therapy to consult him about laetrile.

The Gerson therapy

'I see in him [Dr Gerson] one of the most eminent geniuses in the history of medicine'   DR ALBERT SCHWEITZER.

A German doctor, Max Gerson, originally started to use dietary therapy to cure his own crippling migraine headaches. He continued his researches into the relationship between food and illness and found dietary treatment successful with TB, asthma, arthritis, diabetes, heart conditions and other chronic incurable illnesses.

In 1928 he started treating cancer patients, beginning with three hopeless, inoperable cases of stomach cancer. All three recovered. After some setbacks and failures and years of study and research, his therapy was producing a 50% recovery rate for even far-advanced cancer cases.

In 1946 Dr Gerson became the first physician to demonstrate

recovered cancer patients before a US Congressional Committee, which was discussing a bill to release money for cancer research. This bill, which could have supported extensive research into Gerson's therapy, was defeated by four votes as a result of pressure from the lobby supporting radiotherapy, surgery and drugs.

Gerson states that cancer is a disease of the whole organism where almost all essential organs are involved in the more advanced cases. He emphasises the destructive role played by our denatured, refined food. This food has been grown on soil unbalanced by chemicals, and the crops themselves have been sprayed with other chemicals. We eat, therefore, distorted food from an unbalanced soil.

The Gerson therapy concentrates on *restoring the body's ability to heal itself*.

Gerson illustrated the idea that a healthy body will overcome cancer. He took two rats, one of which had cancer, joined the sick rat to the healthy rat by a blood vessel and sewed them together. In a day or two the sick rat recovered, cured by the bodily defences of the healthy rat whose bloodstream it was sharing. We come back yet again to the strength and effectiveness of a healthy immune system. This is what the Gerson therapy strives to enhance, as well as allowing the body to cleanse itself of toxins. Cancer, says Gerson, develops in a poisoned body, particularly where toxins have accumulated in the liver.

The Gerson therapy sets out to accomplish:

1   Far-reaching detoxification of the whole body over a long period of time.

2   Restoration of various metabolic functions, particularly the immune system, enabling the body to fight the cancer itself.

3   Absorption and elimination, as a result of this restoration, of cancer masses and cells.

4   Healing of the damage done by the cancer, and recovery of essential organs, especially the liver.

It will be seen that this treatment, which is predominantly dietary, *is not aimed directly at the cancer.* It is concerned with the body's accumulation of poisons and lowered ability to defend itself against illness – any illness. This is completely in accordance with the principles of Nature Cure (SEE pages 391–6).

The Gerson therapy seeks to regenerate a diseased liver. The liver is the largest single organ we have, and its many complex activities are absolutely vital to health. Fortunately, this crucially important organ of detoxification has tremendous reserves and it can also heal and rebuild itself.

The Gerson diet is limited to freshly pressed fruit and vegetable juices, raw fruits and vegetables, vegetables stewed in their own juices, stewed fruits, potatoes and oatmeal, a special soup and rye bread. All the above, including the bread, are taken without salt. Gerson has found that the abolition of salt, and the lifting of the potassium level, are essential. All the fruits and vegetables must be organically grown and free from artificial chemicals. Freshly pressed calf's liver juice is taken, and peppermint tea; later fatless, saltless cheese, natural yogurt and churned buttermilk are added. All other foods are forbidden.

Two machines are needed for the juice preparation. No pressure cookers or any other aluminium vessels are to be used for cooking.

Supplements include iodine, potassium salts, vitamin B3 (niacin), royal jelly, liver injections, pepsin, pancreatic enzymes, ox bile, linseed oil and thyroid extract.

Gerson makes the point that after the death of the tumour the elimination of millions of dead cancer cells throws a heavy strain on the liver and kidneys in particular. This process can be too great a shock and the patient may fall into a hepatic coma unless help is given. Coffee enemas are used to assist elimination. Used in this way, coffee has quite a different effect, helping the liver in its enormous task of getting rid of cancerous masses. Castor oil is also given by mouth, and castor oil and camomile tea enemas are given. This frequent and regular elimination of poisonous substances is a vital part of the treatment.

Sometimes, within the first two weeks of treatment, a 'flare-up' may occur. This is a favourable reaction and should be regarded as part of the healing process. It can comprise nausea, headaches and sometimes vomiting and the first flare-up is usually the most violent one. It is the same thing as the 'healing crisis' described in the *Nature Cure* section, and is the body's vigorous attempt to cleanse itself, to heal itself, by producing an inflammation. The sick body cannot do this; only when a body starts to become detoxified is it able to produce a healing inflammation. Gerson gives his patients peppermint tea and extra coffee enemas to help them through this necessary reaction.

Results of the Gerson therapy are poor if the patient has had his pancreas, stomach, adrenals or all of his colon removed. Drugs and radiotherapy, too, will hinder this therapy, for it rests upon the body's inherent ability to heal itself and this ability is damaged or destroyed by orthodox treatments.

It will be seen from the foregoing that the Gerson therapy is not a picnic. It is a far-reaching and ruthless exercise, expensive, time-consuming and demanding. But it works. And, to quote Gerson himself, 'where affection and devotion in the family exists, all difficulties are disregarded for the sake of saving a life.'[30]

The Gerson therapy, if assiduously followed, can achieve recovery from early to intermediate cancer in 90% or more of cases. When the cancer has reached the liver or the pancreas or has spread elsewhere in the body, recoveries can be achieved in 50% of cases, depending on the degree of drug or other damage, and the extent to which the liver is affected. Many of Dr Gerson's patients are still alive today, some 30 years after their treatment (SEE *Recommended reading*).

For more details about the Gerson therapy, please SEE *Information* at the end. *Please note* that this treatment needs professional assistance.

Information
Dietary treatment The diet in the *Guide to Healthy Eating* can control some cancers. This is obtainable from The Natural Health Network, of 51 Rodney Road, Cheltenham, Gloucestershire, and the Cancer Help Centre (SEE *Clinics* below).

There is also a leaflet, *Non-Toxic Cancer Treatment*, by Alex Forbes, obtainable from the same organization.
Autogenic training Please write to The Centre for Positive Health, 15 Fitzroy Square, London W1. Telephone 01 388 1007.
Laetrile For information and supplies write to Craftsman's Workshops, Foye Forge, Fowey, Cornwall. Telephone 072 683 2248. Mon–Fri 8–4.30 pm.

Brightport Limited, 5 Timor Court, Longford Avenue, Southall, Middlesex UB1 3QS. Telephone 01 571 3069.

Cantassium Company Limited, 225 Putney Bridge Road,

London SW15. Telephone 01 870 4251.

Green Farm, Burwash, East Sussex. Telephone 0435 882482.

Nature's Own, 51 Rodney Road, Cheltenham, Gloucestershire.

The Gerson therapy   Please contact The Association for New Approaches to Cancer (ANAC) of 1A Addison Crescent, London W14 8JP (Telephone 01 603 7751) for doctors and other practitioners who use this therapy.

Information is also available from The Gerson Institute, PO Box 430, Bonita, CA 92002, USA;

Dr Contreras, The Del Mar Medical Center, Tijuana, Mexico; Dr H. Nieper, Krankenhaus Am Silbersee, Oertzeweg 24, 3012 Langenhagen 1, West Germany.

ANAC also have a list of doctors and other practitioners in the UK who give other non-toxic treatments for cancer.

Clinics which treat cancer patients using non-toxic treatments
The Nature Cure Clinic, 15 Oldbury Place, London W1M 3AL. Telephone 01 935 2787.

The Natural Health Clinic, 133 Gatley Road, Gatley, Cheadle, Cheshire SK8 4PD. Telephone 061 428 4980.

The Kent Private Clinic, Sandwich, Kent. Telephone 0304 612910.

Cancer Help Centre, Downfield House, 7 Downfield Road, Bristol BS8 2TG. Telephone 0272 313216.

Other approaches:
Herbalism   SEE appendix page 405.

Homoeopathy   SEE appendix page 405.

Spiritual healing   'Should be used in every case' – Dr Alec Forbes. The National Federation of Spiritual Healers, Old Manor Farm Studio, Church Street, Sunbury-on-Thames. Telephone 09327 83164.

Recommended reading
A Cancer Therapy: results of fifty cases by Max Gerson (Totality Books, USA, 1977). Hospitals' and doctors' reports on 50 cancer patients treated by Gerson.

An End to Cancer? by Leon Chaitow (Thorsons 1978).

Other books mentioned in this section
Cancer – The Alternative Method of Treatment by Dr Isaac Bryant (Roberts Pubs. 1980).

Cancer and Vitamin C by Ewan Cameron and Linus Pauling (Weidenfeld and Nicolson 1979).

Constipation

'One good stool is worth seven doctors.'   Surgeon DENIS
BURKITT

Constipation is widespread in the West – it is estimated that
over 15% of the UK population takes laxatives regularly.
Almost all the blame for this can be laid on the way we eat.

What is constipation?

This is not such a silly question as it sounds. Constipation is a
hard stool, not an infrequent one. A hard stool, often broken
up into small pieces and very dry, is difficult to expel. It is hard
because it has been inside the colon for long enough for its
natural water to be re-absorbed by the walls of the intestine. It
is the length of time that the wastes take to work their way
along the gut to expulsion that is important – the 'transit
time'. If you have a long transit time, then you are
constipated, even if you have a bowel movement every day.
This is the crucial factor.

Some doctors still say that it doesn't matter how often you
open your bowels. It is of course impossible to have a fast,
efficient transit of wastes through the body without a regular
bowel movement. So this is an important secondary factor.
But your bowel behaviour depends both on what you eat, and
how much. If you eat like a bird, then you can't expect a large
bowel movement every day. Where would it come from?

There is a lot of argument about whether constipation
actually causes you any harm. Chronic constipation can give
you a muddy skin, bad breath, dull eyes, headaches and
constant fatigue. A permanently overloaded bowel can lead to
piles and even contribute to varicose veins, and can cause
diverticular disease, where the overstrained colon muscle fails
in places and little pouches form in the gut. Food breakdown
products, held in close contact with the bowel lining for long
periods, can be carcinogenic.

There is no substitute for the feeling of wellbeing that
accompanies a regular, easy bowel movement. It's pointless,
however, getting upset if you miss a day occasionally. This
occasional lapse, perhaps because of under-eating or some
kind of stress, is not at all the same thing as long-term intractable constipation.

If we look again at the time taken for the wastes to be pushed along the gut and finally expelled, we can see that there are two things that matter – first, the way the gut behaves as it pushes the wastes along efficiently or slowly, and second of course the nature of the wastes themselves, which makes them easy or hard to shift.

For some hours after we have eaten a meal, rhythmic contractions in the walls of the stomach and small intestine mix the food mass along with the digestive juices, enzymes and bile, and bring the already digested food into contact with the absorbing surfaces of the intestinal walls. Without these contractions, food cannot be properly digested and absorbed and neither will it be passed along the gut. So the effectiveness of these squeezing movements – called peristalsis – is part of a healthy gut and its fast discharge of wastes. When the intestinal muscles are weak and flabby, the wastes are delayed, water is absorbed from them, and they become dry and difficult to expel.

Faeces contain bacteria, water mucus, and of course food wastes. So let's look at what we eat.

It has been conclusively proved that the fibre content of our diet – that is, whether the natural fibre is refined out or left in – has a major influence on the state of our bowels (SEE *Fibre*). People in the Third World eat about twice as much fibre as we do, and they have a much faster transit time. Tribal Africans, living on whole grains and other whole foods, have a transit time of about 30 hours. For the average Westerner, it can be from 3 days (young people) to the very long time of 2 weeks (the elderly). Fibre, then, is the most important food to consider when talking about constipation – but *not the only one*.

It is generally accepted now that fibre should be used as a treatment for constipation, and I quote below from some information which surgeon Neil Painter, of Manor House Hospital in London gives to his patients about the richest natural source of fibre – bran.

'Add bran to cereals, porridge or soup, especially pea soup [or to home-made bread – JP]. Bran takes at least 24 hours to work so it is useless for the relief of occasional constipation. Bran often causes flatulence so only two teaspoons should be taken with each meal for the first two weeks. The amount you need depends on the quantity of fibre in the rest of your diet. Take the above dose for two weeks and then increase it until the motions have the consistency of toothpaste and *are passed without straining*. Bran is best taken before meals, or with the first course, otherwise the stomach may become over-filled.

'After two weeks of taking six teaspoons a day find the correct amount of bran by trial and error, even if you need several tablespoons a day. Then take this dose for life. This safe and natural way of keeping the bowels open is also cheap.'

Many people find that they can take their entire daily allowance of bran with their breakfast cereal. You can get bran from your health food store or from some chemists; Boots the chemists stock it. Coarse bran is thought to be more effective than fine. There are also several cereals on the market now which contain bran, including of course All-Bran, and these are effective to varying extents; unfortunately they often have a lot of added sugar, which is bad for you. You can get bran tablets from your health food store or from your doctor.

Although bran is the best source of fibre, it is not the only one. There is dietary fibre in all whole cereals, wholemeal bread, fruits, vegetables, nuts and seeds. (Please SEE the *Fibre* section for a table of the fibre content of some foods.) The fibre in carrots, cabbage and other vegetables contains B vitamins, in particular pantothenic acid and B1, and whole cereals and wholemeal bread can also offer the B vitamins and minerals which are so important for the intestinal muscles, as we shall see later.

For some older people who cannot tolerate bran on its own, naturopath Alan Moyle recommends wholemeal bread, unrefined sunflower oil and sunflower seeds, prunes, figs, beetroot, mushrooms, honey, molasses and a little spinach in the diet. He also advises one dessertspoonful of molasses once a day, taken in water, to encourage a good bowel action. Adjust this amount to suit yourself.

Going back to the discussion of the intestinal squeezing action, peristalsis, this depends on the health of the stomach and intestinal muscles. These muscles need the same nutrients as any others – notably the B group of vitamins for optimum function. Deficiencies of the B vitamins choline, niacin, inositol and B6 can contribute to defective peristaltic action, and when a deficiency of the important B vitamin, pantothenic acid, was induced in volunteers, constipation was one of the symptoms they developed.[1] A deficiency of the mineral potassium can cause the peristaltic contractions to slow down and deficiencies of the B vitamins, together with those of calcium, magnesium and potassium, were found in patients with spasm of the large bowel. Protein contributes to good muscle tone, so a shortage in the diet will encourage flabby, weak intestinal muscles.

Because the gut depends for its healthy muscle action on these B vitamins and minerals, foods with a high content of these nutrients act as gentle natural laxatives: brewer's yeast and wheat germ, honey and molasses. Dried or stewed fruits often help and cider vinegar has proved effective for some people. Yogurt taken every day helps soften the stools. Some people have a regular bowel movement without much fluid in their diet, but others find they need more.

Constipation can also be caused by inadequate bile flow, which allows undigested fats to react with calcium and/or iron, forming a hard soap. Although lecithin and unrefined oils may put matters right for the time being, you should consult your practitioner on this.

Some antibiotics make you constipated, and diuretic drugs can cause constipation by robbing the body of potassium and water.

Constipation can also result from the over-use of laxatives, and these medicines should only be used as a last resort. It is very easy for a flabby bowel, trying to cope with the wrong diet, to get dependent on a laxative. After one dose, your bowel will react very strongly and the rectum will empty completely. It may take several days to fill up again, and during this time many people panic and take another dose. The bowel action, therefore, can become abnormal and forced and the muscles are eventually unable to function naturally, needing larger and larger doses.

At least one laxative, mineral oil, is very harmful, interfering with the absorption of the vitamins A, D, E and K and excreting them in the faeces.

Proper chewing of your food is vital – particularly with a high-fibre diet. Starches are partly digested in the mouth and people who chew their food thoroughly are less likely to be constipated. Other factors are lack of exercise, poor posture and breathing; a very important cause is emotional and physical tension. Some very sexually repressed people tend to be constipated. It is believed that people who do not want to give themselves or reach out to other people are likely to hold on to their body wastes as well.

Don't put off going to the lavatory. After a meal, there is a natural relaxation of the sphincter, the ring of muscle round the anus, so get used to visiting the lavatory after eating; don't worry about results. They will come.

Additional therapies
Acupuncture: SEE appendix page 405.
Deep breathing: the Knowles System has an exercise specifically for constipation; SEE appendix page 405.
Exercise, anything that works the stomach muscles: SEE appendix, particularly Yoga, page 405).
Herbalism: SEE appendix page 405.
Homoeopathy: SEE appendix page 405.
Osteopathy: SEE appendix page 405.
Relaxation: SEE appendix page 405.

Cystitis

Cystitis is an inflammation of the bladder, either from infection or from irritation caused by deposits in the urine. Although it is rarely dangerous by itself, it can be extremely painful and debilitating, and is often associated with kidney trouble. There are no figures for this painful and distressing women's illness, which may be as widespread as the common cold.

The bladder is the outlet for urine, which is produced by the kidneys. The bowels deal, not with tissue wastes like the kidneys, but with undigested food. They can stop working for weeks at a time and we stay alive (but unhappy). Failure of the kidneys, however, can be fatal in a few days.

The kidneys and bladder form part of the urinary system so that many infections can travel down from the kidneys to the bladder, or from the bladder up to the kidneys. The rising figures for kidney failure (over 7000 a year) do not take into account those people with chronic kidney troubles of a less dramatic kind.

Blood enters the kidneys and flows through at the incredible speed of about 2½ pints a minute. The kidneys remove the waste, modifying and re-absorbing part of it and passing the rest along the ureter to the bladder so that it can be excreted from the body.

The bladder holds the urine as it trickles in from the kidneys, the muscles remaining at rest until the volume of urine is enough to stimulate them.

Many conditions predispose towards cystitis. Women on the Pill are often more susceptible to urinary infections. Weak muscles due to advancing age may encourage the urine to stay for too long in the bladder. The ureter may become narrow, making the passage of urine difficult, or pressure from an enlarged prostate gland may result in incomplete emptying. Internal irritants such as kidney stones or gravel may cause trouble. Sitting on cold, damp grass or stone can often precipitate an attack.

'Honeymoon cystitis' is a common complaint. Frequent sex stimulates bacterial growth in the urethra which carries urine from the bladder to the outside. This simple condition can often be helped by drinking a couple of tumblers of water immediately after intercourse and then emptying the bladder as soon as possible.

Acute cystitis
Symptoms are severe local pain and a frequent desire to pass urine, even just after emptying the bladder. Urine may be thick, dark and stringy, containing pus and even some blood; there is a scalding pain during and after urination and sometimes pain in the lower back as well. Patients feel very ill and often have a rise in temperature.

If you have these symptoms, go to a qualified naturopath or nutritionally aware doctor (SEE appendix page 405) as soon as possible. It will be necessary for him also to find out if you have any kidney troubles as well.

Chronic cystitis
This may follow an acute attack, especially if the original cause is not removed. In this case the symptoms are less severe and

there will probably be no rise in temperature, but this exhausting and depressing illness can continue on and off for many years.

Nutritional treatment

Bacteria co-exist in great numbers in a healthy bladder. When an infection arises, from a bacterial imbalance or from outside, the body's defences will go into action to overcome it. Similarly, if the bladder is affected by an accumulation of toxins or a catarrhal inflammation due to chill, the body will cleanse itself if given the chance. The dietary treatment described below is designed to assist these curative reactions. Even if your symptoms are slight, or even absent for a time, don't wait for an attack. Start the dietary treatment at once. Treatment in the chronic phase will reduce the severity of the next acute attack, if and when it comes. Naturopathic treatment is aimed at improving the state of health of both kidneys and bladder, and indeed of the body as a whole. This treatment will help kidney disorders such as nephritis and pyelitis, which are likely to affect the bladder.

Drugs, on the other hand, will often result in kidney damage. Anyone on a course of drugs must consult a qualified practitioner, preferably a naturopath, for advice. The diet will minimize withdrawal symptoms and cut down the pain, and painkillers are not recommended, so try and stick it without.

Some people may worry about the fruit in the diet, thinking that it may have an acid effect. But the acid in fruits is given off very rapidly by the body after digestion and the residue is alkaline.

Elimination diet   (to be followed for ten days)

On rising   a full tumbler of half-and-half unsweetened apple juice and carrot juice. If you do not have a mechanical juicer, grate some raw carrot finely on to a double thickness of muslin, fold the muslin over and twist it to express the juice.

Breakfast   ripe melon or pears or sweet grapes (not citrus fruits, rhubarb or plums). Follow with about one-third of a pint of yogurt, home-made or from a health food store (SEE *Yogurt*). This may be sweetened with a little honey.

Mid-morning   mix a teaspoonful of a yeast and vegetable extract containing vitamin B12 (from your health food store) into a cup of hot water; this may be taken hot or cold as liked. Vecon, which is rather salty, is best avoided for the time being.

Lunch a raw salad consisting of shredded raw carrot, shredded raw beetroot, watercress or shredded raw Dutch white cabbage. Immediately after shredding the ingredients, mix in a dressing of natural yogurt with a teaspoonful of honey added, flavoured with chopped parsley and chives or finely grated onion. Add a portion of lactic cheese. Follow with a ripe apple.

Teatime one cup of dandelion coffee or pure unsweetened grape juice.

Supper salad of lettuce and celery. Portion of melon sweetened with a teaspoonful of honey.

Later one tumbler of raw carrot, raw beetroot and apple juice, mixed.

Stick strictly to this diet for the time recommended. It is designed to cleanse the blood and tissues and provide natural vitamins and minerals in balanced proportions.

You may experience 'false hunger' for a few days, but this will pass off.

For the next three weeks, follow the diet outlined in the *Food Therapy* section (pages 396–401). Please bear in mind that yogurt, home-made or from a health food store, is believed to help urinary infections, so eat about one-third of a pint every day. (As before, avoid salty drinks such as Vecon.)

After this three-week Food Therapy plan, take a fruit-only diet for the next three days.

This should be of ripe, raw fruit only, selected from grapes, melon, pears or apples, three times a day, taken with half a glass of mixed carrot and beetroot juice.

Following this fruit break, repeat again the Elimination diet followed by the Food Therapy plan.

If at any stage in this regime an acute attack develops, with-hold all solid food immediately (SEE *Fasting* pages 159–63). Attacks are possible while the body throws off its poisons and this process is further explained in the *Nature Cure* section (pages 391–6), so don't worry; if an attack comes during your dietary treatment, it is a part of the healing process, like the colds and other eruptions described under *Nature Cure*.

During your fast take only a glass of water or diluted carrot juice every two or three hours. Rest and keep warm. You will help yourself to recover, and minimize your pain, by hot water treatment. Immerse your pelvis in hot water, or use a towel wrung out in hot water to cover your abdomen, putting a dry towel over that to keep in the warmth. This water should not scald; test on the back of your hand to make sure it's not too hot. A little vegetable oil rubbed into the skin will avoid too much reddening. Alternate hot compresses with cold ones. The hot compress should be left on for several minutes, and the cold compress for about half a minute only.

After you have continued this fast for three to four days, the inflammation should have gone down and your temperature, if raised, should have returned to normal.

For the next three days eat only ripe, raw, sub-acid (not citrus) fruit, selected from grapes, melon, pears, peaches or apples. Following this, go back to the Elimination diet and Food Therapy Plan.

Vitamin C is used by some naturopaths in the treatment of cystitis. It combats infection and can be very useful in urinary conditions. With the Elimination and Food Therapy diets, take 1g a day. With the fast and the fruit diet, take 2g a day.

Drinking lots of fluid is often recommended for cystitis. But naturopath Clifford Quick comments that 'the urinary tract bears no resemblance to a domestic draining system and attempts to "flush out" disease with large amounts of fluid are more likely to overload the system than to assist cure.' Over-working the kidneys can result in the retention of fluid. The dietary here contains enough fluid, both in the drinks and in the foods themselves.

Before you undertake your Food Therapy, it will be necessary for you to know how and why it works. Please, therefore, read the *Nature Cure* section first.

Please note that the dietary treatment is on general lines only, and that you may also need additional vitamins and minerals. For individual guidance on both your Food Therapy plan and any supplementation, please consult a naturopath or a nutritionally aware doctor.

Additional Therapies

Acupuncture: SEE appendix page 405.
Herbalism: SEE appendix page 405.
Homoeopathy: SEE appendix page 405.
Osteopathy (for possible lesions): SEE appendix page 405.
Water treatments: ask your naturopath if you need any further advice.

Recommended reading
Nature Cure for Cystitis by Clifford Quick (Thorsons 1979).

Diabetes

What is diabetes?
Basically, diabetes mellitus is a condition where glucose cannot effectively be used by the body. This malfunction has many effects.

To understand diabetes, we must trace what happens to carbohydrates when we eat them.

When carbohydrates (sugar is a carbohydrate) are digested, they are changed into simple sugars and in particular into glucose. In this form they pass into the blood and the blood sugar goes up.

The blood sugar must now be lowered, and the only agent which can do this is insulin. There are cells scattered throughout the pancreas gland in little clumps (islets) and these cells produce insulin. This hormone is released into the blood and encourages the glucose to enter the liver, thus lowering the blood sugar to normal levels again. When the glucose enters the liver, it is broken down to produce the body's readiest form of energy. The liver stores any excess, or it is deposited round the body as fat.

In diabetes, this lowering of the blood sugar does not happen. The reason it does not is usually, though not always, a lack of insulin.

One of the results of this defect is that the glucose circulating in the blood does not enter the liver. The liver therefore gets short of the raw material for energy. So, while there is a lot of unuseable glucose going round in the bloodstream, the liver cannot reach it, and is forced to break down fats and proteins from the tissues.

Because of the liver's emergency action, the body is deprived of both fats and proteins, and the person loses weight and becomes exhausted. Toxic ketones (acetone and related substances) appear in the blood, making it acid. Other secondary effects include bad breath and cold hands and feet.

When the blood sugar level, uncorrected by insulin, gets too high, sugar spills over into the urine. The kidneys, trying to excrete all this sugar, call upon large quantities of water from the rest of the body. Otherwise the diabetic's urine would be treacle. This is why he experiences a terrific thirst and frequent urination. Without treatment, diabetes of this severity leads to coma and eventually to death. Most diabetes is less serious than this.

We have seen that a main factor is usually a lack of insulin. Insulin can be present in the blood of a diabetic – in fact he may produce more than a normal person – but it is useless and cannot work properly because of antagonistic factors also present in his blood.

There are two kinds of diabetes.

The juvenile-onset type – now called type 1 – usually happens to children or young people. Its onset is sudden and the symptoms are severe. The patient is very thin and either does not produce any insulin at all or hardly produces any.

The maturity-onset type is now called type 2. It usually happens to middle-aged people, often accompanies obesity, and is strongly hereditary. Symptoms are mild or non-existent. Insulin is being insufficiently produced, or it cannot be properly used by the body. Three out of four diabetics are type 2. The disease progresses more slowly than in type 1, but it can lead to serious complications, especially in fat people.

The older we get, the less efficient is our mechanism of storing away sugar, which probably explains why the incidence of diabetes rises with age. There is diabetes in about 5% of English adults under 50, and in about 15% of those over 50. There are 600 000 known diabetics in the UK, and probably another 600 000 people who have mild diabetes without knowing it; a Bedford survey showed that 12% to 14% of the adult population possessed an abnormal glucose tolerance – a sign of mild, or incipient, diabetes.[1] It is the sixth ranking cause of death in the West, and its incidence is rising.

Diabetes is a complex group of diseases and it is believed that there is much more to it than a raised level of blood sugar and a defect in the insulin mechanism. When you consider its deadly complications, the toll of diabetes is high.

As well as the immediate symptoms already listed, diabetics run the risk of heart disease. This is a major cause of death among them. It may be that diabetes itself increases the risk of heart damage. This brings with it the danger of a stroke. Blood vessel damage is very common in diabetics. Some of the circulatory problems may be due to increased platelet adhesion. Platelets are tiny discs which stick together when the blood needs to clot after you have cut yourself. In the diabetic – and often in the person with too much fat in his blood – these platelets clump together when they are not required to do so and this impedes the free circulation of the blood. Plugged arteries cause poor circulation and there can be impaired sensation in the limbs and haemorrhaging of the blood vessels in the eye (retinopathy) leading sometimes to blindness.

Kidney damage often accompanies diabetes, and in the long-term diabetic neuritis can lead to impotence as the nerves leading to the penis are affected. There is no effect on a woman's sex life, but a diabetic needs close medical supervision while she is carrying her baby.

At a meeting organized by the British Diabetic Association (1 July 1980), Professor Harry Keen of Guy's Hospital, London, stated that blindness due to diabetic changes in the eyes is the commonest cause of blindness in the West. Half of those diagnosed as diabetic in youth will be dead before the age of 40, partly because of the kidney failure associated with diabetes. In older men, diabetes increases the risk of heart attack two to three times and in diabetic women as much as five to seven times.

Treatment

Insulin has saved the lives of many thousands of diabetics. But it is not an exact match of the insulin which would be produced by a particular human body. And it is not, of course, measured out in exact response to specific changes in blood sugar levels, as would happen naturally.

When injected, it will exert its effect whether or not food has been eaten and whether or not there has been any change in the blood sugar. So a delay in eating, when you are taking insulin injections, will lead to low blood sugar as the insulin acts regardless of the state of your digestion. This is why you must stick to the eating plan drawn up for you by your doctor.

Too much insulin, too little, missing a meal, or eating the wrong food, cause low blood sugar (hypoglycaemia). This must immediately be relieved by taking some sugar or a glucose sweet. Otherwise you may go into a diabetic coma and may even die. Every diabetic should be allowed to experience the early warning signs of hypoglycaemia so that he recognizes them and knows what to do.

Insulin dosage must be carefully worked out. Many diabetics need more insulin than their bodies would normally produce, and probably insulin antagonists in their blood are interfering with its action. It is important to know that oral contraceptives and the diuretic chlorothiazide can lessen the effects of insulin.

Insulin must be injected because it is inactive by mouth. Its principal sources are slaughtered animals, pork and beef, and because of this some patients occasionally become allergic to one particular type. Side-effects from insulin include skin rashes and itching and swelling of the face and throat.

Some researchers believe that the arterial damage accompanying diabetes may arise from the insulin injections themselves, but because diabetics would formerly have died without insulin, it is difficult to test this idea.

Work has now been done to persuade bacteria to produce insulin virtually identical to human insulin. This synthetic product is currently being tested at Guy's Hospital, where it is performing well. There is also a very small machine being developed which can supply the body with insulin only when the rise in blood sugar requires it. The US National Center for Disease Control, however, reports (*New Scientist*, 25 February 1982) that there are several unexplained deaths among users of these pumps.

Many patients with mild diabetes do not need insulin. Their condition can be controlled with drugs and diet, or just with diet alone.

Drugs   There are two main groups of antidiabetic drugs – the sulphonylureas and the biguanides.

The *sulphonylureas* are thought to lower blood sugar levels by making the pancreas produce more insulin; they also increase the latter's effectiveness. Any of them may produce a fall in blood sugar, especially in the elderly and in those with impaired kidney or liver function. They may affect thyroid function in patients with serious thyroid disorders. Acetohexamide (marketed as Dimelor) can produce headaches, stomach upsets, vertigo, nervousness and disturbed liver function. Tolbutamide (Rastinon) can produce skin rashes, weakness, headaches, blood disorders, jaundice and intolerance to alcohol, and chlorpropamide (Diabinese) has much the same possible side-effects.

The biguanides increase glucose uptake by the muscles when insulin is present, and they reduce the release of glucose by the liver. The commonest biguanide prescribed now is metformin (Glucophage). This can produce anorexia, nausea and vomiting with, less commonly, skin rashes and weakness. Phenformin (Dibotin) can produce appetite loss and a bitter taste, nausea and vomiting, and diarrhoea; these side-effects are common. Loss of weight and fatigue are also possible. Deaths have been reported due to alterations in blood acidity in patients taking phenformin but no concrete relationship has been proved.

The British Nutrition Foundation Bulletin No. 18 states that diabetes is associated with obesity, high blood fats, too much insulin in the blood, and possible high blood pressure, and adds that these symptoms may be due *as much to diabetic drug therapy* as to diet. [2]

Diet by itself is often enough to control mild diabetes, and this approach is of course harmless. Indeed, an American study[3] found that the combination of diet and the drug tolbutamide, was no more effective than just diet alone. This study also showed that the death rate from heart disease in those diabetics taking tolbutamide was *2.5 times higher* than in those not taking the drug.

American nutritionist Adelle Davis writes[4] that anti-diabetic drugs for mild diabetes are not effective unless some of the cells of the pancreas are still producing some insulin. These drugs often cause liver damage and cannot build up the pancreas, so they are in effect beating a tired horse. She states that unless nutrition is markedly improved, more and more cells in the pancreas are put out of action until eventually insulin has to be used. Adequate nutrition, on the other hand, helps the body to produce its own insulin and can lower the injected insulin dose.

Neither animal insulin nor drugs are a *cure* for diabetes. They act only to control the symptoms and do not influence the disease itself. While insulin and drugs are controlling the blood sugar, all the associated long-term degenerative changes are allowed to continue while the unfortunate patient thinks he is controlling the whole illness. The need for insulin to control blood sugar is recognized. But additionally, the diabetic is running a greater risk from heart and artery disease and other damage, which the orthodox doctor generally does nothing about.

Diet For many mild diabetics, the standard diabetic diet is enough to control their illness.

Refined carbohydrates – in particular, table sugar or sucrose – are rapidly absorbed into the bloodstream and therefore call upon the quick release of insulin to bring down the blood sugar level to normal again. The standard diabetic diet is low in carbohydrates, especially sucrose, so that this immediate, heavy demand for insulin does not occur and the pancreas is protected. The less carbohydrate eaten, the less insulin the pancreas has to produce so the less work it has to do. A low-carbohydrate diet will also keep weight down.

But research in recent years is uncovering more and more links between nutrition and all the chronic degenerative diseases, bringing to the fore a more sophisticated, deeper approach to the relationship between diabetes and food. It has been found, for instance, that a diet high in the natural fibre found in unrefined carbohydrates is better for the diabetic than the standard low-carbohydrate diet.

Before going into this, and other nutritional research, in detail, we can look at some of the possible reasons for diabetes.

Why diabetes?

It is a commonly held view that a cause cannot usually be found for diabetes. Rarely, a virus infection may have destroyed the insulin-producing mechanism in some young people, and diabetes occasionally follows mumps. Too much cortisone has caused both diabetes and inflammation of the pancreas. We have seen that the diuretic chlorothiazide can damage the islet cells which produce insulin so that diabetes follows.

The contraceptive Pill impairs glucose tolerance, thus making a woman more vulnerable to diabetes, When a group of women were tested after taking the Pill for a year, their blood sugar levels were higher than before they started taking it. [5]

Some diabetics inherit their disease, perhaps through a defect in their ability to use carbohydrates, and some food allergies are implicated in diabetes.

It has been said that our refined Western diet is partly responsible for the high – and rising – incidence of diabetes among us. The lack of fibre in our diet (SEE *Fibre* pages 35–42) is blamed and leading fibre authority Denis Burkitt in his book *Don't Forget Fibre in your Diet* states that diabetes decreases and may even disappear in peoples eating a traditional wholefood diet.

Between 1941 and 1954, when the use of high-fibre National flour was compulsory, the diabetic mortality rate in Britain fell by 54%.

Our rocketing consumption of one particular carbohydrate – refined white sugar – is probably one of the factors in diabetes. We have seen that all refined carbohydrates, especially sucrose, pass quickly into the bloodstream. The pancreas is forced to respond by rapidly pouring out insulin. Too much sugar over-stimulates the pancreas until it is exhausted and cannot produce any more insulin. Result: diabetes.

When the Yemenites are in their native land, the incidence of diabetes among them is 0.06%. When they migrate from the Yemen to Israel, and start eating more sugar and less bread, the incidence rises to 2.6%.[6]

Nutritionist John Yudkin in his book *Pure White and Deadly* suggests that fat consumption may be partly responsible for diabetes. (This may explain the high level of blood fats associated with it.) This theory is difficult to test because when people eat a lot of fat they almost always eat a lot of sugar, too. But Dr J.L. Mount, in his authoritative work *The Food and Health of Western Man*, writes, 'Over-nutrition and that derived particularly from the consumption of fats, sugars and refined carbohydrates is the most important nutritional aetiological factor in maturity onset diabetes.'

Really fat people have a very high level of insulin.[7] This high production of insulin demands a lot from the pancreas, which again may get exhausted, and refuse to produce any more. Many obese people can control their diabetes simply by losing weight, thereby relieving the pancreas of its extra burden.

Gorging huge meals will make you fat. But it's also risky if you are a potential diabetic. The metabolic stress carries with it high blood sugar and high demands for insulin, with the eventual possibility of pancreatic exhaustion.

The condition of low blood sugar, or hypoglycaemia, is

more common now (SEE *Low Blood Sugar* pages 340–5). It can follow eating a meal with a lot of refined carbohydrates, including sugar. The symptoms, which appear two to three hours after eating, are pallor, sweating, nervousness, tremor and hunger. This may be a prelude to diabetes, because it is thought to involve a stressed pancreas and poor control of insulin release.

Nutrition and diabetes: an up-to-date approach

Diabetes is two diseases. Speaking about it, Dr Evan Shute, Director of the Shute Foundation for Medical Research in Canada, said, 'one disease is high blood sugar, treated by diet and insulin and all that sort of thing. All that does is to usher in the ugly second half of the disease, degeneration of blood vessels, and this is what kills. This is what knocks out the eyes and the kidneys and the heart and produces gangrene.'[8]

There has been a lot of recent work on the many ways of using nutrition in diabetes, both to lower the insulin and tablet dosage and to minimize or cut out the ugly complications. Of course, many diabetics would die without their injected insulin or anti-diabetic drugs. But in view of the potential harm in this medication, the more the dosage can safely be lowered, the better.

Current nutritional research into diabetes is taking in a wide range of vitamins and minerals.

For unknown reasons, diabetics are unable to turn carotene, the precursor of vitamin A, into a form of A that can be used by the body. They are advised to take vitamin A in its preformed state – in fish liver oils, or as a supplement.[9]

In laboratory animals, diabetes can be produced very quickly by making them deficient in vitamin B6. This deficiency means that an amino acid, tryptophan, which needs B6 to be correctly used by the body, will turn into xanthurenic acid. This acid can interfere with the carbohydrate-insulin balance in many ways, thus creating diabetes. The mineral magnesium is needed to help the B6 to work, and a high intake of saturated fats increases the body's need for both B6 and magnesium.

Diabetics have lower blood levels of B6 than normal and when a group was given this vitamin as a supplement[10] some of their symptoms disappeared. Vitamin B6 is also intimately concerned with arterial health, and arterial damage can be massive in the diabetic. In the *Journal of the American Geriatrics Society* Dr R. Levine writes that 70% of the deaths in diabetic patients are the direct result of blood vessel disease.[11]

Another B vitamin helpful in diabetes is folic acid. Diabetics given 5mg of this vitamin daily noticed an improvement in both eyesight and general circulation after four weeks.[12]

Lecithin is an excellent source of the B vitamins choline and inositol which are important for arterial health. It helps the body to make use of B6 and magnesium and contains plenty of the essential fatty acid, linoleic acid. Linoleic acid, according to some Dutch research,[13] may protect against retinopathy and it also seems to protect diabetics against heart attacks. Lecithin is made by the body and is also available as a supplement (SEE pages 121–3).

Vitamin C has been found valuable in the treatment of diabetes. Dr George V. Mann, writing in *Perspectives in Biology and Medicine* for winter 1974, recommends extra vitamin C for the diabetic. He explains that we all need insulin for another purpose – to transport vitamin C into certain cells. Impaired insulin output, therefore, will lead to impaired transport of vitamin C, which can cause blood vessel abnormalities and make the already defective circulation worse. Natural insulin output has often increased when diabetics have taken supplementary vitamin C, and one man was able to stop his insulin injections altogether by taking 4g a day.

Vitamin E is very valuable for diabetics. Dr Evan Shute of the Shute Foundation states that no diabetic is being treated at all unless he takes vitamin E. This vitamin is excellent for lessening some of the devastating vascular damage accompanying this condition. Writing in *The Complete Book of Vitamins*, Shute's brother Dr Wilfrid Shute recommends 800 to 1600 I.U. of E a day to prevent the massive arterial degeneration in diabetes which can even lead to gangrene and the amputation of a limb.

Swedish tests have established that vitamin E is also effective for another circulatory disease, intermittent claudication, often found in diabetics. There was less pain and patients were able to walk greater distances after treatment. It is effective against diabetic retinopathy, too. In all these circulatory problems, vitamin E helps to stop the platelets in the bloodstream from clogging together when they should not.[14]

When 300 to 600 I.U. a day are given, vitamin E can also help diabetics to decrease their insulin requirements.

The bioflavonoids (also known as vitamin P) can inhibit the formation of diabetic cataracts, and garlic may lower high blood sugar (SEE *Garlic* pages 114–15).

The main mineral being used for diabetes is chromium. Chromium works together with insulin in the metabolism of glucose; it is essential before the body can use sugar. Chromium deficiencies induced in laboratory animals impaired their ability to use sugar, and added chromium corrected this problem. A report drawn up by the Royal College of Physicians (*The Medical Aspects of Dietary Fibre*) suggests that diabetes can be improved by feeding chromium and adds that diets with their natural fibre intact contain more chromium. The report warns that refined, heat-processed foods may lead to a deficiency of chromium and a greater susceptibility to diabetes.[15] This is yet another recommendation for the whole grains and raw foods in a wholefood diet.

Consultant Alec Forbes tells me that brewer's yeast, which has plenty of chromium, will help many diabetics and some of his elderly patients who take brewer's yeast have been able to stop their drugs. Most of them however have to stay on their diet. Brewer's yeast helps to lower the blood fats and this too is valuable in diabetes. Liver also has plenty of chromium.

Another mineral implicated in diabetes, although not in such a major fashion as chromium, is potassium.

Laboratory animals develop high blood sugar if they are deprived of potassium. Diabetics are often short of this essential mineral. 'Brittle' diabetics, who see-saw very easily from very high to very low blood sugar, lose this instability when they are given potassium, together with extra protein, B2, niacin, pantothenic acid, C, and lecithin.[16] Potassium in the blood will also rise if magnesium is added to the diet. Because they tend to be short of potassium, diabetics should not eat highly salted foods. Too much salt drives out potassium; for a full description of this please SEE the section on *Salt*, pages 57–61.

Shortages of protein, pantothenic acid and vitamin B2 in laboratory animals can reduce the output of insulin, thus interfering with the glucose-coping mechanism in another way. Large amounts of these nutrients – in particular pantothenic acid – will stimulate insulin production. [17] Insulin is made up of amino acids combining to create a lightweight protein structure. Some of these amino acids cannot be made by the body and need to come from the diet, otherwise the person will not be able to manufacture insulin.

The most significant recent discovery in diabetes research has been the importance of fibre.

We have seen that diabetics were formerly advised to stick to a low-carbohydrate diet so that little strain was put on the body's mechanism for producing insulin. Recently, however, it has been found that eating a diet with plenty of *unrefined* carbohydrates is very helpful for the diabetic. This turns the traditional view upside-down.

In his book *Don't Forget Fibre in your Diet* Denis Burkitt states that a high-fibre diet induced a remission of diabetes in about 85% of the patients tested. Eating high-fibre foods slows down the rate of glucose absorption, whereas refined carbohydrates speed it up. This slow absorption of the foods means that insulin is not needed as quickly or in such large amounts. Some patients given high-fibre diets can lower or even discontinue their insulin; for the type 1, more serious diabetic, the insulin can usually only be lowered however and not discontinued. The *British Medical Journal* for 15 December 1979 states that dietary fibre modifies carbohydrate absorption and metabolism in both normal and diabetic individuals. Fibre fills you up more quickly, too, and you tend to eat less – obesity is common in diabetes.

In Lexington, Kentucky, diabetic volunteers ate a high-fibre diet with wholemeal bread, fruit and vegetables. After 14 days, 5 of the 13 men were able to discontinue their drugs, and 4 of the 5 men taking insulin in modest amounts could stop their injections. In a follow-up study 15 months later, 7 of the 10 men then examined still continued on the wholefood diet, without any drugs. [11] This diet not only offered the benefits of natural fibre in the wholemeal bread, but also the nutrients in fruits and vegetables. It has been claimed that diets based on raw foods can allow type 1 diabetics (the severe type) to reduce their insulin dose by 50% to 100%. [19]

The standard dietary advice to diabetics in the past has left them with little carbohydrate and sugar but a lot of fat. High blood fats are associated with diabetes, however; and in view of this, together with the arterial damage and possibility of high blood pressure, a medical Working Party[20] recommends that dietary advice in diabetics should take high blood fat levels into account. It is believed by some researchers that insulin can be cut even further if the diabetic reduces his fat intake as well. A wholefood diet is low in fat.

With all this new nutritional research guiding doctors, they can now start to tackle some of the devastating complications of diabetes, as well as cutting down on the insulin and other drugs which may even be partly responsible for them.

Note: if you are a diabetic and you wish to try a better nutritional approach, *please first consult a qualified naturopath* (SEE appendix, page 405) *or a nutritionally aware doctor, and put yourself in his hands.* Your insulin injections or drugs have been carefully worked out, as has your diet. Should you take foods or supplements which are likely to lower the amount of medication you need, you must be carefully monitored. Your blood sugar, for instance, could fall dangerously low if you go on a high-fibre diet without reducing your insulin accordingly, and you must not cut back on the insulin before the fibre begins to take effect.

Additional therapies

Exercise: mild exercise lowers the blood sugar and can even reduce your insulin need. Please check with your practitioner, especially if you have eye troubles (also consult him about the care of your feet), SEE appendix, page 405.

Herbalism: SEE appendix, page 405.

Homoeopathy: SEE appendix, page 405.

Recommended reading

Diabetes Explained by Dr Arnold Bloom, MPT 1971.

The British Diabetic Association, 10 Queen Anne Street, London W1M 0BD, (telephone 01 323 1531) supply dietary and other advice for diabetics, together with cookbooks and various leaflets.

Other books mentioned in this section

Don't Forget Fibre in Your Diet by Denis Burkitt (Martin Dunitz, USA, 1979).

Pure White and Deadly by John Yudkin (Davis Poynter 1972).

The Food and Health of Western Man by J.L. Mount (Precision Press, 1979).

The Complete Book of Vitamins by Wilfrid Shute (Rodale Press, 1977).

Fatigue

Flat out

It's a familiar feeling. Your muscles ache after an extra set of tennis, or your head is spinning when you finally close that file. Or perhaps you have said goodbye to visiting friends or relatives and, turning back to the house, you feel flat and suddenly tired.

When you have been pouring out physical, intellectual or emotional energies, you expect to feel tired. Physical fatigue is a weary, aching body. If the lactic acid formed during exertion is not removed efficiently from the muscles, they do not function properly and get stiff and painful. Long journeys, noise, extremes of temperature, cramped working conditions with poor lighting and ventilation – or any other stresses – will also deplete your vitality. A good night's sleep, or perhaps a holiday, will dispel all this, and you are ready to tackle things again.

But persistent, crippling fatigue is something different. The bone-weariness that weighs a person down all day, from the morning when he hears the alarm to the time he falls into bed again and tries, perhaps unsuccessfully, to sleep. This kind of fatigue will not yield to sleep and rest and is a constant nagging presence, taking away the joy of living and making everything an effort.

Chronic fatigue can bring with it headaches, insomnia, irritability and difficulty in concentrating, digestive troubles including flatulence, palpitations, occasional dizzy spells, frequent urination, and constipation alternating with diarrhoea. A person may not have all, or any, of these symptoms, but he will always feel a vast tiredness and fatigue affects the whole person. This can be called nervous exhaustion, neurasthenia or – to use a Victorian term – prostration.

When you feel this kind of fatigue, you must first question your state of health. Fatigue can be caused by several specific illnesses including anaemia, thyroid disorders, diabetes, emphysema, arthritis and rheumatism, high blood pressure, liver dysfunction, allergy, inadequate digestion; or it may be hormonal, i.e. related to pre-menstrual tension or the menopause. Fatigue is a side-effect of many drugs, too.

General fatigue, unrelated to definite illness, is a sign of the body's inability to fight back any more against constant stress and tensions, bad living habits and the resultant undermining of health.

Fatigue causes impaired digestion; the digestive system does not have the energy to work normally. Efficient elimination through the bowels, kidneys, skin, lungs, mucous membranes and bloodstream is also impaired when a person is really fatigued. There is less energy for this process; the body therefore accumulates more toxins and the result is lassitude, indecision and mental and physical exhaustion unaffected by rest. The body's attempt to discharge these toxins can clearly be seen in the colds which sometimes accompany fatigue. As well as giving the body a chance to rest by confining the person to bed, a cold can produce a runny nose and phlegm – channels through which the system can discharge some of its wastes.

Fatigue and drugs

A person who is chronically tired will often ask his doctor for a tonic, although the doctor probably knows that this is a pretty pointless exercise. Millions of pounds are spent every year on tonics, many of which are useless. Some tonics contain laxatives and some caffeine, a stimulant drug. If you are always tired a laxative won't help, and caffeine will only flog tired nerves, causing more exhaustion after its effects have worn off. A tonic is only good for you if you are determined to feel better, whatever it contains.

Sleeping pills will force you into an unnatural sleep. They cut out the dreaming which is a valuable part of natural sleep, and cause a hangover the morning after. They carry the dangers of side-effects, including addiction.

If your medical practitioner has assured you that there is nothing organically wrong, you can assume responsibility for your own fatigue. You can look into your life and find out what is causing you to be permanently tired so that you can do something about it. Fatigue is a sign which each person must learn to recognize and interpret for himself; you are the only one who can feel it and you cannot prove its presence to your doctor. Now is the time to do something about it before it develops into a real illness. 'Fatigue', says naturopath Harry

Clements, 'is the first step in the making of practically all forms of disease.'[1]

Stress

A long period of chronic worry can cause nervous exhaustion. Negative emotions – rage, anxiety, frustration, fear – are stresses and will result in fatigue, especially if they are bottled up. Readers may be interested to turn to the section on *Stress*.

Boredom and depression are exhausting too. A job which you do not enjoy will tire you far more rapidly than work you find rewarding. World authority on stress Hans Selye believes that a good night's sleep will follow a rewarding day which is winding to a peaceful close. A day spent on a frustrating task which does not satisfy you and which you cannot finish will keep you awake.

If you are using your body incorrectly through permanently tensed muscles, poor posture and lack of exercise, then you are likely to feel tired (SEE *Additional Therapies* at the end of this section for exercise and relaxation).

Nutrition and fatigue

The commonest single cause of fatigue is iron-deficiency anaemia. Things are not as simple as this however – iron needs other nutrients in order to be properly used by the body. Copper facilitates iron uptake, vitamin E helps maintain the circulation which distributes the iron, and zinc makes iron more available to the tissues. Iron cannot be absorbed without vitamin C. You can get anaemic symptoms from a deficiency of manganese, and it can also be caused by shortages of the B vitamins, notably B6 and folic acid. Pernicious anaemia can be caused by a lack of B12.

Another common cause of fatigue is low blood sugar. Briefly, the over-consumption of refined sugars and refined starches puts a strain on the pancreas, which secretes insulin to deal with them. As time goes on the pancreas may over-react to a large intake of sugar by pouring out too much insulin. The blood sugar level, instead of being adequately controlled, is then forced down too low by the over-abundance of insulin. This makes the person more exhausted than ever, and he craves more sugar to give him some quick energy. Eating this sugar will put up his blood sugar and the whole vicious circle starts all over again. These heavy demands on the pancreas can be a forerunner of diabetes. (For more information, SEE the section *Low Blood Sugar*.)

Low blood sugar can follow a breakfast of, say, doughnuts and sweet coffee. The blood sugar is sent soaring by the refined sugar and starches in this meal, but it soon drops to a low level and the person feels tired and wobbly and needs more coffee to pull him round. To use the carbohydrates in this breakfast, the body needs a number of B vitamins, notably B1. These nutrients have been partly removed from the flour and sugar in the doughnuts and coffee during the refining process. When you eat foods from which these nutrients are missing, the carbohydrates cannot be properly metabolized and a by-product, pyruvic acid, accumulates in the tissues and causes fatigue. Refined sugars and carbohydrates, therefore, give the body raw materials for plenty of energy, but they do not supply the vitamins which would enable that energy to be used. Fats and proteins supply energy too, but we cannot use the energy stored in these nutrients either unless there are enough vitamins (principally the B vitamins) and minerals present to activate it. (Minerals help the enzymes to change body fat into energy.) These vitamins and minerals are found in unrefined starches and sugars.

The best safeguard against all this is a good breakfast. That old tag about a cooked breakfast being the best is nonsense. After all, you could fry a couple of bootlaces and call it a cooked breakfast. It's the content that matters. Protein, wholegrain cereals, wholemeal bread, a little molasses or dark brown sugar, some milk and yogurt and some fruit – these are the best for you (SEE *Food Therapy* section pages 396–401). A good breakfast produces a slow, steady rise in blood sugar and sustains you throughout the morning. It also helps you to cut down on your calories for lunch and supper; the earlier in the day you take your calories, the more are used up and the fewer stored as fat. To say that energy depends only on the number of calories we eat, therefore, is a pretty crude way of looking at it.

All unrefined cereals and unprocessed sugars such as brown sugar and molasses will give you energy safely without a letdown afterwards. Honey, however, can be quite lethal if you suffer from low blood sugar (SEE *Low Blood Sugar* pages 340–5). The carbohydrates in fruits and vegetables are also energy sources to some extent. All these foods are found in a whole food diet (SEE *Whole Foods* pages 101–6).

The best energy-producing foods are liver and brewer's yeast. Both have lots of B vitamins. The liver is very rich in iron and copper and brewer's yeast has plenty of potassium; a lack of this mineral can cause fatigue too.

Specific vitamins to help with fatigue are vitamin C, all the B vitamins especially B1 and pantothenic acid, and probably also pangamic acid, also called vitamin B15. The Russians, who have researched pangamic acid, give it to their athletes; it is said to increase stamina and to help the transport of oxygen round the body. Lecithin (SEE index) can also be useful for fatigue. This does not mean that these isolated substances will give you energy by themselves. But, used as part of an excellent diet, they may help your body to function a little more efficiently. You may have a high individual need for some of these nutrients.

Dealing with chronic fatigue

First, see a naturopath (SEE appendix page 405) or doctor to make sure that your fatigue is not due to an illness for which you need treatment.

If your tiredness is a result of bad living habits over the years, including bad nutrition, then it can be reversed.

One of the best treatments is rest. Of course, rest in bed is valuable. But you should give your *whole body* a rest – and that means a fast. This takes the workload off the digestive and eliminative system. When you are deeply tired, a fast can have an almost miraculous effect.

We have seen that one result of fatigue is the retention of toxins – called by the naturopath 'auto-intoxication'. It is believed that all forms of disease are caused, or encouraged, by auto-intoxication.

Fast, therefore, for one to three days – please read the *Fasting* section first – and stay in bed. If you cannot fast, then eat as lightly as possible; the *Food Therapy* section will give you a dietary plan. Another good way of helping your system to cleanse itself is to eat nothing but fruit for one day every week, drinking nothing but fruit juices and water. If you can, add to this one rest day every month in bed, fasting on fruit juices and water only.

Continue after your fast by following the dietary plan

outlined in the *Food Therapy* section, eating as lightly as possible and remembering to include brewer's yeast and lamb's liver.

However good your food is, it will not nourish you unless you can digest it properly. People often do not chew their food enough and this is a major cause of fatigue. You cannot digest your food, particularly the starches, unless it is thoroughly chewed.

Avoid stimulants such as sugary foods, tea and coffee. These are just whipping a tired horse, and you will be drawing on your reserves until there aren't any left.

Before you decide upon your dietary treatment, it would be sensible for you to read the *Nature Cure* section. Please note that the dietary advice given here is on general lines only, and that you may also need additional vitamins and minerals. For individual guidance on both your dietary plan and any supplementation, please consult a naturopath or a nutritionally aware doctor.

Energy drink
This drink contains virtually all the nutrients which help us to feel energetic. If you wish, you can sprinkle the ingredients on your cereal in the morning and take it that way instead.

A glass of milk or more to taste
one-third of a teaspoon of powdered vitamin C (about 1g)
1 or 2 teaspoons of powdered skimmed milk
1 teaspoon of lecithin granules
half a teaspoon of brewer's yeast
Optional extras: natural yogurt, molasses or dark brown sugar
one egg (several naturopaths recommend taking egg yolk only), orange juice, soya powder.

Mix together with a fork or in a blender, and sip slowly.

Additional therapies
Acupuncture: SEE appendix page 405.
Deep breathing, will relax and revitalize you: SEE appendix page 405.
Exercise, any exercise that you enjoy will give you more stamina and energy: SEE appendix especially *Yoga*, page 405.
Herbalism: SEE appendix page 405.

Homoeopathy: SEE appendix page 405.

Osteopathy: SEE appendix page 405.

Relaxation, much fatigue is caused through chronic muscular tension and negative thinking; SEE appendix, especially *Autogenic Training*, page 405.

Heart and Artery Disease

The killer disease

The Western world has an epidemic on its hands – heart and artery disease. Four out of every ten men will die from coronary heart disease (CHD) and two out of every ten women. Women are less vulnerable (a protective effect may be exerted by the female sex hormones) but the incidence for them is rising, too. Younger and younger men are succumbing to CHD. Arterial degeneration is part and parcel of heart disease, and of 3000 US soldiers under 30 killed in the Korean war, 50% showed some damage to their coronary arteries and 25% marked changes. For middle-aged people, between 45 and 64, the incidence has almost *doubled* in 17 years. Heart disease kills over 100 000 people a year in Britain and is the commonest fatal disease for Western man.

The incidence of CHD is less in the country areas of southern and eastern Europe, and low in Italy. It is higher in northern and western Europe, very rare in China and uncommon in rural India.

Although heart disease now is the greatest epidemic mankind has ever known, it has not always been so. When the electrocardiogram came into general use during the 1920s, CHD was rare.

What is heart and artery disease?

The heart is a pump and the blood vessels supply it with fuel. Keeping the heart muscle going is the most important part of staying alive.

The blood going into the right side of the heart, the right ventricle, is pumped into the lungs, where it gives up carbon dioxide and acquires fresh oxygen. From here it goes back to the left ventricle, which pumps it round the body. After its tour of the body it returns to the heart again and the whole process repeats itself.

The heart muscle is stable, adaptable, resilient and very strong. It depends entirely on its supply of nutrients – principally oxygen – in the blood coming to it through the coronary arteries. This vital blood supply can be impaired in either quantity or quality. The quantity of blood depends on the health of the arteries, and its quality upon nutrition.

Arteries get furred up. Almost all adults in the West are afflicted by artery damage. Atheroma ('porridge') is the name given to the greasy deposits lining the artery walls. These deposits stimulate scar tissue to form around them and the eventual condition is called atherosclerosis, meaning a fatty scar. Atheroma damages the coronary arteries most seriously, and when it affects the arteries to the brain it can result in a stroke.

An unhealthy arterial lining is scarred with cholesterol and calcium so that, as well as fats clogging the arteries, there are mineral deposits. These cause the hardening and loss of elasticity known as arteriosclerosis. Because of the damaged blood vessels, blood cannot move smoothly along and tends to clot; this is a thrombosis. Obstruction of a coronary artery is coronary thrombosis. Sometimes debris breaks off the artery walls, wandering round the body perhaps to plug a smaller artery somewhere else. Rarely, a large artery may begin to tear at a weak spot.

When the coronary arteries have been narrowed and made less efficient in this way, the blood supply to the heart is affected. When the body is under stress, the heart is asked to do extra work and it will therefore need extra blood. If the blood supply is impaired enough, the heart will either stop for lack of oxygen or the part of it supplied by that particular damaged artery will die. (Clotting, added to arterial damage, can also cause a heart attack or a stroke.)

Blocking of the coronary arteries, which starves the heart, is the commonest cause of heart failure. When part of the heart muscle dies because its associated artery is blocked, this is called myocardial infarction. The patient may die at once, or his heart may start beating in the wrong way, or it may slowly fail so that he eventually dies. Some people recover from one heart attack but succumb to a second one; some will have a series of attacks, and a few only one, and nothing more for the rest of their lives. A person can suffer the death of part of his heart muscle without having had an obvious heart attack.

Angina pectoris means 'pain in the chest'. The patient has probably been asking a lot of his heart through unaccustomed exercise or other stress. Because the arteries are damaged and cannot open up properly, enough oxygen cannot reach the heart and this causes pain. Once the heart is allowed to relax its extra efforts, the pain will stop. Angina can sometimes be caused by intense cold, which makes a coronary artery go into spasm. The angina sufferer usually has a whole series of attacks.

Causes

As with most chronic degenerative conditions, cardio-vascular disease has many possible causes. These are believed to be:

1 diet
2 obesity
3 lack of exercise
4 cigarette smoking
5 stress
6 body type; sex, age; inherited factors
7 associated disease – high blood pressure, high blood fats, diabetes, gout
8 The Pill. Professor Martin Vessey states that there is a definite relationship between venous thrombosis, stroke and coronary thrombosis in young women and oral contraceptives.

New hearts for old

In the *Evening Standard* for 2 September 1980, Dr Peter Draper, Director of the Unit for the Study of Health Policy at Guy's Hospital, made the headlines with 'Stop This Heart Transplant Epidemic'. In the first half of 1980 there had been a number of highly publicized heart transplants, but Dr Draper argued that the number of patients who are suitable for heart transplants, and would survive a reasonable length of time after the operation, is insignificant compared with the thousands who die every year from heart disease. He was supported by Alastair Mackie, Director-General of the Health Education Council, who commented that however good coronary surgery may be, it will always be limited to very few people; and the condition of many heart sufferers *can be prevented.*

Heart transplants are dramatic – but very expensive. And of course you not only have to have a suitable patient, you also need a spare heart. The new heart of the most famous transplant patient, Dr Philip Blaiberg, was taken from a 20-year old man. But after only 12 months inside Blaiberg, it was more severely affected by artery damage than his old one had been after more than 60 years.[1] Accelerated hardening of the arteries is a real risk after heart transplant operations, probably triggered in some way by the antibodies involved in the body's attempts to reject tissue which is not its own.

There are two hospitals in England carrying out heart transplants, Papworth and Harefield. At Papworth Hospital, 41 heart transplants have been carried out since 1 January 1979 and 24 patients are still alive. At Harefield, 41 heart transplants have been carried out since 31 January 1980 and 19 patients are still surviving. This means that out of 82 patients, 39 – almost half – have died during the three years and ten months since the transplants have started (written on 28 October 1982). A heart transplant operation, including post-operative care, costs about £20,000.

In a coronary by-pass operation, the surgeon puts in vessel grafts which bypass blockages in the coronary arteries feeding the heart. Studies show that up to 20% of these grafts clog up during the first year after surgery, and that those who have this operation rarely live any longer than those who don't.[2]

A purely mechanical heart is being researched for insertion into the patient's body, and pacemakers, which force the heart to keep going, are commonplace now.

Some drugs

Digitalis and related drugs such as digoxin and digitoxin cause the heart muscles to work more efficiently and reduce the heart rate. Side-effects can be appetite loss, nausea and vomiting, diarrhoea, stomach pains, headache, drowsiness and fatigue. in *Medicines: A Guide for Everybody* Peter Parish warns that digitalis and related drugs cause symptoms of intoxication when taken in high doses, and can even prove fatal.

Disorders of heart rhythm can be treated by quinidine (Quincardine, Auriquin). Its use should be preceded by a test, since many patients are hypersensitive to it. Even small doses can cause ear noises, vertigo, visual disturbances, headache, confusion, skin rashes, swelling of the throat, vomiting, cramps and diarrhoea. Asthma and breathing arrest may occur, and the blood pressure may fall rapidly, causing collapse. It can cause irregular heartbeat and death.

Amyl nitrite and glyceryl trinitrate (nitroglycerin, trinitrin, Sustac) have been used for years for angina pectoris. They dilate the blood vessels, improving the blood flow, and reduce the workload of the heart so that it needs less oxygen. High doses reduce the passage of blood to and from the heart to such an extent that a person may faint if he remains standing after taking the drug.

Beta-receptor drugs block the receptors which make the heart beat faster. They can make heart block worse, and can cause constriction of the bronchial tubes in asthma, bronchospasm and bronchitis. They can trigger off heart failure in patients who are near to it and their sudden discontinuance has caused heart attacks.

A drug to lower blood fat levels, clofibrate (Atromid-S), was the subject of long-term trials by the World Health Organization. The newspaper *General Practitioner* reported in its issue of 22 August 1980, 'Deaths up to 25% in Clofibrate Trial' and went on to describe a major long-term trial using the drug clofibrate in which 25 per cent more of the men given the drug died than died in a control group. This resulted in a clofibrate ban in West Germany and Norway, and tighter restrictions on its use in the UK. It is *still being prescribed* here for certain illnesses.[3]

The heart and nutrition

We have seen that there are many factors influencing the health of the heart and arteries and that diet, however important, is only one of them. The area of nutrition and heart disease is fraught with argument; some people even deny that there is any relationship between the two. A balanced view is that heart and artery disease have many causes. We must not over-simplify the issue by believing that all cases of CHD have a solely nutritional origin. Commenting on the arguments about causes, Ian Kennedy said in his 1980 Reith Lectures *Unmasking Medicine* that, 'Indeed, if we are to wait until the perfect controlled experiment has demonstrated that it is factor X which is the real killer, preventive medicine will have to await the millenium.' Preventing heart and artery disease is too important to wait that long; it is literally a matter of life and death.

To improve the cardiovascular health of people in general would be less dramatic than a heart transplant and less toxic than a drug. Nutrition plays a vital part in the arrest and even the reversal of heart and artery disease, and we can all do something about what we eat.

Heart development and nutrition begin before birth. Dietary deficiencies induced in laboratory animals can result in a vast number of deformities, including a deformed heart and blood vessels.

Fats   Most of us believe that the fat cholesterol is a frightful villain, existing only to line our arteries. Cholesterol is in fact an essential substance, both made inside us (mainly by the liver) and eaten in our food. It is found in saturated fats; these are mostly the fats from meat and dairy products which are hard at room temperature. It is true that cholesterol, circulating in the bloodstream, will sometimes settle down on the artery lining and cause arterial plaque. So the argument runs: avoid eating cholesterol-rich foods, and you will avoid getting a cholesterol lining.

This works to some extent – but it is sometimes found that cutting out cholesterol completely simply encourages our bodies to manufacture more of it. So it looks as though we can't win.

Cholesterol, however, is not an arch-fiend. It is a substance which, in certain circumstances, can behave in a harmful way inside us. A high blood level of cholesterol *can* be dangerous, and most research is concerned with lowering it. But many people who never develop CHD have a high blood cholesterol. And a high blood cholesterol, moving along with the bloodstream, is not the same thing as arteries lined with porridgy cholesterol deposits. So there must be a reason why this fat should put us in real danger by forming lumps and attaching itself to our blood vessels.

Cholesterol only clogs up the arteries when it is allowed to do so through incorrect nutrition. The right food means that the bloodstream will deal with cholesterol in the right way, passing it smoothly along.

'The evidence shows', writes Roger J. Williams in *Nutrition Against Disease*, 'that high fat consumption, when accompanied by plenty of the essential nutrients which all cells need, does *not* cause atherosclerosis or heart disease.' It is true that under ordinary dietary conditions laboratory animals will accumulate cholesterol deposits if they are fed a lot of saturated fats. But if they are fed the same amount of fats (61.6% of the total diet), *plus plenty of protein, minerals and vitamins*, no pathological changes are seen in the principal aorta artery or in the heart. (They do get obese, however.[4]) These findings are supported by work at the Tufts University School of Medicine.[5] Further, a study of the Masai tribe in Tanzania showed that, although they eat almost nothing but milk and meat, both with plenty of saturated fat and cholesterol, there was no artery or heart disease among them. Significantly, their diet also contains plenty of vitamins and minerals.[6]

Fats, therefore, are an important factor in heart disease, but other nutritional factors matter just as much.

We have also been led to believe that polyunsaturated fatty acids protect the heart. Is this true?

There is little doubt that in favourable dietary conditions *unrefined* polyunsaturated fats and oils do indeed lower the blood cholesterol. This effect depends to some extent on the presence of other nutrients, including protein and vitamin B6. Definite evidence is lacking that polyunsaturates will lower the incidence of actual deaths from heart disease.

But, like too much saturated fat, too much polyunsaturated fat is harmful. Increasing the amount of polyunsaturates puts up the body's need for the antioxidants – substances which are naturally present in these fats and oils. This would not matter if the polyunsaturates were in their original unrefined state, complete with their anti-oxidants (vitamin E and selenium) and other vitamins and minerals. In refined oils, however (and in refined white flour too), these anti-oxidants are processed out. (Please SEE the *Fats* section pages 23–35 for further information.)

Ceroid pigments are an early accompaniment of cardio-vascular disease. These harmful brown deposits are prevented from forming by vitamin E and other anti-oxidants. A diet high in *refined* polyunsaturates, therefore, will not only increase the body's need for the vitamin E and other nutrients which are the fat's natural accompaniments but, because it does not supply these nutrients, it will encourage the formation of ceroid pigments.

Not only have the refined oils been stripped of their natural anti-oxidants; they have also been heated to very high temperatures during the refining process. Discussing research into this, Roger J. Williams writes, 'The indiscriminate eating of polyunsaturated vegetable oils . . . must be strongly condemned. The above data are highly suggestive that unheated [i.e. unrefined] vegetable oils . . . are protective against atherosclerosis. Heated oils – oils that have been subjected to temperatures of 215 degrees centigrade for 15 minutes or longer – are another source of danger to the cardio-vascular system.'[7] Refined oils are commonly held above this temperature for several hours during processing. He goes on to warn that most commercial 'polyunsaturated' vegetable oils are possibly productive of atherosclerosis and should be avoided by the consumer.

Fat consumption has risen over the past 70 years. So has the incidence of heart and artery disease. There is very probably a connection. But it's no good simply substituting lots of poly-unsaturated fats and oils for the saturated fat in our diet. We must make sure that as many of our polyunsaturated fats as possible are unrefined – and that means sticking to unrefined, 'cold-pressed' oils and wholemeal bread. (Unhydrogenated margarines are obtainable from some health food stores.) And we must also cut down our *total* consumption of fat. Cutting total fats in the diet has been clearly shown to cut the risk of heart disease.[8]

A recently researched group of fatty acids from fish oils (EPA and DHA – SEE *Fats*, page 23) has been shown to lower high blood cholesterol levels, prevent platelets from over-stickiness and raise the amount of HDLs in the blood. Some doctors, therefore, are recommending cod liver oil now for heart and artery disease.

All the nutrients are involved in a healthy cardiovascular system. Before we look at some others, let's deal with two suspect foods – sugar and salt, and with everybody's villains, alcohol and tobacco.

Sugar   The scientist most responsible for giving sugar a bad name is John Yudkin. He writes in *The Lancet* (2: 155, 1957) that too much sugar is statistically associated with artery disease and heart attacks. Refined sugar seems to be more harmful than white flour and its products.

Sugar can be blamed indirectly for heart and artery disease.

A high consumption of sugar makes you fat. Obesity increases the work the heart has to do, thus making you more vulnerable to heart disease. (This is probably a less potent risk, however, than high blood pressure or diabetes, which often go with heart disease.) This theory is difficult to test because people who eat a lot of fat usually eat a lot of sugar as well; in rich foods the two go together. Indeed sugar and fats may act upon each other. When sugar is added to an already high-fat diet, the blood cholesterol will go up still more. So don't add sugar to your Cornish cream.

Sugar is generally believed to be only a contributory factor in the direct causation of heart disease. A Medical Research Council report concludes that the evidence in favour of a high sugar intake as a major factor in the development of heart attacks is extremely slender (*Lancet*, 2: 1965, 1970).

Salt Salt has also been implicated, somewhat tenuously, in heart disease. It appears that too much salt can put up the blood fats.[9] Since a lot of salt can induce high blood pressure, which makes heart disease more likely, it can be blamed indirectly as well. Too much salt also creates a deficiency of the mineral potassium. Potassium is essential for heart action, and the greatest harm from a severe potassium deficiency is its effect on the heart.

Alcohol, coffee, tobacco People who drink a lot of alcohol often have high blood fats; alcohol readily changes into saturated fat, and can cause the amount of blood fat to double.[10] Those who drink five cups or more of coffee a day are more likely to develop heart disease,[11] and heavy cigarette smokers are five times more likely to die from coronary disease than non-smokers.[12]

On the positive side, let's look at the nutrients most involved in keeping the heart and arteries healthy.

Lecithin This soap-like substance (SEE *Lecithin* pages 121–3) is made by the liver. It is also available as a supplement. To manufacture lecithin, the body needs methionine (an amino acid), sugars, fats, and the B vitamins B6, choline and inositol. Lecithin protects against artery damage by preventing fatty arterial deposits and inhibits blood clotting. When an ounce of lecithin a day was taken by volunteers for three months, their blood cholesterol levels dropped.[13] Some patients with coronary thrombosis were found to have low blood levels of lecithin.[14]

Vitamin E   According to Dr Wilfrid E. Shute, cardiologist at the Shute Foundation for Medical Research in Canada, vitamin E is a safe answer to angina pectoris. He has used it for many thousands of heart patients and in *The Complete Book of Vitamins* he writes, 'That vitamin E will save lives from myocardial infarction and from heart failure must now be accepted by all physicians.' American nutritionist Dr Richard A. Passwater states that a vitamin E deficiency produces 'marked alterations in heart metabolism'.

Vitamin E decreases oxygen need, helping the heart muscle to function when less oxygen is reaching it through narrowed arteries. Shute states that it also speeds up the opening of collateral circulation round damaged veins and arteries and that for this reason it is valuable after a heart attack. Mexican tests showed a reduction of angina pectoris with a combination of vitamin E and the mineral selenium.

Blood must be able to clot, otherwise we would bleed to death. But for some people their blood clots too readily. They can develop spontaneous clots inside the blood vessels, and if the clot lodges itself somewhere lethal this can lead to a stroke or heart attack. Anticoagulants, which keep the blood from clotting too much, can cause dangerous bleeding, but vitamin E has the same action and is harmless. Blood platelets, involved in clotting, sometimes clump together in a web right across a blood vessel, and vitamin E reduces this to some extent. Surplus platelets are often found linked with heart attack and stroke, after surgery and in Pill takers. They are also suspected of disrupting the electrical impulses which keep the heart beating as it should.

Listing all the cardiovascular benefits of vitamin E, it

1   conserves oxygen
2   opens up collateral circulation
3   contains anti-clotting factors
4   reduces blood cholesterol
5   strengthens the walls of the small blood vessels.

Incidentally, the American figures for heart disease are slightly lower now. The margarine companies gleefully claim that this is all due to the swing to polyunsaturated fats. But the Shute Foundation observes that about 30 million Americans are regularly taking extra vitamin E. The choice is yours.

(Large doses of vitamin E can sometimes influence the

blood pressure slightly, so ask your naturopath or doctor for guidance on dosage.)

Vitamin C No heart or blood vessel can stay healthy without vitamin C. It is essential for the building of connective tissue (collagen). High doses of C reduce blood cholesterol levels[15] and this vitamin also inhibits cholesterol build up on the artery walls. Some authorities relate arterial degeneration in general to a deficiency of vitamin C. Heart attack victims admitted to hospital show a severe deficiency of vitamin C in their blood; the vitamin has gone to the heart to help repair it.[16] Vitamin C reduces the post-operative risk of clots, encourages healing and helps relieve the effects of stress.

Cadmium is a toxic metal. Autopsy examinations of stroke victims carried out by Dr Isabel H. Tipton at the university of Tennessee showed that these people had high cadmium levels in their bodies. Vitamin C is an excellent detoxifier of this poisonous mineral.

The Bioflavonoids Sometimes called vitamin P, these substances are closely related to vitamin C and are found with it in foods. They help protect against clotting and arterial degeneration and, with C, have been used to reduce artery damage.

Vitamin B6 This vitamin is intimately involved with arterial health and therefore with a healthy heart. It helps to control the blood cholesterol level and prevent cholesterol from forming arterial plaques. It is highly likely that among heart patients a B6 deficiency is widespread; low levels have been found in human atherosclerotic tissue.[17] Laboratory animals deprived of B6 quickly develop artery damage. In *Nutrition Against Disease*, Roger J. Williams states that a sufficiency of this vitamin has a high priority in the avoidance of artery disease.

If we eat extra fat, we need more B6.[18] So a high-fat diet is not only potentially damaging to the heart and arteries in a direct way. It acts indirectly too by creating a higher need for vitamin B6, vital for cardiovascular health. Refined foods are often denuded of their B6 – and other B vitamins too. It is milled out of white flours, and is also destroyed by the contraceptive Pill.

Folic acid Folic acid given to patients with hardened arteries dilated the smaller arteries, and X-rays showed that these smaller arteries were then able to carry additional blood which was not getting through the clogged major blood vessels.[19]

Thiamine (vitamin B1)   This is another B vitamin essential for a healthy heart. Victims of heart failure were found to have less thiamine in their heart muscle than those dying of other causes.[20] In their book *The Avitaminoses* Doctors Walter H. Eddy and Gilbert Dalldorf state that a thiamine deficiency impairs heart function, increases the build-up of extravascular fluid, and can even cause a heart attack.

Thiamine is used by the body to metabolize refined sugars and starches (unrefined carbohydrates bring their own thiamine). So a diet high in refined carbohydrates can, by causing a thiamine deficiency, contribute indirectly to heart disease.

Niacin

After a person has had a heart attack, the level of free fatty acids in the blood more than doubles. This can cause heart irregularities and yet more injury. Niacin given to patients after a heart attack will lower the free fatty acids and prevent further damage (*Lancet*, 27 February 1975). Writing in the *Medical Tribune* for 12 June 1974, Dr Rowe hoped that niacin would be used routinely for heart attack victims.

The other B vitamins, choline and inositol, are involved with cardiovascular health as well. They help the body to manufacture the substance which helps to clear the bloodstream and arteries – lecithin.

Minerals

Calcium is essential for the heartbeat. Vitamin D is needed by the body to store and use calcium; we therefore need both these nutrients.

In patients with angina pectoris and coronary thrombosis, magnesium injections brought about a dramatic clinical improvement. Blood fat levels also fell to normal in many cases.[21]

The balance of magnesium and calcium is important; if the calcium level is high, magnesium needs to be plentiful too. But although calcium is added to white bread, magnesium is not. This can put up the need for magnesium and a deficiency of this mineral is probably widespread.

Potassium is needed by the heart. This is also a mineral which we tend to lack – it is refined out of our grains, and we do not eat enough of the vegetables and fruits in which it is found. Eating a lot of salt will drive potassium out of the body, too, so we should cut down on salt and eat plenty of whole grains, vegetables and fruits, to ensure that the heart gets plenty of potassium (SEE *Salt* pages 57–61).

Research has found that there are more deaths from heart disease in areas with soft water. This may be because magnesium, calcium and trace minerals are found in hard water. [22]

Copper, manganese, chromium and selenium are trace elements which also help to keep the heart and arteries healthy.
Evening primrose oil   This oil has been given to heart patients with good results (SEE *Evening Primrose Oil* pages 111–14).
Fibre   The dietary fibre found in wholegrain flour, vegetables and fruits protects against cardiovascular disease. Fibre reduces cholesterol absorption from foods and increases the elimination of bile acids. During long-term studies of 337 middle-aged men, it was found that those eating the most fibre had the lowest incidence of heart disease (*British Medical Journal*, 19 November 1977). People on high-fibre diets tend to have lower blood cholesterol levels, and American volunteers lowered their blood fat levels (and lost weight) after only eight weeks on a high-fibre diet.

Among rural Africans, heart disease is almost unknown and it is uncommon in most rural Asian communities. Most of these people eat unrefined grains from which the fibre has not been milled.

One particular kind of fibre is pectin, found mostly in the skin and rind of citrus fruits and in sunflower seeds. It lowers blood cholesterol and increases the amount of cholesterol eliminated. [23]

Prevention – general dietary advice
We have seen that fats, sugar and too much salt are best avoided for a healthy heart and arteries, and that natural fibre should be included. We have also discussed the major vitamins and minerals involved.

But cardiovascular health is not just a matter of cutting out some things and adding others. No essential mineral, amino acid or vitamin can safely be left out when considering nutrition and heart disease.

Can heart and artery disease be prevented by, among other

factors, an informed interest in what we eat? 'In a large measure, yes. The ideal diet would be low or absent in sugar, low in refined carbohydrates, low in animal fat and high in vegetables and fruit, writes Dr James Lambert Mount in *The Food and Health of Western Man*. This is the kind of diet followed by tribes like Los Viejos in Southern Ecuador and the Hunzas in India, who live long and remarkably healthy lives. A study of the Hunzas revealed that 25 people between the ages of 90 and 100 had *no signs of heart or artery disease at all*.[24] Doubtless other factors contribute to this record, but nutrition is among the most important.

Wholefood eating therefore – with its unrefined cereals, low fat, sugar and salt, and high vegetable and fruit content – is the best nutritional protection for the cardiovascular system (SEE *Whole Foods* pages 101–6).

What about meat? Vegetarian eating lowers blood cholesterol.[25] Vegetable protein contains carbohydrates which can manufacture various B vitamins in the gut, including vitamin B6.[26] The Seventh Day Adventists, a strict religious group about half of whom are vegetarians, have a lower than average incidence of cardiovascular disease.[27]

Large meals strain your metabolism and a heart attack can be triggered off by an eating binge. Eat little and often – avoid excess.

Cure?

F.R. Ellis and T. Sanders, writing in *The Lancet* (29 May 1976) describe their dietary treatment of four patients with severe angina pectoris. The patients were put on a vegan diet (without animal or dairy products). All four were cured and able to lead strenuous lives by the fifth or sixth month of treatment.

In her book *Let's Get Well*, Adelle Davis states that when lecithin is given to laboratory animals, fatty deposits on the arterial walls quickly disappear. Roger J. Williams agrees with this, saying that lecithin acts to inhibit or improve atherosclerosis.[28] It seems, then, that it is possible to clear obstructed arteries.

Nathan Pritikin takes patients with advanced heart and artery disease and other chronic degenerative diseases at his Longevity Center near Los Angeles, California.

Patients are carefully tested both when they arrive and when they leave. This painstaking record-keeping means that

Pritikin can justify his claims that his treatment can both halt and often reverse these diseases. The Center has been operating for about five years and has treated well over 1000 patients.

The Pritikin programme involves a strict diet – wholegrains, vegetables, pulses and fruit, with a little skimmed milk. No coffee, egg yolk, refined sugar, added salt, alcohol or tobacco are permitted. Patients are given carefully graded exercises and encouraged to do plenty of walking.

This approach to cardiovascular disease is slowly gaining ground and doctors are starting to find that it works. It has long been advocated by naturopaths.

If you suffer from heart and artery disease, you are advised to follow the *Food Therapy* plan (pages 396–401). This complies with the nutritional guidelines already discussed. Please observe the following modifications:

1   Cut out all cow's milk. American cardiologist Dr Oster has discovered that an enzyme found in cow's milk, xanthine oxidase, can attack the arterial walls, causing the body to lay down cholesterol deposits to cover over the damage. Soya milk is an excellent substitute.

2   Try to cut out meat and dairy products too. This means that your diet will be vegan. You will probably find the section on *Vegetarian and Vegan Eating* (pages 209–16) of interest.

Please also put yourself in the hands of a qualified naturopath or a nutritionally aware doctor. The dietary treatment is on general lines only and you may need supplements and individual guidance. Please read the section on *Nature Cure* pages 391–6).

Many factors enter into heart and artery disease and you are recommended to ask your practitioner about the additional therapies listed below.

Additional therapies

Acupuncture: SEE appendix page 405.

Exercise, physical activity protects against heart disease: SEE appendix page 405.

Herbalism: SEE appendix page 405.

Homoeopathy: SEE appendix page 405.

Osteopathy, general treatment to help circulation: SEE appendix page 405.

Relaxation, in particular Autogenic Training: SEE appendix page 405. Stress is an important factor in heart disease, but hard to measure. Personality plays a part – the pushing, aggressive person who is unable to relax is believed to be more likely to have a heart attack. Stress experienced as negative feelings can cause the blood fats to soar in a few minutes. Please SEE the section on *Stress*, pages 378–81.

Water-therapy: ask your practitioner about this.

Recommended reading
The Pritikin Program of Diet and Exercise by Nathan Pritikin (Bantam Books, 1981).

Other books mentioned in this section
Medicines: A Guide for Everybody by Peter Parish (Penguin 1980).
Nutrition Against Disease by Roger J. Williams (Bantam 1978).
The Complete Book of Vitamins by Wilfrid Shute (Rodale Press 1977).
The Avitaminoses by Walter H. Eddy and Gilbert Dalldorf.
The Food and Health of Western Man by James Lambert Mount (Precision Press 1979).
Let's Get Well by Adelle Davis (Unwin 1975).

High Blood Pressure

Blood pressure
Blood pressure is the force exerted by the bloodstream against the walls of the blood vessels – like the pressure that water exerts against the inside of a garden hose. This force pushes nutrients through the porous capillary walls into the tissues of the body and is therefore vital for the normal nutrition of cells.

The arteries begin at the heart, where they are very wide, and blood pressure is measured in the arm where the pulse of the heart is easily felt. The heartbeat forces blood through the arteries, which get smaller as they reach to the farthest parts of the body and the head. After its beat, the heart rests for a moment and during this momentary rest the elastic arteries, which have expanded to let the blood through, contract slightly.

Measurement of blood pressure comes in two parts. The first part is the systolic pressure – the pressure that your blood exerts against the sides of the blood vessels when your heart is pumping it through. The second, diastolic, pressure is that exerted when your heart is at rest between beats.

The range of normal blood pressure is between 100 systolic and 60 diastolic (expressed as 100/60) and 140/90. Blood pressure can fluctuate considerably – after eating (even after a cup of coffee), when making love, and in response to factors like the time of day. Blood pressure rises in response to any form of stress (strenuous physical effort for instance) so that extra nourishment can pass from the blood into the tissues. Some people's blood pressure rises simply because the doctor is taking it; this is called 'white coat' hypertension.

High blood pressure

Some people have naturally high blood pressure and are perfectly healthy. This is called residual high blood pressure. There is a marked difference, too, between a natural rise in blood pressure in response to the body's extra demands – which will subside when these demands are met – and permanent, unnecessary hypertension.

Pathological high blood pressure, or hypertension, is one of the epidemics of our time. In 1978, 6895 people died from hypertensive disease in England and Wales.[1] About 10% of the young and middle-aged have symptomless raised blood pressure; the over 65s have more. Most hypertension is dubbed 'essential'; this means that it is not connected with disease in any other part of the body, and does no *apparent* damage to the heart or kidneys. Non-essential hypertension is caused by kidney complaints, hormonal disturbances, circulatory disorders and, rarely, tumours of the adrenal glands.

High blood pressure is not considered to be a disease in itself, but a risk factor in other diseases. It exacerbates the dangers of heart attack, stroke, artery disease and kidney trouble.

The symptoms of high blood pressure are often very fleeting; occasional headaches, noises in the ears, giddiness, an inability to stop working and relax, moments of great tiredness, digestive upsets. Eventually there may be haemorrhage in the eyes. When a person has high blood pressure, putting it even higher by violent exercise or other stress can result in a heart attack or stroke.

Hypertension can be caused in several ways.

When the body contains more salt and water than it needs, the volume of blood increases and its pressure goes up as well. In addition, arteries can be plugged with cholesterol; the cholesterol lining the arteries can come from our diet or it can be made by the body, which is then unable to deal with it effectively. High blood pressure encourages the deposits of yet more fatty substances on the walls of the arteries by allowing the blood less room to pass, and these deposits help to put up the blood pressure still more in a vicious circle. Excess fat can press on the arteries, compressing them in beds of fatty tissue and making the passage of blood more difficult.

Arteries can be scarred by inflammation from tainted foods, tobacco, drugs and other pollutants. When the inflammation heals, the scar tissue left behind is inelastic and cannot contract or relax properly to let the blood through. When the finer arteries are scarred there is a risk of arterial rupture. The brain has very small arteries which cannot support the strain and blood leaks out of them; brain haemorrhage is a common end-result of high blood pressure.

An unhealthy bloodstream causes impaired circulation as well as irritation of the artery walls. Impurities in the blood sometimes affect the nervous system of the arteries, which becomes over-sensitive. Toxins can cause nervous contractions of the artery muscles.

A sluggish, toxic bloodstream burdens the kidneys, causing them to be less efficient. Kidney dysfunction slows down the blood filtering through them and higher blood pressure will build up in the rest of the circulation. Kidney weakness is a very common cause of high blood pressure and can be caused by too much tea, coffee, alcohol and condiments; excessive tea drinking in particular is very bad for the kidneys, especially tea which has been 'stewed'.

Stress and tension cause the artery muscles to contract and make the arteries smaller as the body prepares itself to meet the challenge; this natural rise in blood pressure goes down when the person relaxes. A state of constant tension, however, will result in constantly elevated blood pressure.

The permanently narrowed blood vessels which are a part of chronic high blood pressure force the heart to pump against greater resistance and put it under constant strain. A strong heart will try to meet this challenge by growing larger, and the person can end up with hypertensive heart disease, or an enlarged heart.

We can see that the immediate, local factors influencing blood pressure include the efficiency of the heart, the health of the bloodstream and the elasticity and width of the arterial walls.

'The patient with high blood pressure . . . must adjust to the facts that he will have to go on taking the tablets for ever and that the benefits are long-term.' (From a leaflet published by the Chest, Heart and Stroke Asociation).

Drugs used to treat high blood pressure relax the blood vessels, either directly or by blocking the nerves leading to them. Diuretic drugs are also often used, to reduce any overload in the circulation by stimulating the kidneys to excrete excess water and salt from the body.

Drugs to relax the blood vessels can block the beta-receptors, the nerve endings which bring about a rapid heart-beat. These drugs, called beta-blockers, result in a reduction of the volume of blood being pumped by the heart and therefore in less work for the heart to do. Vasodilators are used to improve the circulation, but are of limited value.

Beta-blockers include acebutalol (marketed as Sectral), atenolol (Ternormin), labetolol (Trandate), metoprolol (Betaloc, Lopresor), pindolol (Visken), propranolol (Inderal), oxprenolol (Trasicor), sotalol (Beta-cardone, Sotacor). They can trigger off heart failure in patients already near to such a state and may make heart-block worse; they may constrict the bronchial tubes, and sudden discontinuance of these drugs has caused heart attacks. They should not be given to pregnant women, people with asthma, bronchospasm and bronchitis, or patients taking oral anti-diabetic drugs.

Diuretic drugs can cause a deficiency of potassium, which may affect the heart and can be extremely dangerous. They can also produce muscle weakness, constipation, appetite loss and gastro-intestinal irritation, sensitivity to light and dehydration. They may increase the risk of gout.

Other drugs for hypertension include clonidine (Catapres, Dixarit) which reduces the blood pressure, slows the heart rate and has a sedative effect. It can cause dry mouth, drowsiness, itching, impotence, swelling of the throat and face, nausea and dizziness, and constipation. It must not be stopped suddenly. Hydralazine (Apresoline) works in a way which is not understood. It has to be given in large doses and has severe adverse effects, including a disorder like rheumatoid arthritis and skin rashes. Prazosin (Hypovase) acts directly on the muscle walls of blood vessels, causing a reduction in peripheral resistance. It may produce a severe fall in blood pressure *in its recommended dosage.* Methyldopa (Aldomet; Dopamet) can cause drowsiness in the first few days of treatment. Other possible side-effects include diarrhoea, dry mouth, nausea, depression and nightmares, oedema, stuffy nose, dizziness, fever, failure to ejaculate, blood disorders and liver damage.

Guanethidine (Ismelin) lowers the blood pressure, often causing diarrhoea at the start of treatment. It can also cause dizziness and weakness which clear up as treatment continues. Other side effects are a slow pulse, breathlessness, fluid retention, nausea, vomiting, pain in the cheeks, stuffy nose, blurred vision, muscle pains, trembling, dermatitis, failure to ejaculate, frequency in passing urine and depression. Bethanidine (Esbatal), which lowers the blood pressure by working on the nerve endings to the blood vessels, can produce adverse effects the same as those produced by Guanethidine, but rarely depression. It does not produce pain in the cheeks.

Space only permits me to mention one more drug for high blood pressure – reserpine (Serpasil). Side-effects, which are alleged to be mild, can include lethargy, stuffy nose, nightmares, stomach upsets and diarrhoea, vertigo, breathlessness, weight increase, skin rashes. High doses can cause flushing, insomnia, redness of eyes, a slow pulse, occasionally Parkinsonism and severe depression which may lead to suicide.

Discussing hypertensive drugs, Dr Robert Downs of the Southwest Center of Healing Arts, Albuquerque, USA expresses doubts about the action – quite apart from the side-effects – of these drugs. We have seen that any restriction in the arteries, for whatever reason, will challenge the heart to pump more blood in order to sustain the vital blood flow to the tissues. This will put up the blood pressure. Dr Downs is of the opinion that since a rise in blood pressure is an attempt on the part of the heart to increase the flow of blood, it is wrong to cut across this increase by suppressing the body changes needed to bring it about. This suppression, by robbing the body of the increased blood flow it needs, will also rob the tissues of vital nutrients carried to them by the blood.

Dr Downs states that hypertensive drugs, given over a long period of time, could be one of the reasons why their recipients complain of loss of recent memory. The blood is not carrying nutrients to the tissues because it is being prevented from doing so and these people 'have the symptoms of premature senility because they [the drugs] have defeated the purpose of the body's elevation of blood pressure.'[2]

It should also be borne in mind that the diuretic drugs which expel excess salt and water from the body also expel other minerals, including potassium, and can cause a potassium deficiency. Since this causes fluid retention, these drugs are in fact encouraging the very condition they set out to remedy. Further, in 39 patients with mild high blood pressure, diuretics caused a rise in blood fat levels, making heart damage more likely. Blood pressure was down – but cholesterol was up.[3]

Essential hypertension is a strain on the body. We have seen that it is possible to interfere with body processes in order to force the blood pressure down and that this may lead to further complications. This approach also has no effect on the root causes of hypertension.

But there is another way – slow, but safe. The body will heal itself, if given the chance; this is one of the fundamental tenets of Nature Cure. By correct nutrition and other alternative therapies, you can give it that chance, and bring the blood pressure down to a level which is right for the individual.

The drugless approach to high blood pressure

Please note that no hypertensive patient who is taking drugs should change his treatment unless he is under the guidance of a qualified naturopath (SEE appendix page 405) or a nutritionally aware doctor.

High blood pressure 'is a change in the function of the body in response to any of a number of causes,' writes naturopath Leon Chaitow in the magazine *Here's Health*, 'all of which can be reversed, removed or at least improved, if the individual has the will to change the way of life responsible early enough.'[4]

It is assumed by orthodox doctors that blood pressure rises inevitably as we get older, but Chaitow states that he has examined many patients in their 70s and 80s whose blood pressures were equivalent to that of a healthy young adult; the common factor in many of these people was a vegetarian or vegan diet or one low in animal protein.

Here, then, is the dietary approach.

A good start is a short fast of one or two days. This is usually enough to bring down the blood pressure a little. Please read the *Fasting* section (pages 159–63) first, drink only when you are thirsty, and rest in bed.

After this, turn to the *Food Therapy* section (pages 396–401) and follow the diet outlined there. Please bear in mind that the best foods for high blood pressure are vegetables, either raw or short-cooked to conserve the vitamins and minerals as much as possible. Fruit is also very helpful, but if you have an acidic condition such as rheumatism or stomach acidity, it will be best to leave out the very acid fruits such as lemons, grapefruit and all other citrus fruits, rhubarb and plums and their juices. Concentrate on plenty of salads, cooked vegetables and fruit. Eat just a little vegetarian protein, and cut back drastically on salt, sugar and fats. Starchy foods should be eaten in small quantities. Keep your diet as dry as you can, only drinking when you are thirsty. If you drink a lot of water you can bring about a certain increase in the blood pressure. You should take the fresh or dried fruit breakfast, leaving out the cereal or bread as part of your starch reduction. Snacks should be fruit only.

For one day every week during your Food Therapy regime, take fresh raw fruits only. This partial fast is also very beneficial.

During this dietary treatment, you may feel very tired for a time, and perhaps you will experience some depression. These are signs that the nervous system is relaxing and that your whole body is reacting to the lifting of both nervous stress and the strain imposed by the wrong foods. Once these feelings have passed, the healing will have begun and your vitality will return.

Get as much rest in bed as possible; sleep if you can during this time. Rest will almost always bring down the blood pressure. It is important to incorporate a relaxation and/or a breathing technique in your treatment as well and these are described later.

It is now widely accepted that too much salt can put up the blood pressure, and low-salt diets are commonly prescribed for hypertension. Things are not as simple as this, however. The mineral potassium helps the body to excrete any surplus of salt, and human volunteers kept on diets *deficient in potassium*, rather than high in salt, retained so much salt that they developed hypertension.[5] Although the development of high blood pressure through a potassium deficiency, rather than salt excess, has been little studied, it has been found that if foods rich in potassium are eaten or a potassium salt is taken, high blood pressure drops to normal provided it is due to excessive salt.[6] This is confirmed by research at the London Hospital Medical College.[7] The diet outlined in the *Food Therapy* section is low in salt and high in potassium.

This dietary is also low in fat. Too much fat in general in unhealthy (SEE *Fats* pages 23–35) and too much saturated fat will encourage the build-up of cholesterol in the arteries which makes them narrower and forces up the blood pressure as a result.

In the *British Medical Journal* for 15 December 1979, some research on dietary fibre and high blood pressure is described. Volunteers were divided into two groups; the first group were people who habitually ate a high-fibre diet, and the second group a low-fibre diet. On examination at the start of the experiment, those in the first group had an average lower blood pressure than those in the second. During the experiment, the first group cut down on their high-fibre eating and the second increased it. At the end, the first group had increased their blood pressure and the second group, simply by eating more fibre, had decreased it. The dietary treatment set out in the Food Therapy section has its full complement of natural fibre, and you are recommended to add bran should you so desire.

Dr Ellen Grant of the Charing Cross Hospital has worked with migraine patients who were also hypertensive. 25% of her patients were not only cured of their migraine when they gave up foods to which they were found to be allergic, but recovered from their high blood pressure too. This indicates that hypertension may sometimes be due to a food allergy.

The B vitamin choline has been used to treat essential hypertension.[8] Garlic also can lower high blood pressure; it is believed to act by dilating the blood vessels and it also protects against the high blood fats which can attach themselves to the linings of arteries.

Zinc is a major factor in the control of hypertension. It is displaced by the toxic mineral cadmium, which accumulates in the kidneys. Vitamin C, as well as working against pollutants such as cadmium, helps to lower blood cholesterol and is a mild natural diuretic.

Other supplements used for hypertension include the vitamin B complex (especially choline), vitamins E and P, potassium salt, kelp powder or tablets. Recent research into evening primrose oil indicates that it can lower mild high blood pressure (SEE *Evening Primrose Oil* pages 111–14).

Too much alcohol can send up the blood pressure, as can cigarette smoking. Obesity can be a cause of hypertension, and the blood pressure will often come down when the person's weight is normal again (SEE *Obesity* pages 363–74).

Before you undertake your Food Therapy, it will be necessary for you to know how and why it works. Please, therefore, read the *Nature Cure* section first (pages 391–6).

Please note that the dietary treatment is on general lines only, and that you may also need additional vitamins and minerals. For individual guidance on both your Food Therapy plan and any supplementation, consult a naturopath or a nutritionally aware doctor.

Additional therapies

High blood pressure and stress reduction: An article in the *New England Journal of Medicine*, states that investigators using a variety of techniques, including yoga, Transcendental Meditation and biofeedback, observed blood pressure reductions in many patients.[9]

Medical journalist Audry Carli, writing in the American magazine *Bestways*, described research with 21 hypertensive patients. 11 of these patients were given hypertensive drugs. The remaining 10 were given the same drug, plus lessons in a relaxation technique.

The group taking drugs had an average drop in systolic blood pressure of 1.1 points. The group taking drugs and also practising relaxation had an average drop of *13.6 points.*

A person who is chronically tense and who cannot relax, even when he has the opportunity, is a prime candidate for all the circulatory ills, including high blood pressure.

Readers with hypertension are strongly advised to learn to relax. One well-known meditation and relaxation technique, transcendental meditation, has been stated twice in *The Lancet* to be effective in lowering high blood pressure[10] but there are several other ways of learning to relax; for instance, Autogenic Training, yoga, Biofeedback. (Please SEE appendix, under *Relaxation* page 406).

Acupuncture: SEE appendix, page 405.

Deep breathing, it has been found by naturopath Russell Sneddon that patients who practise deep-breathing exercises as well as following a naturopathic diet show a greater drop in blood pressure than those on the diet only; SEE appendix page 405.

Exercise: a carefully paced programme of mild exercise is very useful. *Do not overstrain yourself*, and let your practitioner know what you are doing. Walking is probably the best for you.

Herbalism: SEE appendix page 405.

Homoeopathy: SEE appendix page 405.

Osteopathy, can be of some help in relaxing you: SEE appendix page 405.

Water therapy, consult your practitioner.

Recommended reading
Nature Cure for High Blood Pressure by J. Russell Sneddon (Thorsons 1979).

Hyper-active Children

It is difficult to be sure about the incidence of hyper-activity. In the US it is thought that between 2 and 4 million children are affected but in the UK, partly because the diagnosis is made less readily, the hyper-active label is much less common. Like all behavioural disorders, too, it is hard to pin down. In one study carried out on the Isle of Wight however the term was applied to one out of every thousand children.[1]

All children fidget and grizzle from time to time, especially when they are bored or tired. But the hyper-active child is in a constant whirl of disruptive, compulsive activity which he cannot control. He is clumsy, aggressive and reckless, rushing from one thing to another and unable to concentrate for long or tolerate failure or frustration. He sleeps badly and in extreme cases – hyperkinesis – his IQ is not reflected in his school work. From time to time he will stop this manic behaviour and plunge into exhausted depression and lethargy.

Hyper-active children are usually boys, of a normal or high intelligence. The family probably has a history of allergy, and usually only one child will be affected. His diet almost always contains large amounts of food additives. The condition may also be connected with incomplete brain development, certain hereditary conditions, complications in pregnancy or labour or severe meningitis in infancy; another strongly supported, theory is that it may be genetic. There seems to be confusion over whether or not hyper-activity is, strictly speaking, linked with allergy. It can be associated with low blood sugar (SEE *Low Blood Sugar* pages 340–5). Children often grow out of this condition, but they may be left with learning difficulties.

Drug treatment
There are several drugs used for hyper-activity.

Amphetamines are stimulants, but when given to a hyper-active child they can have a calming effect. The amphetamine Dexedrine (dexamphetamine, dexamphetamine sulphate, dextroamphetamine sulphate, Dexamed) is sometimes prescribed. Side-effects include nausea, diarrhoea or constipation, difficulty in urination, headache, dry mouth, trembling, rapid heartbeat and chest pains, inability to concentrate. Higher doses can produce worse side-effects, and *dependence occurs easily*.

Another drug used is Ritalin, or methylphenidate. This too, stimulates the nervous system but can have a calming effect. Side-effects include appetite loss and nausea, dry mouth, dizziness, headache, insomnia, nervousness and palpitations.

The use of both Dexedrine and Ritalin for hyperactivity is being questioned now by medical authorities.

It is obvious that none of the drugs being used for hyper-activity have the slightest effect on its causes. The idea of giving drugs, with their possible side-effects, to children for long periods of time is quite horrifying.

'It may be regrettable that we have waited until the 1970s to ask the mass of chemicals: Are you harmful to touch and breathe, eat and drink?'   DR BEN F. FEINGOLD, *Why Your Child is Hyperactive.*

Dr Ben Feingold, chief allergist at the Kaiser Permanent Medical Center in San Francisco, California, has pulled together the growing body of evidence linking hyper-activity with food. Dr Feingold prefers not to treat his hyper-active patients with drugs.

Noticing that some people who are allergic to aspirin also react to food containing natural salicylates (closely related to this drug), Feingold designed a 'salicylate-free' diet. Banned foods were apricots, prunes, peaches, plums, raspberries, grapes, oranges, cucumbers and tomatoes, together with foods to which chemicals had been added which themselves contained salicylates. Dr Feingold went on later to exclude foods containing additives, including monosodium glutamate (a flavour enhancer), tartrazine (a yellow food dye) and cyclamates (artifical sweeteners); this last he found responsible for five different skin conditions.

Dr Feingold believes that some people are born with a defect that makes them react abnormally to certain food additives and other food constituents. Because of the rapid growth of the modern food industry, we are simply not able to cope with all these food additives and, whether the patient is an adult or a hyper-active child, he lacks natural body defences against them. (Dr Feingold does not claim, however, that chemicals in foods are the only cause of this condition.)

Since the last century, when organic chemistry began, about 3 million chemicals have been created in the laboratory, and some are put into our food. These chemicals have never existed in nature. In this and in many other ways we have polluted our air, water and food in a little over 100 years. Is it surprising that some of us cannot adapt?

When a food additive is tested, it is tested singly, for a limited period, on laboratory animals, and for cancer and other cell damage only. When the same additive is eaten in our food, it is eaten together with other additives, for long periods – and *by human beings*. There are many ways to damage a human being besides giving him cancer. Causing behavioural change is one of those ways. How much disruptive, aggressive behaviour may be due to our food, which not only contains chemicals some of us cannot stand, but is deficient in the nutrients essential for a healthy nervous system? Some food chemicals affect the way the body absorbs trace minerals, too, so they may be causing mineral deficiencies.

Dr Feingold has established that people can be sensitive to almost every food additive there is. Trouble can even be caused by the artificial colouring on a vitamin tablet. So his dietary treatment consists of two lists of forbidden foods – those which contain natural salicylates and those which contain food additives. He also advises many of his hyper-active children to cut down on white sugar, honey and molasses.

Dr Robert Downs, of the Southwest Center of the Healing Arts, Albuquerque, USA has also treated many hyper-active children by using dietary measures instead of drugs. He believes that other environmental pollutants are involved as well, in particular lead. There is some evidence that hyper-activity can be linked with a high lead level in the body[3] and that, when lead is present in these amounts, the nervous system cannot regenerate properly.[4] Downs recommends that hyper-active children should be tested for both mineral deficiencies and lead levels, and uses vitamin C, calcium, magnesium, zinc and other substances to help the body to excrete lead.

Dr Downs takes the Feingold concept a stage further. He agrees that an additive-free diet is usually an excellent starting point in the treatment of a hyper-active child, but comments that the Feingold diet can sometimes be high in white sugar and that white flour is also allowed. He states that his hyper-active patients usually have abnormal blood sugar behaviour (either insulin malfunction or high/low blood sugar). This condition is made worse by refined sugars and starches such as white flour, but is helped by unrefined whole grains and wholemeal bread (SEE *Low Blood Sugar* pages 340–5). In an interview in the American magazine *Bestways* for July 1980, Dr Downs describes his approach to hyper-activity, saying 'case after case has indicated that these kids are so reactive to the refined carbohydrates, that even once one gets them straightened out and controlled, if a sugary food is introduced into their system they go "bananas" for 24 hours.' He finds that hyper-active children are usually short of magnesium and zinc (magnesium is needed for proper nerve functioning), and that those with learning disability (hyperkinesis) are usually low in manganese too. He ensures that each child has a high intake of the B vitamins, niacin in particular, and suggests that fluorescent lighting can irritate the nervous system.

Dr Allan Cott, psychiatric consultant to the New York Institute of Child Development, gives large doses of the vitamins B3, B6, C and E to his hyper-active patients. Like Dr Downs he has found that they often have a blood sugar disturbance. He points out that eating refined sugars and starches will starve the body of the B vitamins, as these nutrients are used in their metabolism. (Unrefined carbohydrates bring their own B vitamins with them.)

Recent research into the oil of the evening primrose plant shows that it can be very effective in some cases. The Hyper-active Children's Support Group, listed at the end of this section, has further information – SEE also *Evening Primrose Oil* pages 111–14.

It is difficult to arrange controlled trials to test the effects of food additives on children, but some research has been done. In a laboratory test, food dyes were found to significantly impair the learning performance of 40 hyper-active children; about half the children were affected.[5] The researchers state that the dosage used was about *50 times smaller* than the maximum allowable daily intake recommended by the American Food and Drug Administration. A separate controlled double blind study and a series of open trials have confirmed that about half the children given the Feingold diet show a decrease in hyper-active symptoms, but 'the mechanism for and the magnitude of this effect remain in question',[5]

Further work revealed that 20 of 22 hyper-active children tested with food additives did not respond. But when the dose was raised, 17 out of those 20 reacted with adverse effects.[6] Clinical trials by American doctors James O'Shea and Seymour Porter reported that 13 out of 15 hyper-active children reacted when they were given skin injections of food additives and airborne allergens.

At the University of New Mexico, doctors Gordon K. Hodge and Richard T. Linn have been using biofeedback to help hyper-active children. Results so far seem to show that this technique (SEE appendix page 405, *Relaxation*) increases the attention span of these children and gives them confidence in their ability to control themselves. Professor Martin Herbert, director of the Child Treatment Research Unit at the University of Leicester, believes that behaviour modification (ignoring bad behaviour and rewarding good) can be helpful for hyper-active children.

To sum up, there are many possible factors involved in hyper-activity – physical, psychological and social – of which diet is one. Dr Feingold himself emphasises this and further studies are obviously needed.

Fortunately, several British doctors now are aware of the dietary approach. In a letter to me Dr Hugh J.E. Cox states that when he treats a hyper-active child on a prescribed diet the results are quite striking. He has not treated large numbers of such children, but cannot recall any patient that has not responded in some degree.

Dr Stephen Davies, another leader in the treatment of hyper-active children in this country, points out that the condition is multi-factorial and emphasises the high probability of an overload of toxic metals, in particular lead, in the body. He always carries out mineral analysis on the hair of these children (SEE end). Many mineral deficiencies, together with a shortage of the B vitamins, are involved. He advises the mothers of these patients to stop using aluminium cookware and to cut down on refined carbohydrates and fats. Food allergies (SEE *Allergies to Food* pages 219–29) and additives, skipped meals, lack of sleep, sensitivity to fumes including car fumes and domestic gas, are some of the possible causes.

Dr Davies treats the mothers too with nutritional therapy. In a letter to me he writes that most women with hyper-active children 'have been labelled as neurotic, worriers, inadequate, anxious, by their own family doctors, and actually weep when they find a doctor who will listen to them, who understands, who does not dismiss them as "loony".'

Information
The Hyper-Active Children's Support Group Formed in November 1977, the HACSG is voluntary and its aims are:

1 To help and support HA children and their families (not financially).
2 To encourage formation of local groups where mothers may get together for mutual support and understanding.

3 To urge the medical profession and the health and education authorities to take more interest in the day-to-day problems of HA children and adolescents.

4 To promote urgent research into the causes of HA whether it be linked to chemical food additives, nutritional deficiencies, food allergies and/or environmental pollution.

5 To press for early and proper diagnosis of HA, research into other possible treatments and management of this condition; and to disseminate information to all interested parties.

There are HACSG groups all over the country now. They publish a book list, their diet (based on the Feingold diet) and newsletters. If you would like to contact them, please write to Mrs I.D. Colquhoun, Mayfield House, Yapton Road, Barnham, West Sussex, PO22 0BJ, or the Secretary, Sally Bunday, 59 Meadowside, Angmering, Sussex BN16 4BW, enclosing a stamped and addressed 9in × 4in envelope and marking your letter 'Information only required'. Readers who would like a copy of the diet should send £2 and mark the envelope 'Diet Please'. Membership of the Group costs £3 per annum. I am told that the HACSG has had more than 35 000 enquiries since its inception.

Hair analysis: The following laboratory provides a 21-element hair analysis and dietary survey with a comprehensive computer printout, interpreting the significance of both sets of results in non-medical language:

Mineralab UK, 59 Dunnings Road, East Grinstead, West Sussex RH19 4AB (telephone 0342 311810).

Recommended reading

Why Your Child is Hyper-active by Dr Ben F. Feingold (Random House, USA, 1975).

Growing up with Good Food (nutritional advice) by the National Childbirth Trust, ed. C. Lewis (Unwin 1982).

Low Blood Sugar
(Hypoglycaemia)

Low blood sugar is a condition showing itself in so many ways that it is the hypochondriac's latest fad. Some medical authorities believe that it is widespread and on the increase and some say that it hardly exists at all. A 1966 survey of the US Department of Health, Education and Welfare showed that 66 000 out of 134 000 people examined were hypoglycaemic. On the other hand, in 1973 the American Medical Association labelled it a 'non-disease'.

There are two sorts of low blood sugar. The first is organic – caused by a diseased liver, pituitary, adrenal or pancreas, or a tumour of the abdomen. This is very rare.

The second kind is functional; this 'reactive' hypoglycaemia may be transient and is the one we are concerned with. The conditions in the body predisposing to it may be hereditary but reactive hypoglycaemia itself is not.

Although it may be associated with several other illnesses, hypoglycaemia is not a disease. It is a disorder of the blood sugar metabolism. The carbohydrates which we eat are changed into glucose which we use for energy. Normal blood contains about 0.1% of glucose and numerous mechanisms interact to control this level. The amount of glucose (blood sugar) is constantly fluctuating; it goes down during hard exercise or other stress, during pregnancy or before a menstrual period. Food and drink put the blood sugar up. The main hormone concerned with keeping the blood sugar constant is insulin. Insulin removes some excess glucose from the blood by combustion and stores the rest in the muscles and liver in the form of glycogen for use later.

The pancreas produces insulin. If this gland over-reacts, too much insulin is poured into the bloodstream, lowering the blood sugar too fast and too far, and causing the symptoms of hypoglycaemia.

The symptoms of low blood sugar are often so slight that most of us experience one or more of them at some time, but usually the condition is quickly corrected by the body's sugar-regulating mechanism. Some people have naturally low blood-sugar levels, without any symptoms, and this is harmless.

Hypoglycaemic symptoms can be grouped under changes in the nervous system including the brain, psychological changes, and changes in the circulatory, glandular and digestive systems. The brain is particularly vulnerable to any sudden swings in the blood sugar level, because it needs glucose to function. It has no reserves of this nutrient and depends upon a constant supply from the bloodstream. Symptoms include yawning, fatigue, insomnia, forgetfulness, confusion and inability to concentrate, sudden ravenous hunger, trembling, anxiety, depression, irritability, high or low emotional states, dizziness, palpitations, slow co-ordination, hot and cold sweats, headaches, crying spells. There can be twitching of the eyelids or other parts and a craving for tea, coffee, sugar or other stimulants. Low blood sugar can be associated with skin and digestive disorders, diarrhoea or constipation, over-breathing or shortness of breath, cold hands and feet, tingling lips and fingers, blurred or double vision. In children there can be asthma, allergies, hay-fever or hyper-activity. In severe hypoglycaemia, the patient risks brain damage. He may have an epileptic fit or may even die.

Low blood sugar can cause potassium loss and water retention. It is accompanied by a low level of calcium in the blood (this happens before a menstrual period) which can lead to muscular cramps and spasms. The hypoglycaemic is very vulnerable to stress – the condition itself is a stress on the body. Hypoglycaemia often goes with loss of temper; when his blood sugar plummets the person cannot control himself, and an impairment of the glucose supply to the brain can cause a personality change. Many sufferers have gone the rounds of psychiatrists in vain.

The typical hypoglycaemic hates the idea of breakfast. He will make do with a cup of coffee containing several spoonfuls of sugar and perhaps a cigarette. He gets ravenously hungry for sugary foods and will sip sweet coffee throughout the day to keep himself going. He may wake up in the night feeling hungry.

It can be seen that low blood sugar has so many symptoms and most of them are so vague and fleeting that this condition is hard to diagnose.

Causes
We have seen that low blood sugar is caused by the pancreas

pouring out too much insulin. Eating refined, sugary foods for many years can damage the body's ability to handle sugar properly. These foods are digested quickly, the pancreas releases too much insulin to deal with the sudden influx of blood sugar and the person craves more sugar to bring the level up again. The adrenal glands (which secrete factors to control the insulin reaction) and the liver may also function less efficiently. The caffeine in coffee acts like sugar, over-stimulating the pancreas, and causing low blood sugar which leads to fatigue and to another cup of coffee as a pick-me-up. Alcohol and tobacco can bring about low blood sugar too (a hangover is a hypoglycaemic reaction). Eating a food to which you are allergic, especially a cereal, can also result in low blood sugar (SEE *Allergies to Food* pages 219–29).

Severe dieting and fasting *on water only* can bring about low blood sugar. Any other severe, continued stress such as lack of sleep or depression, can cause it by exhausting the adrenal glands so that they control insulin output less effectively.

Numerous drugs can cause hypoglycaemia: analgesics including aspirin, anti-inflammatory drugs, anti-coagulants, antibiotics, diuretics, stimulants, tranquillizers and hormones including the Pill. Too much insulin given to a diabetic can lower the blood sugar too fast and too far.

Associated diseases

Hypoglycaemia can be a forerunner of diabetes. The pancreas, which has been over-reacting and pushing the blood sugar down too low, finally gets exhausted and cannot produce enough insulin, so that the blood sugar rises too much and causes diabetes. Many cases of diabetes could be prevented by proper treatment of its precursor.

Insulin promotes the storage of starch and fat. The person with low blood sugar craves sugar. The insulin produced in response to this sugar causes fat to be stored or spilled over into the blood. With a fat person, the pancreas can react more and more quickly until he gets low blood sugar, with its attendant craving, more quickly than a person of normal weight who is eating the same food. Migraine sufferers often have low blood sugar during an attack. Headaches associated with hypoglycaemia are particularly common after stress.

P.L. Meiers, writing in *Orthomolecular Psychiatry*,[1] states that low blood sugar is present in up to 70% of patients with schizophrenia. It can also be associated with asthma, hay fever, and arthritic conditions.

Diagnosis

The symptoms of hypoglycaemia are so many and varied that almost all of them can be caused by real diseases. Diagnosis, therefore, is very important (SEE Information at end).

The best way to uncover this condition is to use a six-hour glucose tolerance test. According to naturopath Martin Budd in his book *Low Blood Sugar (Hypoglycaemia) – The 20th Century Epidemic?* the more usual two-hour glucose tolerance test is useless; any significant reactions invariably occur *after* two hours. He also supports other practitioners who believe that the incidence of hypoglycaemia is rising, saying that out of 210 patients selected and tested with a six-hour GTT, 92% showed hypoglycaemia. The patient comes into the surgery with an empty stomach except for some water, and the glucose level of the blood is measured. Then he is given a sugar solution or some food. His blood glucose is tested again if he experiences any symptoms or, failing that, it is measured again after four, five, and finally six hours to determine exactly how his body handles sugar. It is important to measure not only the amount of the blood glucose fall, but the speed of its fall, and to decide whether the figures taken are right or wrong for that individual. A urine test is also taken. This GTT is not infallible in showing up hypoglycaemia, and there are other tests.

Dietary treatment

For much of this information I am indebted to Dr Andrew Lockie.

Turn to the *Food Therapy* section (pages 396–401) and follow the dietary, with the following modifications. Take small meals, and every two hours take a snack as well, such as crispbread and cottage cheese, a glass of milk or yogurt, nuts, seeds, some dried or fresh fruit, unsweetened fruit or vegetable juices, herb tea (especially juniper tea), or grain coffee (obtainable from a health food store). Have a small protein snack before going to bed and a glass of milk on waking.

For the first two weeks, omit all flesh foods, honey (thereafter limited to two teaspoons a day), full fat cheese, grapes, plums, figs, bananas, prunes, raisins, dates, lentils, kidney beans, potatoes, unsweetened fruit juices. Limit these foods thereafter.

Avoid at all times all the foods forbidden in the Food Therapy plan together with all medications containing caffeine, cough syrups and laxatives. Cut out salt completely and use kelp or Ruthmol (obtainable from a health food store).

This treatment is aimed at giving the body a steady supply of unrefined carbohydrates, fats and proteins which it can break down into glucose but which do not produce such a high blood sugar level and over-stimulate the pancreas.

Supplements

Zinc is involved in the regulation of insulin release, and a chromium deficiency alters glucose tolerance; chromium is one of the nutrients being used to treat diabetes, where there is usually insufficient insulin rather than too much. The stress of low blood sugar causes adrenal exhaustion and the mineral potassium is excreted in the urine. There may therefore be a deficiency of potassium. Manganese and magnesium are also concerned in the body's handling of glucose.

Dr Robert Downs of the Southwest Center of the Healing Arts, Albuquerque, USA finds that his hypoglycaemic patients are usually short of the B vitamins and have inadequate protein stores. A shortage of the B vitamin pantothenic acid leads to a decrease in adrenal efficiency and an inefficient sugar metabolism; it also influences the insulin-glucose balance. The range of B vitamins helps to normalize sugar metabolism. Vitamin E helps the circulation and encourages the uptake of glycogen (formerly glucose) in the muscles and vitamin C is essential when the body is under stress; it is also valuable for controlling insulin production. In addition to these supplements, Dr Downs uses B15, lecithin and niacin to help the circulatory problems which can be associated with low blood sugar.

A deficiency of the B vitamin folic acid, which works with an enzyme to metabolize sugar, can aggravate hypoglycaemia. Dr Robert Herman, writing in *Biochemical Medicine* for 1978, treated his hypoglycaemic patients with folic acid.

Finally, avoid continued stress and exhaustion. Try to exercise daily and stop before you get tired. Get enough sleep and relaxation.

Information

The six-hour glucose tolerance test is not standard. Most GPs are not familiar with it or with the diagnosis of hypoglycaemia. If you wish to find a practitioner who understands this condition and will be able to test you effectively for it, please write to:

The Secretary, The Basingstoke Clinic, 54/56 New Market Square, Basingstoke, Hampshire

or

The Honorary Secretary, Research Society for Natural Therapeutics, 94 Banstead Road South, Sutton, Surrey SM2 5LN;

or consult a naturopath (SEE appendix, pages 405).

Additional therapies
Acupuncture: SEE appendix page 405.
Herbalism: SEE appendix page 405.
Homoeopathy: SEE appendix page 405.

Recommended reading
Low Blood Sugar (Hypoglycaemia) – The 20th Century Epidemic? by Martin L. Budd (Thorsons, 1981).

Migraine

A migraine headache can vary from relatively mild to disabling. It may be accompanied by a wide range of symptoms, particularly disturbances in seeing, speech and feeling, which indicate that the brain is affected. Blood circulation is disturbed, the circulation in the brain and scalp, where the blood vessels first contract and then relax, becoming abnormally wide and stretched.

Migraine was described in about 180 AD by a Greek physician as a *hemicrania* (half-skull) headache, and this word was eventually changed to migraine. In the UK there are over 5 million migraine sufferers – about 10% to 12% of the whole population. Women outnumber men by 2 to 1, but children of both sexes are equally affected. Incidence levels off in middle age and declines in old age. The strain of governing our country can be deduced from the fact that 21% of Members of Parliament have migraine.

There are several kinds of migraine.

1 *Classical migraine* There is a warning of an attack – an 'aura'. Perhaps there will be blurred vision, zigzagging lines or lights, red, watery eyes, facial numbness, pins and needles in the arm or face, flushing, pallor, speech disturbances, vertigo, muscular weakness, queer tastes or smells; another warning is a feeling of unusual well-being.

These signals are usually followed by nausea and vomiting, and the headache arrives soon after the warning symptoms. It is usually, but not always, in half the head. The attack can last from a few hours to several days.

2 *Common (simple, or minor) migraine* This headache is less elaborate, with little or no warning. Attacks are just as frequent as for classical migraine.

3 *Migrainous neuralgia* This is uncommon and usually found in men between 20 and 40 years old, during the spring or the autumn. It is over one eye and the Americans call it a 'cluster headache'.

4 *Abdominal migraine* Usually confined to women and children, this headache can be triggered off by travel sickness or excitement; the digestion is also affected.

5 *Facial migraine* This is less painful, and of shorter duration, than other kinds of migraine.

6 *Basilar migrain* This is a pain over the back of the head. The attack can include giddiness, double vision, slurred speech and even loss of consciousness due to less blood being supplied to the brain.

These are the main forms; there are of course many headaches which are not migraine.

Drug treatments
Migraine is the most unpleasant of all headaches, and orthodox medical science can offer only palliatives and not a cure.

Drugs can be used either to prevent migraine or to cope with an attack once it has started.

Methysergide (marketed as Deseril) is used to prevent an attack. According to Doctors Behan and Reid writing in *The Practitioner* for February 1980, about 36% of patients suffer side-effects. These include nausea, drowsiness, muscle pains, lack of co-ordination, skin rashes, psychic disturbances and serious circulatory disorders. It can produce rebound headaches on withdrawal.

Clonidine (marketed as Dixarit) is also used as a preventive. It can induce dry mouth, drowsiness, constipation, impotence, itching, swelling of the throat and face, nausea and dizziness; at the start of treatment, clonidine may slow down the heart rate.

Pizotifen (marketed as Sanomigran) can cause drowsiness, dizziness, nausea, appetite and weight increase, flushing of the face, muscle pains and mood changes.

Propranolol has been tested and the results described by Behan and Rein in the issue of *The Practitioner* mentioned above. These studies suggest that it is of value in preventing migraine, and they did not show up any side-effects over the period of the tests. (A letter also published in the same issue, however, mentions side-effects ranging from high blood pressure to rapid heartbeats and more headache after discontinuing this drug, prescribed on this occasion for hypertension.)

Sedatives, anti-depressants and beta-blocker drugs are also given to prevent migraine.

To stop an attack once it has begun, several drugs are used containing ergotamine. The side-effects of this substance are so severe that about one-third of patients are unable to take it. It tends to aggravate nausea and vomiting and can produce a toxic state of increased, more painful headache. It is 'highly addictive' (Dr Marcia Wilkinson, Princess Margaret Migraine Clinic, London). Rarely, it causes cold, white fingers and muscle cramps. Preparations containing ergotamine are Bellerga, Cafergot, Effergot, Femergin, Lingraine, Medihaler-Ergotamine and Migril.

Drugs to stop vomiting are sometimes used as well and, because migraine can be linked with a women's hormonal fluctuations, hormones are sometimes used to treat it. Dr Ellen Grant of Charing Cross Hospital is against hormone treatment, saying that the symptoms may stop, but liver dysfunction is caused; she believes that symptoms may re-appear later in a different, more severe way.

The relationship between migraine and liver function is currently under study by Dr Grant and workers from the Marie Curie Foundation.

There are other drugs for migraine, but chemotherapy for

this illness is very limited due partly to the ineffectiveness of the drugs and partly to their toxicity.

Factors associated with migraine
Migraine and food   Some migraine sufferers cannot cope with certain natural substances in their food. These substances are not food additives.

Tyramine, for instance, is present in alcoholic drinks, many fruits and vegetables, yogurt, cheese, pickled herrings and yeast drinks such as Marmite. Another natural chemical, phenylethlamine, is found in chocolate and another, octopamine, in citrus fruits. Almost any food, it seems, can trigger off a migraine attack.

Fatty and fried foods can make matters worse by increasing the absorption of these chemicals into the bloodstream. This means that you can eat foods containing migraine precipitants quite happily for some time without any ill-effects and then, by eating something fatty as well, you make absorption of the precipitant easier and get a migraine attack. Hormonal fluctuations in women can also decide whether a food will cause a migraine or not, and some anti-depressant drugs interact with some foods, encouraging its onset.

Here are the main foods which have been found to trigger off a migraine attack, in the order of their frequency:

chocolate, cheese and other dairy products, citrus fruits, onions, fatty and fried foods, meat especially pork, tea and coffee, seafood.

An article in *The Lancet* of 5 July 1980, reported that two-thirds of a group of severely migrainous patients were found to be allergic to certain foods. In these 23 patients, elimination of those foods from the diet resulted in relief (complete in most cases) from the migraine, usually within two weeks. Some food allergies show themselves immediately, but some only show themselves when you *stop* eating the causative food. This happens because, over a long period of time, your body has changed its reaction to the allergen food. Instead of reacting adversely, it has come to actually *need* the food and when you stop eating it you will get withdrawal symptoms which you can only cure by eating the allergen again (SEE *Allergies to Food* pages 219–29). Thus some people will say that to eat, for example, some chocolate is the only way to stop a migraine from developing. They are in effect suffering from withdrawal symptoms when they feel a migraine coming and by eating the chocolate they are taking more of the food which is causing the trouble in the first place, and at the same time stopping their withdrawal symptoms. Again, it is possible to be addicted to coffee (or rather to the caffeine in it). If you do without your 'fix' of coffee for a few hours, you can get a headache which is a withdrawal symptom as your system begins to throw off the coffee. Another cup of coffee will stop the headache for you, but, of course, it's better to learn to do without your addictive food altogether.

Additionally, many additives put into foods by the manufacturers and processors can trigger off a migraine attack – the sodium nitrate used in preserved meats or the monosodium glutamate added to Chinese food can have this effects.

There is a connection, too, between migraine and low blood sugar.

After you have eaten a meal, your blood sugar rises and insulin from the pancreas brings it back into line again. Sometimes, however, the insulin overdoses things and brings your blood sugar down too low, particularly if you eat a lot of refined carbohydrates. Low blood sugar also happens simply because you are hungry.

Adelle Davis quotes 35 migraine sufferers who were linked up to electroencephalograms for five hours during their migraine headaches. The lower their blood sugar dropped, the worse their headaches became. The headaches were present when they woke up in the morning and their blood sugar was very low; this was particularly noticeable if they had not eaten much the night before. A high-protein diet without refined sugars and starches and a snack taken before going to bed brought permanent relief. [1]

To keep your blood sugar level reasonably stable, eat little and often and cut out refined carbohydrates, taking whole carbohydrates such as wholemeal bread and jacket potatoes (please SEE *Low Blood Sugar* pages 340–5).

Migraine and vitamin therapy There is a relationship between headaches, including migraine, and nutritional deficiencies. Iron deficiency can cause headaches, and they can also be caused in volunteers eating a diet short of either vitamin B6 or pantothenic acid. [2] The headaches associated with menstruation have been successfully treated with calcium and vitamin D, and vitamins B1 and B2 have been used to treat migraine. Adelle Davis advises her patients to take calcium and B6 between headaches to stop them from occurring. American writers June Biermann and Barbara Toohey[3] recommend taking half a gram of vitamin C and one B-complex tablet after every meal, three times a day. If this treatment works on your migraine, test it by stopping it for a week to see if the headaches return. It will work within a few days if it's going to work at all. Dr Miles Atkinson advises his migraine patients to avoid any allergenic foods such as chocolate or cheese. He also gives supplements of riboflavin, niacin, pantothenic acid, B6, vitamin C and whole dried liver.[4] This treatment has had some success.

Migraine and other factors

It is often thought that conscientious, hard-working, anxious people are prone to migraine. This is not borne out by recent studies.[5] Some migraine sufferers, however, are found to be aggressive, demanding and mistrustful. But which comes first, the chicken or the egg? If you had frequent, crippling migraine headaches, would your serenity be intact?

We have seen that some migraines are connected with a woman's hormonal fluctuations – her pre-menstrual tension or the menopause – and some are undoubtedly caused by the Pill.

Dr Ellen Grant of Charing Cross Hospital finds that the best way to treat women for migraine is to take them off the Pill. She alleges that the widespread use of the Pill is the reason why migraine is on the increase. In her experience, it is about three years after a woman starts taking it that she turns up at the migraine clinic. (A few women, however, have fewer migraines when they go on the Pill.) After taking her patients off the Pill, Dr Grant instructs them in elimination dieting and the avoidance of trigger foods. She states that 85% of her patients become headache-free.

Nicotine can trigger off a headache. About half women migraine sufferers and 70% of men migraine sufferers are smokers. Some people can even get an attack from inhaling other people's smoke. Again, if you are addicted to your cigarettes, missing one will bring on a headache which is a withdrawal symptom.

Other factors increasing the risk of migraine are lack of

sleep or other stress, hot dry weather, bright lights, eye strain, travelling, injuries to the head and neck, high blood pressure. There is disagreement as to whether it runs in families.

The naturopathic approach

Naturopaths say that some migraine attacks are caused by an accumulation of toxins in the body, reacting on the tissue fluids. These fluids supply nourishment from the bloodstream to the cells and drain away wastes into the lymph system. A rise in the content of the tissue fluids, caused by the build-up of toxins, will affect the brain and its arteries, causing increased pressure and pain. Some people are more sensitive to tissue fluid changes than others and they retain toxic wastes longer.

Anything affecting the nervous system will be reflected in the less efficient functioning of vital processes and their slowing up, and this of course includes the flow of tissue fluids. All negative feelings as well as all physical toxins will influence these processes.

Looked at in this way, migraine is a reaction to the pollutants in our food and other stresses, including nervous fatigue and negative feelings. The nausea and vomiting are nature's way of making sure that we do not put any more food into the body until the fluid pressure has had a chance to go down.

Migraine and food therapy

For the general dietary advice outlined here, I am indebted to *The Causes and Treatment of Headaches and Migraine* by naturopath Harry Clements, which contains much useful information for the migraine sufferers.

It is not enough to cut out the foods which may trigger off a migraine. By eating refined denatured foods, we are losing essential nutrients which are processed out of them and depriving the body of the resources it needs in order to stabilize itself and throw off a malfunction such as migraine.

We have seen that refined carbohydrates (white sugar and white flour and their products) can exhaust the mechanism that deals with blood sugar levels so that low blood sugar is encouraged, and that this condition is often associated with migraine. The B vitamins, necessary both for nervous and vascular health and therefore vitally concerned with the prevention of migraine, are burned up when the body assimilates refined carbohydrates. Unrefined carbohydrates on the other hand bring with them their own B vitamins.

Refined carbohydrates, therefore, must be cut out of the diet. To begin with, too, all starches and sugars must be left out. Starches and sugars of all kinds tend to encourage the over-retention of tissue fluids and tissue wastes, and we have seen that this can be a cause of migraine.

Follow, therefore, the *Food Therapy* general plan (pages 396–401), but omit all high-starch foods (cereals, bread, potatoes) and added sugars to begin with. For instance, take a breakfast of fruit alone, without any cereals or bread. Grapefruit is suitable, and delicious. Do not eat any bananas at this stage; they are very starchy.

Continue to omit starches and sugars but otherwise follow the Food Therapy plan until your headaches become less severe. Don't worry about the small amounts of starches and sugar contained in other foods.

As your condition improves you can add some unrefined starches to your diet in the form of bananas, or potatoes cooked in their skins. Still keep away from bread of all kinds, and all other foods containing wheat flour, whether refined or unrefined.

When you reach this stage, please bear in mind that migraine sufferers often obtain further relief when they take care not to mix high-starch and high-protein foods at the same meal. It will help you to read the section on *Compatible Eating* for a full explanation of this.

Eventually, you can start eating starches again in the form of wholemeal bread and other unrefined cereals and their products, and jacket potatoes.

Before you undertake your Food Therapy, it will be necessary for you to know how and why it works. Please, therefore, read the *Nature Cure* section first (pages 391–6).

Please note that the dietary treatment is on general lines only, and that you may also need additional vitamins and minerals. For individual guidance on both your Food Therapy plan and any supplementation, please consult a naturopath (SEE appendix page 405) or a nutritionally aware doctor.

Additional therapies
Acupuncture: SEE appendix page 405.

Biochemic Tissue Salts for migraine headache (at your health food store): SEE pages 107–8.

Herbalism: SEE appendix page 405.

Homoeopathy: SEE appendix page 405.

Osteopathy: SEE appendix page 405.

Relaxation, in particular Autogenic Training: SEE *Relaxation* in the appendix, page 405.

Recommended reading

The Causes and Treatment of Headaches and Migraine by Harry Clements (Thorsons 1980).

Multiple Sclerosis

'There is no cure for clinically established MS' (*British Medical Journal,* 14 December 1979, 1571).

'There is a CURE for multiple sclerosis' (Frederick Robert Klenner, B.S., M.S., M.D., Fellow of the American Association for the Advancement of Science, The Royal Society of Health (London), Hon. Fellow of the International Academy of Preventive and Orthomolecular Medicine, etc. *Cancer Control Jnl.* 2, 3.

There are about 50 000 people in the UK known to be suffering from multiple sclerosis. If you include those who have a form of MS so mild that they are unaware of it, the total figure is probably 75 000.[1] It is the single greatest cause of disability in young adults, affecting people mainly between the ages of 20 and 45, and commoner in women than men. Perhaps partly due to better diagnosis, its incidence is increasing.

What is MS?

MS is a disease of the central nervous system. Nerve fibres throughout the body are protected by myelin sheaths. In MS, these protective coverings develop lesions which interfere with the normal transmission of nerve impulses. After an initial swelling the destructive process stops, but these lesions can only be repaired to a limited extent, and some myelin will have been altered or destroyed, leaving scar tissue (the word 'sclerosis' means scar).

The symptoms of MS reflect the damage being done to the nervous system. They are muscular weakness and lack of co-ordination with loss of balance and slow, slurring speech. There can be strong, jerky movements of the arm, leg and eye muscles, double vision or blindness on one side, difficulty in bladder control, dizziness, numb or tingling limbs or loss of sensations and feelings of cold. There may be an 'intention tremor' which means that the hand will shake violently just as an object is about to be grasped. Fatigue and loss of stamina are very common, together with depression. The so-called 'MS euphoria' is rare.

No two cases necessarily start in the same way; symptoms can develop acutely and at apparently random intervals. Some patients have periods of many years when the symptoms all but disappear before coming back worse than before, and others have a steady progression of nerve damage, leading to incapacity. If the lungs and heart muscles become affected by the paralysis spreading through the body, the disease will be fatal.

Some people have mild, 'benign' MS without ever bothering to do anything about their fleeting symptoms, and the disease may not be revealed until examination of the brain and spinal cord after death.

MS is labelled incurable. But it follows a course of attack, disability and a partial recovery, with remissions that can be long-standing or even permanent. The fact that these remissions occur means that the body is fighting the illness and, for the time being, winning.

Possible causes

There are various geographical patterns connected with MS. Several investigations show that when the soil and food samples in an area contain more lead than average, the MS incidence is higher too. Lead poisoning produces symptoms similar to MS. The number of cases increases further north and near the equator incidence is very low. It is very rare in the Far East. This, it is thought, may be due to the fact that people in the north eat a lot of saturated fats whereas those further south eat more polyunsaturated oils. It has also been noted that more rye and wheat are eaten in the north; many MS victims are allergic to rye and wheat. MS even appears to be connected with the seasons; peak periods for its onset are late summer and autumn.

The *British Medical Journal* for 21 March 1964 states that MS patients who resume smoking after a break in the habit get worse; there is lead and arsenic in tobacco, and it is suggested that cigarette smoke may carry more lead to the lungs than pipe smoke does.[2] According to Dr David C. Poskanzer of Harvard Medical School's Departments of Preventive Medicine and Neurology, your chance of getting MS is higher if you have had your tonsils removed. There is a possibility, but not a strong one, of a genetic factor. Some doctors believe that MS is caused by a virus.

MS is often linked with allergy to food. The body attacks its own cells through a fault in the immune system (auto-immune reaction). There is no doubt that MS is often related to stress in various forms – accidents, emotional upsets, exhaustion and so on.

MS is becoming increasingly linked with nutrition and the orthodox medical profession is catching up with their more nutritionally-aware colleagues. Writing about MS in the magazine *Here's Health* for October 1978, naturopath Leon Chaitow says, 'we must recognize that in the history of medical science no single chronic disease has been successfully prevented or cured without recourse to nutritional or environmental factors' (more about this later).

Orthodox treatment
This consists of drugs to control or suppress symptoms. Drugs are given to help with the bladder problems, tranquillizers and pain-killers are often used, and the corticosteroids ACTH will bring down inflammation and can be very useful in an acute relapse. Writing in the *Cancer Control Journal*, vol 2, No. 3, however, Dr F.R. Klenner states that all patients deteriorate after the use of ACTH, which he considers destructive; he goes on to allege that the continued use of this drug in MS 'borders on malpractice'.

However harmful or benign these drugs may be, the most important point is that they do nothing to arrest or reverse the disease itself.

Nutrition and MS

'Of all the efforts made at treating MS with a variety of modern drugs and techniques, the use of nutrients and the careful observation of diet have shown the most promising results. One might even say that such measures have shown the only results.' Editorial, *Cancer Control Journal*, vol. 2, No. 3.

It is not true that there is no answer to MS. It is not true that all the sufferer can do is to take his pills and wait for a slow death or a miraculous, inexplicable remission. Several doctors and naturopaths now are using nutrition to treat this horrible disease and many patients have either improved or recovered.

What is debatable is whether nutrition and other natural therapies can bring about a 'cure', or only a permanent remission. One of the dietary pioneers in MS, Dr Joseph Evers, claims that he can cure the disease but not the patient. He explains that the MS sufferer's 'inborn metabolic errors' must be compensated for by a strict adherence to a healthy diet for the rest of his life. Dr E.K. Ledermann describes a woman with MS whom he treated with diet and homoeopathic medicines.[3] He writes, 'the excellent permanent cure must be attributed to Natural Therapy which the patient continued, having adopted its principles as a way of living.'

If you had MS, however, would you care whether your improvement was a cure or a permanent remission?

Here follows a brief description of some successful nutritional treatments. It is by no means exhaustive. Addresses, etc., are given against the numbered references at the end of the section.

Roger MacDougall Playwright Roger MacDougall was diagnosed in February 1953 by Sir Charles Symonds at the National Hospital for Nervous Diseases as suffering from MS. Sir Charles was one of the world's leading neurologists. MacDougall was eventually unable to use his legs, arms and fingers. His voice and eyesight were affected and he could not stand erect at all.

Twenty-two years later, MacDougall went back to the neurologist who, at the original examination in 1953, had beeen Sir Charles's assistant. He examined MacDougall again. Every reflex, every muscle, every movement, was normal. 'I can't fault you', he said. At the extremity of MacDougall's field of vision, the specialist found a small trace of juddering of the optic nerve. At the worst period in his illness, MacDougall was virtually blind.

Today, Roger MacDougall is over 70 and he is living a normal, active life – as I saw for myself when I met him in London. How did he achieve what he describes a 'a remission which I firmly believe to be self-induced'?

With medical help, MacDougall designed for himself a diet free of gluten, low in sugars and animal fats, and high in unsaturated fats. He emphasises in his booklet *My Fight Against MS* that foods missed out must be replaced with other acceptable foods which will make good the nutrients you would otherwise lack, and he also helped to put right any deficiencies by taking vitamins and mineral supplements. His diet, therefore, is not just gluten-free.

The MacDougall diet does not work for all sufferers. A small percentage have experienced no improvement. It takes, too, a long time to halt and reverse MS. It was *four years* before enough movement returned to MacDougall's fingers for him to do up a button.

Dr Joseph Evers The German physician Joseph Evers has treated many thousands of MS patients with a nutritionally-based programme. He maintains that if the disease is caught in its early stages the patient can achieve a 100% remission, which is maintained as long as he stays on the diet. The success rate goes down according to the length of time the condition has been active. Evers does not believe that the damaged parts of the myelin sheath can ever be repaired, but that the body will restore a degree of normality, given the chance. He warns that there will be fluctuations in symptoms during treatment.

The Evers diet allows the following foods: raw fruit, raw root vegetables, unpasteurized milk, butter, raw oat flakes, wholemeal bread, raw eggs, honey and water. All vegetables and fruits must be organically grown, and emphasis is placed on sprouting grains (SEE *Sprouting Seeds and Grains* pages 133–5). No potatoes or green salads are allowed in the early stages of treatment, and nicotine, coffee, cocoa, tea, sugar, salt and all other condiments and sweets are banned. Natural wine and brandy are allowed occasionally, and can be taken if there is violent pain or sleeplessness.

For the constipation which often accompanies MS, Dr Evers recommends plenty of whole fruit, with linseeds or soaked prunes before each meal. His treatment also includes cold showers, daily exercise, massage, yoga and plenty of rest.

Asked to conduct a controlled trial, which would have meant giving one group of sufferers the diet and denying it to another, Dr Evers refused, saying that he did not wish to deny his treatment to anyone. He has however made available the case histories of more than 13 000 of his MS patients, treated over the past 30 years. In a sample of over 400 such patients, 42% showed improvement.[4]

Dr Are Waerland This Swedish doctor recommends a fast of three to five days on diluted fruit or vegetable juices at the start of treatment, followed by two weeks on a raw cleansing alkaline diet. After this, a large mixed vegetable and green leafy salad is taken daily and the other main meal is fruit. Sprouting wheat is taken with the salad and one slice of wholemeal bread a day is allowed. Lunch is a mixture of whole grains called five-grain kruska, with a little cottage cheese and a jacket potato. Vegetable broth, unpasteurized sour milk, yogurt and dried fruit are included. Dr Waerland also incorporates exercise, water treatments and massage.

Dr Michael Crawford Dr Crawford of the Nuffield Laboratories of Comparative Medicine in London has researched into MS and diet, using his extensive knowledge of dietary fats.

In accordance with their specific need for cell division, unborn and very young babies need a lot of polyunsaturated fats. Human breast milk contains a high ratio of these fats for the growing baby when he most needs them. The period of growth before and just after birth is the time when the nervous system is most likely to be vulnerable to dietary shortages; 60% of the solid matter of the brain and 70% of the myelin sheath are made up of polyunsaturated fats. It has been suggested that cow's milk, substituting for human breast milk and containing about a quarter of its essential fatty acid content, may be relevant to the incidence of MS.

The essential fatty acid, linoleic acid, must be provided in the diet and is found only in polyunsaturated fats (SEE *Fats* pages 23–35). Once absorbed into the body, linoleic acid is changed first to gamma linolenic acid, and lastly prostaglandins are made from the second conversion stage, gamma linolenic acid. They act like hormones, as regulators of body processes and as messengers. They help to keep the immune system healthy, and there is almost certainly something very wrong with the immune system in MS patients. They also help to control platelets, small discs which clump together at the site of a wound to stop the bleeding. In MS and certain other other conditions these platelets clump together unnecessarily and cause circulatory difficulties.

The conversion of linoleic acid to prostaglandins is slow and inefficient, even in a healthy person, and research suggests that this process may be further delayed or disturbed in MS patients. The levels of essential fatty acids in the blood of some MS sufferers are usually found to be abnormally low, but this is not always the case; very high levels also exist. Commenting on these two extremes, Dr Crawford suggests that 'we are probably seeing some evidence of neurological damage, in effect biochemical debris, as these results were usually only obtained in severely affected cases.'[5] It is thought that this fat imbalance, which seems to be a general part of MS, is likely to be the result of metabolic or nutritional disturbances during the early period of life, both before and just after birth, when the brain and nervous system are still growing.

Dr Crawford emphasises the importance of linoleic acid for a healthy nervous system and brain, and in his dietary recommendations a good supply of the essential fatty acids predominates. He recommends liver and other offal, fish, dark green vegetables and raw salads with a seed oil dressing, fresh fruit, other lean meats, whole cereals and wholemeal bread. Sugar and hard saturated fats are cut to a minimum. Dr Crawford gives his patients individual attention, and tries to find out exactly what is happening inside the patient before deciding finally on what he should eat.

Dr F.R. Klenner Dr Frederick Robert Klenner uses megavitamin treatment (SEE *Orthomolecular Therapy*) on his MS patients. This consists of very high doses of the B vitamins thiamine, niacin, choline, B6, calcium pantothenate, B12 and B2, with vitamins C and E, liver injections and lecithin, calcium and magnesium and other minerals. His patients also follow a high-protein diet, with drug therapy.

Max Gerson The late Dr Max Gerson instituted an intensive nutritional therapy to cure all chronic degenerative diseases, but principally cancer (SEE *Cancer – the Gerson Therapy* pages 277–81). This treatment, which revitalizes and detoxifies the body rapidly and profoundly, has also been used to treat MS and there have been many successes. This is a tough and demanding regime, but a strikingly successful one.

MS and allergy

Many MS sufferers are allergic to rye and wheat, and we have seen that there is a high incidence where these cereals are staple foods. Incidence is low where rice is the main cereal. In one survey, diets free of whatever food the sufferer was found to be allergic to gave favourable results in about 31% of the cases tested.[6] (About 24% of these peopole were also found to be short of fat.)

MS and low blood sugar

Abnormally high or low blood sugar was found in every one of 126 MS patients examined by Dr E.M. Abrahamson (*New York State Medical Journal*, 1 June 1954). He used a diet to correct the sugar level, together with injections of calcium, and obtained good results.

Individual supplements

Evening primrose oil This plant is well-known to herbalists and the oil from its seeds is the subject of much current research. It contains a high proportion of gamma linolenic acid. We have seen that linoleic acid changes into gamma linolenic acid inside the body, and many practitioners now are short-cutting this often cumbersome process by giving the oil as a supplement. They have also tried sunflower oil (containing the original essential fatty acid, linoleic acid), but have found evening primrose oil, with both gamma linolenic and linoleic acid, more helpful.

Please SEE the *Evening Primrose Oil* section (pages 111–14) for more information, including where to get the oil.

Minerals One correlate of MS appears to be a low zinc level in the body. MS is more common in inland regions than in coastal areas, where more seafoods, containing zinc, are eaten. This mineral is needed to help turn the essential fatty acids into prostaglandins.

Calcium, magnesium and zinc orotate are being prescribed and copper, manganese, iron and selenium may also have important roles to play.

Vitamin B13[7] This vitamin-mineral bridge, orotic acid (B13) is being used for MS, particularly on the continent. Part of the success of Dr Evers' therapy may be due to the fact that the raw root vegetables he recommends contain B13. This substance is used by the body in the metabolism of folic acid and B12, and it transports nutrients past the brain barrier. It has been suggested that a high fever in childhood, perhaps undiagnosed encephalitis, can produce a scarring of this protective membrane and that, combined with nutritional deficiencies (especially mineral) this may be a precursor of MS.

Other vitamins   Virtually all the B vitamins are recommended for MS. Thiamine and niacin[8] and B6 with hydrocortisone[9] have brought improvement. When taken with essential fatty acids, B6 and zinc, vitamin C helps to form prostaglandins.

Any diet rich in essential fatty acids needs the anti-oxidants vitamins C and E to prevent the oxidation of polyunsaturated fats into dangerous substances.

Early diagnosis
It is vital to get an early diagnosis of this disease so that treatment can be started early. Your doctor will not help you by trying to conceal the truth from you; nutritional treatment must be started at once. Please consult a naturopath (SEE appendix page 405) or a nutritionally aware doctor and place yourself in his hands.

The *Nature Cure* section of this book (pages 391–6) will help you to understand your treatment and the *Food Therapy* section (pages 396–401) will give you an example of the ideal basic therapeutic diet.

Information
Organizations   Action for Research into Multiple Sclerosis (ARMS), 71 Gray's Inn Road, London WC1X 8TR (Telephone 01-961 4911 or 01-965 5733, ext. 627).
ARMS Telephone Counselling Service, 01-568 2255 (England and Wales), 041-637 2262 (Scotland), 24-hours a day 7 days a week all-year service for anyone suffering from MS or their family and friends. Manned by trained counsellors who have personal experience of the disease.
Multiple Sclerosis Society of Great Britain and Northern Ireland, 286 Munster Road, London SW6 6AP (Telephone 01-381 4022).

Clinics etc   Nature Cure Clinic, 15 Oldbury Place, London W1M 3AL (telephone 01 935 2787).

The Natural Health Clinic, 133 Gatley Road, Gatley, Cheadle, Cheshire SK8 4PD (telephone 061 428 4980).

The Kent Private Clinic, Sandwich, Kent (telephone 0304 612910).

Dr Paul Evers' MS Clinic, Langschweid–Sorpesee, 5768 Sundern, Hachen, Germany.

MS and other Metabolic Diseases clinic: Sanatorium Romrod, Am Jungfernbrunnen, 6326 Romrod 1, Germany.

Dr F.R. Klenner, 217 Gilmer Street, P.O. Box 840, Reidsville, North Carolina USA 27320.

Gerson therapy   Please contact The Association for New Approaches to Cancer (ANAC) of 1A Addison Crescent, London W14 8JP (telephone 01-603-7751) for doctors and other practitioners who use the Gerson therapy.

Additional therapies

Acupuncture: SEE appendix page 405.

Exercise, classes for MS sufferers: contact ARMS for information. Yoga for Health Foundation give special courses for MS sufferers; SEE Yoga under *Exercise* in the appendix, page 405.

Herbalism: SEE appendix page 405.

Homoeopathy: SEE appendix page 405.

Relaxation: fatigue in MS is devastating. You must rest every day. SEE appendix page 405.

Recommended reading

Multiple Sclerosis – A Self-Help Guide to its Management by Judy Graham (Thorsons 1981).

Help Fight MS – Dietary Therapy with Polyunsaturated Fatty Acids from Dr Evers' Clinic – SEE Clinics.

The First Clinical Ecology Cookbook by Rita Greer, whose husband recovered from MS. Cooking without gluten and other common allergens. Obtainable from Ms Greer at 44 Wallisdean Avenue, Portsmouth, Hampshire, price £3 including postage.

My Fight Against Multiple Sclerosis by Roger MacDougall, obtainable free on receipt of a 9in × 6in stamped and addressed envelope from Regenics Limited, 25/27 Oxford Street, London W1R 1RF.

Recipes: apply to Judith Harding at ARMS.
Good Food, Gluten Free by Hilda Cherry Hills, (Roberts Publications) 225 Putney Bridge Road, London SW15 2PY.
Contact ARMS for further information and books.

Obesity

We are becoming a nation of fatties. About half the people in this country weigh more than is good for them.[1]

To be fat – very fat – is asking for trouble. The obese get more diabetes, arthritis, gout, heart and artery disease, high blood pressure, kidney and thyroid disease, hernia, colitis, peptic ulcer, bronchitis, gall bladder disease and cancer and they have a higher mortality rate. They may have problems during pregnancy and difficulty in breathing properly. With the burden of excess weight to carry around, they are under constant strain and age more quickly.

How fat is fat?
If you are fat you know it. From having trouble doing up your jeans (they must have shrunk in the wash) to billowing around like a jelly, not daring to look at your reflection, you know when you are putting on fat.

If you want to be sure, strip naked in front of a full-length mirror and judge for yourself. Are you the size *you* want to be? To be a little plump may suit you very well and it is quite different from the acres and pounds of uncontrolled flesh which make life so difficult, and so dangerous, for your hardworking body.

But thin is beautiful . . . isn't thin what we are all supposed to strive for? American biochemist Roger J. Williams comments that there are plenty of people who function better when they are heavy and goes on to say that 'the fight to be normal . . . *is in itself a disease*'[2] (my italics).

Having said all that, I assume that you still want to slim down, or you would not be reading this section.

Ways of being fat

Scales are deceptive, and so is the whole question of *weight*, rather than size. The water content of the body varies from 45.6% to 70.2% and this swing is closely linked in women to the menstrual period. Men's bodies contain about 20% more water than women's. As well as being affected by the amount of body fluid, weight can also mean not more fat, but more muscle.

What body type are you? You may be round and soft (endomorph), angular and muscly (mesomorph), slender and delicate (ectomorph) or a mixture, like most of us. Your body type will strongly affect the way you deal with fat. The paperclip-thin young model is probably an ectomorph and if you're not you're never going to look like her.

A calorie is a unit of energy (the amount of heat needed to warm a kilogram of water by 1°C). One way of measuring our food is in terms of calories, which give us energy. If we take in more calories than we need our bodies will store the extra as fat. Some of us however can burn this extra energy by boosting heat production or oxygen consumption. There is, therefore, a difference between people who store their extra calories and those who can get rid of them using, it is thought, the recently researched brown fat cells for this extra boost.

There are other individual differences, too. Some people have abnormalities in their body processes which encourage obesity. People with low blood sugar, for instance (SEE *Low Blood Sugar* pages 340–5) feel exhausted and wobbly and crave sugar. This sugar intake is met by insulin which lowers the blood sugar again to its normal level after a brief lift. With repeated sugar intake the pancreas (the gland which produces the insulin) does its job more and more efficiently so that the sugar in the blood is lowered more and more quickly, making the sugar craving and the exhaustion worse. Low blood sugar causes potassium loss and water retention, so that the person will get waterlogged.

Dr Ted Randolph in the USA and Dr Richard Mackarness in Britain believe that compulsive eating can be an addiction developing from a food allergy (SEE *Allergies to Food* pages 219–29). The offending food causes low blood sugar.

Many fat people do not deal with fat properly, storing too much of it, and the same can sometimes apply to the way they deal with protein and glucose. The glands associated with obesity are the pituitary, the thyroid, the adrenals, the pancreas and the sex glands. We are all slightly different in every way, including the ways in which these glands function. Oral contraceptives also cause some women to put on fat.

The number and size of your fat cells is determined during your first few months of life. Obese people have a higher number and the cells are bigger. But these cells can, of course, remain empty.

Many of the foregoing are hereditary characteristics; there are also a few very rare diseases which will cause obesity. If you are grossly obese, please consult your doctor. It is a good idea to let him know in any case about your plans for slimming.

The average fatty
The connection between obesity and refined foods can be traced all over the Western world.

Obesity starts in the cradle and fat babies make fat people. Infant foods are sometimes sweetened (less now), but breast milk contains *no added sugar*. We have more fat school-children than ever before, and children are particularly vulnerable to junk food advertising on TV. The annual budget for advertising confectionery on British commercial television is more than £20 million.

We love sweet foods, but carbohydrates and sugar provide calories which can be quickly absorbed and accumulated, as every fatstock farmer knows. Fats and proteins can make you fat, too. As we saw earlier, all you need for fatness is a greater intake of calories, or energy, than your output (taking into account, of course, your biochemical individuality). The chart on page 366 shows the number of calories consumed in an hour of exercise.

Naturopaths believe that, because our food is refined and lacking in nutrients, some people overeat in an instinctive attempt to take in enough essential substances. It is thought, too, that the thin person you envy so much may simply have a bowel so clogged with impurities that its capacity to absorb is impaired.

So advertising, our sedentary lives, and our rubbishy food, encourage us to get fat. But need we really eat so much? Can we sidestep this deluge of sugary foods?

There is a neural control centre – working rather like a

9: How exercise can help

Level*	Walking	Running	Sports & Games
Level A (about 175 cals per hr.)	Ambling, strolling (1½–2½mph)	—	archery, billiards, bowls (green), boule, cricket, croquet, golf, rifle-shooting, sailing, table tennis
Level B (about 270 cals per hr.)	Slow, easy walking (2½–3½mph)	—	badminton, bowling (ten-pin), canoeing, dancing, diving, rowing, softball/baseball, surfing
Level C (about 355 cals per hr.)	Standard walking (3½–4mph)	gentle jogging (3–5mph)	basketball, bowling (cricket), cycling, fencing, gymnastics, hockey, judo, karate, lacrosse, orienteering, rambling, skating, sub aqua swimming, tennis, trampolining
Level D (about 435 cals per hr.)	Brisk striding walk (4–5mph)	slow running (5–6mph)	climbing, football, skiing, swimming
Level E (about 740 cals per hr.)	Sprint walking (6–7mph)	standard running (7–8mph)	boxing, handball, rugby, squash, water polo, wrestling

* **Remember that you would use up approximately 60 calories if you rested for an hour. All these figures include this value for resting metabolism.**

Chart supplied by BUPA.

switch – in our brain called the appestat which tells us when we have had enough. But this mechanism is concerned with *hunger*, and not *appetite*. What we feel when we see food advertised is not usually hunger, but appetite. True hunger is an unfamiliar sensation to most of us in the West.

Fat people are used to eating, and they ignore the appestat which is trying to tell them that they have eaten enough. They munch on regardless of a full stomach.

Do you *want* to be fat?
Compulsive eating has a function. What does it do for you?

Writer and psychotherapist Susie Orbach, who has worked extensively with women who are trying to reduce, has found that fat can be an escape from life or a shield against it. If you're fat, you won't attract men, so you won't have to worry about your sexuality. If you don't try, you can't fail (*Fat is a Feminist Issue* by Susie Orbach). The fat person is often afraid of being thin, because it means coming out of her shell of excess flesh and being what part of her would like to be. The challenge is too much for some people, who need to understand that being thin – or any other state for that matter – does not carry with it an obligation to be perfect.

Compulsive eating can be used to suppress rage and allay anxiety and fear. One of our primitive, hidden fears is of starvation and I recall a recent cinema ad which exhorted patrons to buy a hot-dog in the interval 'just in case you get hungry later'.

As well as being ashamed of her body and unable to control her food addiction (and of course all this applies to men as well), the compulsive eater is doubly unhappy because she does not even enjoy her food. From being obsessed with food, she becomes obsessed with dieting. She just exchanges one pre-occupation for another, with food her constant enemy. Since her appestat has been shouted down long ago by her negative feelings, she never goes without food long enough to experience the sensation of hunger.

What controls hunger?

The appestat, a mechanism located in the mid-brain, is nature's way of controlling your food intake in both directions. We have seen that it can be overruled, and it is of course as vulnerable to poor nutrition as any other part of the body. If you deprive a laboratory rat of vitamin B1, its appestat will not function properly and it will cease to eat. The damage will be worse with a deficiency of vitamin A. There is a case of a ten-year old English boy with a faulty appestat who ate vast quantities of food, vomiting most of it back. A malfunction can also lead to anorexia, where a person can literally starve to death. Lack of exercise will put the appestat out of order, so that animals confined for killing and fattening up will eat a lot; gorging will unbalance it too. We have a similar mechanism to control thirst and this can be damaged as well.

It is probable that high-quality nutrition over a long period

10: Recommended weight in relation to height

Height without shoes		Recommended average weight without clothes		Weight range	
in	*cms*	*pounds*	*kgs*	*pounds*	*kgs*
Men					
62	158	123	56	112–141	51–64
63	160	127	58	115–144	52–65
64	163	130	59	118–148	54–67
65	165	133	60	121–152	55–69
66	168	136	62	124–156	56–71
67	170	140	64	128–161	58–73
68	173	145	66	132–166	60–75
69	175	149	68	136–170	62–77
70	178	153	69	140–174	64–79
71	180	158	72	144–179	65–81
72	183	162	74	148–184	67–84
73	185	166	75	152–189	69–86
74	188	171	78	156–194	71–88
75	191	176	80	160–199	73–90
76	193	181	82	164–204	74–92
Women					
58	147	102	46	92–119	42–54
59	150	104	47	94–122	43–55
60	152	107	48	96–125	44–57
61	155	110	50	99–128	45–58
62	158	113	51	102–131	46–59
63	160	116	53	105–134	48–61
64	163	120	54	108–138	49–63
65	165	123	56	111–142	50–64
66	168	128	58	114–146	52–66
67	170	132	60	118–150	54–68
68	173	136	62	122–154	55–70
69	175	140	64	126–158	57–72
70	178	144	65	130–163	59–74
71	180	148	67	134–168	61–76
72	183	152	69	138–173	63–78

From 'The Facts about Obesity', by kind permission of BUPA.

can repair the damage. Fighting obesity without the help of a properly functioning appestat is like running up the down escalator.

We have already seen that hunger can be affected by factors other than the appestat. Like breathing, which is automatic most of the time and yet can be altered when we choose, hunger can be influenced by excitement and whereas some people 'can't eat a thing' when they are worried, others will stuff themselves.

In general, however, those people who obey the body-wisdom of the appestat will maintain their ideal weight in a flexible and healthy way.

Why can't we diet successfully?

It is not too difficult to *lose* weight. It is almost impossible to keep it down. Why is this?

A dictionary definition of the word diet is to 'restrict oneself to special food, especially in order to control one's weight' *(Concise Oxford Dictionary)*. This definition has an emergency, temporary feel about it. A diet is something which comes to an end, like a rainstorm or a headache. A recent survey found that 97% of people on slimming diets were back to their original fatness in about a year after completing the diet. If to complete the diet is to stop following it, then we will eventually regain our original girth all over again.

When energy intake is reduced with a restricted diet, there is usually weight loss and much jubilation. But the body can adjust to this lower level of calories, even by reducing its basal metabolism (rate of internal workings) so that in effect it needs less food. This could be an explanation for the weight plateau which occurs when a diligent slimmer finds her weight loss slowing down or stopping altogether. A person who sheds only part of her excess weight, or fat, may find such a half-and-half stage difficult to get through.

The reason for the quick weight loss at the beginning of the diet is usually loss of excess body fluids, and not fat – another reminder that to talk about 'weight' rather than actual fat is, although perhaps more delicate, less to the point.

When a dieter restricts her calories, she quite often restricts her nutrients too, throwing her body out of metabolic balance so that, as soon as regular eating starts once again, she will put fat back on again with lightning speed.

Crash diets

A crash diet is shock treatment for the body. Worse still, many slimmers lead a yo-yo existence, rushing from diet to diet with a period of compulsive stuffing in between. This is a severe strain. By over-eating a lot you can overtax the enzymes responsible for splitting down fats, and you will therefore lay down fat all the more easily, even on a very low-fat diet.

Let's look at some crash diets.

High protein Too much protein throws too much work on the kidneys. It brings about a Specific Dynamic Action, which causes the metabolic rate to rise by 20% or even 35% so that the extra heat made 'burns up' tissue. This is an extreme induced version of some people's natural way of dealing with excess calories. This diet may also cause calcium loss, and is not a desirable way to lose weight.

Low carbohydrate Often low in nutrients, this diet can be constipating, and will cause excessive fatty acid release. Some people, too, need more carbohydrates than others.

High carbohydrate For a person with a tendency to low blood sugar this can be a strain on the pancreas.

High fat This is nauseating and often causes diarrhoea, when nutrients are lost in the evacuation of fluids.

Low fat We all need a little fat, but we all eat too much of it. So this one is probably the best and low-fat eating is part, at any rate, of the way of eating recommended by naturopaths. However, the essential fatty acids in unrefined oils are needed to form lecithin, which burns up fat (SEE *Fats* pages 23–35).

Please remember that there is absolutely no fad or crash diet which is nutritionally adequate.

Slimming aids

Fat people prefer pills. They can eat them.

But slimming pills won't necessarily make you thin. Professor John Yudkin treated one group of fat people with pills and the other without. Those without got thinner.

Yudkin points out that slimming foods bear a label stating that they are effective only as part of a calorie-controlled diet. This, of course, would also apply to a suet pudding.

There is some doubt about the long-term effects of the synthetic bulkers (not usually dietary fibre) in many slimming foods. Slimming biscuits and toffees often contain sugar which, particularly in sticky sweets, is bad for your teeth and bad for you (if you want to know how bad, read the *Sugar* section).

The slimming business is booming with pills, 'low-calorie' foods, meal replacements, starch blockers and other glittering promises. But the same principle applies. Nobody is going to eat them for ever, and quite rightly; they're probably nutritionally unsound.

If you have a maths degree then perhaps you go in for calorie counting. But if you were to painstakingly count all the calories you eat, missing out the equivalent of only three peanuts a day, your mistake could theoretically result in a gain of 88 lbs over 20 years.[2]

Goodies, not calories

Let's look at *good nutrition* and obesity, instead of wringing our hands over calories.

When we eat refined, denatured foods, we are impairing the body's ability to dispose of unwanted fat. A deficiency of the B vitamin pantothenic acid means that fats will burn at only half their normal rate. Stored fat cannot be turned into energy without vitamin B6, and E is also needed to make use of fats. The major function of lecithin is to emulsify fats and unrefined oils help us to slim as well. People on very low protein diets can get fatter than those getting enough; this is because proteins are needed to burn other proteins.

The rules for keeping slim, therefore, are the same as the rules for keeping healthy. First of all – very important – over half your food should be raw, fresh fruit and vegetables. Use wholemeal bread and wholegrain cereals. Eat some proteins (the best are lamb's liver and other organ meats, seafoods, some poultry, cheese and eggs, milk, unsalted nuts, soya, pulses and legumes). Cut down on or cut out all sugars, and go easy on salt and fats. Use Biosalt, cider vinegar and unrefined oil as a base for your salad dressings, or just squeeze on some fresh lemon juice. Start sprouting grains and use lecithin and brewer's yeast; kelp and spirulina are also recommended for slimming (SEE index for page references to sections on all these; also SEE the *Whole Foods* section pages 101–6). Don't let yourself get ravenously hungry. It didn't work before and it won't work now. Eat fruit between meals for a snack – it's delicious and good for you (and low in calories too).

This is an eating plan and not a dietary cage. You will break the rules occasionally – we all do. But don't worry about it. If this way of eating is quite foreign to you, then start gently. In particular you will find it necessary to chew your food more thoroughly now, because it contains natural fibre.

Dietary fibre is found in whole cereals including wholemeal bread and in vegetables and fruit, especially if they are not peeled. Because it puts back what has been taken out of our food, it has far-reaching beneficial effects on our health (SEE *Fibre*) and the bulk in a slice of wholemeal bread will satisfy your hunger more than three slices of the supermarket white sliced.

Compatible eating
This way of eating is fully discussed on pages 151–5. It can be valuable for those with digestive problems and has been found useful for controlling weight.

We are *when* we eat.
We all know the person who never has breakfast, skips lunch, and then has a huge supper and stays fat and unhealthy. This 'one large meal a day' habit is very bad for you, putting up the blood pressure and blood fats. Anyway, it's the wrong way around.

Researcher Ronald Gatty took two groups of people. He fed each group the *same number* of calories – but the first group took their calories for breakfast and the other for supper (for experimental purposes only, one meal a day was taken). The first group lost weight, the second put it on.[3]

So the time of day strongly influences the way our bodies deal with food. A protein-rich breakfast causes a slow, steady rise in blood sugar, keeping you alert for the whole morning, and you can plan your eating on a smaller scale after that. I have found that some wholegrain cereal with a little wheat germ, bran and milk is delicious, and I add plenty of fresh raw fruit and a few sprouting seeds (SEE *Food Therapy* section pages 396–401). If you decide to use granular lecithin this can be added too.

Gatty also points out that our biological rhythms include a 'night-eating syndrome' when we sit and nibble in front of the television. Make a delicious raw salad for the evening – it takes so much chewing that any 'night-eating syndrome' is quite vanquished.

Fasting

Since many people find going without food relatively easy, you may decide to fast, or eat fresh fruit only, for one day a week. This repays a terrific bonus in well-being and energy and will of course help your weight loss. If you wish to do this, please read the *Fasting* section first (pages 159–63).

Side-stepping the obsession

I hope I have shown you that it's *nutrients* that matter, not calories; *health*, not size. Wholefoods eating cuts out empty calories, provides your body with what it needs to dispose of fats, increases your energy and gives you back the natural fibre which satisfies your appetite. It also keeps your appestat in good condition. You will lose weight on it, but your weight loss will be gradual, and therefore safe. Because you will benefit from this way of eating, you will stick to it without worrying about the occasional lapse. Anyway, it tastes better.

Enjoyment of what you eat is a vital part of eating less and appreciating better quality foods. If you are too tense to eat slowly and with enjoyment, you will find relaxation valuable. Should you prefer to slim in a group, you might like to contact your local Weightwatchers (SEE *Additional therapies* for both).

As you progress you will find it easier and easier to distinguish between artificially stimulated appetite and your natural instinct, hunger. Listening to your body telling you its needs is what health, and your natural body size, are all about.

Additional therapies

Acupuncture: SEE appendix page 405.

Exercise: SEE appendix page 405.

Herbalism: SEE appendix page 405.

Homoeopathy: SEE appendix page 405.

Relaxation, Autogenic Training is a specific for obesity: SEE appendix page 405.

Weightwatchers since their inception in 1963 have been helping people to lose weight and keep it off in a healthy way. There are about 1200 classes all over Britain – please write to Weightwatchers (UK) Limited, 635–637 Ajax Avenue, Slough, SL1 4DB or get in touch with your local group.

Books mentioned in this section
Fat is a Feminist Issue by Susie Orbach (Hamlyn 1978).
The Body Clock Diet by Ronald Gatty (Gollancz 1980).

Pre-menstrual Tension

Menstruation
Your monthly period is mainly controlled by four hormones;
FSH (follicle-stimulating hormone), LH (luteinizing
hormone), oestrogen and progesterone. The balance of these
hormones changes with the various phases of the menstrual
cycle, and their production is controlled by the pituitary gland.
The whole thing is masterminded by the hypothalamus, inside
the brain.

The cycle begins when, influenced by the hypothalamus, the
pituitary releases FSH into the bloodstream. The FSH goes to
the ovaries and encourages an egg cell, or follicle, to develop,
and an ovary to produce oestrogen. This oestrogen stops the
pituitary from producing any more FSH – no more egg cells
are needed to ripen now, one is enough. The oestrogen also
influences the uterus, which prepares itself to receive the egg.
The oestrogen causes the release of the hormone LH and this
sends the ripe egg into the fallopian tube. This is called
ovulation and happens about half-way through the cycle.

The hormone progesterone is released now which
encourages the uterus to build up more lining. This release is
controlled by prolactin, a hormone whose main function is
milk production. If the egg is fertilized, more progesterone is
released and the egg develops. But if the egg is sterile it
disintegrates. Since some of the progesterone is being supplied
by the egg itself, the level of this hormone now falls, causing
the womb lining to fall away and menstruation to start.

What is PMT?
Symptoms of PMT (pre-menstrual tension) occur in 40% of
otherwise healthy women, starting about ten days before

menstruation. It's even possible to get pseudo-PMT after your menopause. Physical symptoms include water retention; this water may be taken from the bowel and you may therefore be constipated. You can put on from four to seven pounds before your period. Ankles and feet may be swollen and rings do not fit. You may have a headache, due partly also to hormonal changes, and tender breasts are very common. Some women suffer from migraine now. You may get general aches and pains, feel clumsy and uncoordinated and feel cravings, usually for very sweet foods. You may also be very tired (due probably to a drop in blood sugar or a mineral imbalance) and this is sometimes followed by bursts of tremendous energy. Depression and irritability are common, with mood swings, and you may feel very tense. Less common are skin outbreaks and spontaneous bruising. Statistics show that most violent crimes including suicide attempts committed by women taken place at the time of a menstruation or just before.

Causes

Most doctors believe now that PMT is caused mainly by a hormone imbalance. As we have seen, the menstrual cycle is a very complex, delicately-balanced process. It is possible that some of the symptoms may also be connected with other hormonal disturbances in the body.

Extensive research is being done at St Thomas's Hospital in London, where it has been found that nearly half the women with PMT who were tested had progesterone deficiencies. 40% of them had more oestrogen than normal, too.

A deficiency of the vitamin B6 can affect brain function, leading to irritability and depression. Some women may need more than others, and the Pill creates a high need for this essential vitamin. A deficiency of B6 accompanies a faulty metabolism of the amino acid, tryptophan, and women depressed before their periods were found to have this disturbance (*American Journal of Psychiatry*, November 1973); another B vitamin, niacin, also helps tryptophan to be used by the body. It has also been found that, in the week before menstruation, calcium levels in the blood go down.

As well as these biochemical changes, a woman's attitude towards her period affects her cycle. Orthodox Judaism forbids sex during the period and when it has ceased a woman must go to the mikvah (ritual bath) and be ritually cleansed. This may give rise to the idea that menstruation is dirty and shameful and be the underlying reason for some of the problems associated with it. Stress, too, has a marked effect on the menstrual cycle.

Drug treatments

Tranquillizers, anti-depressants and diuretics (for water retention) are often prescribed for PMT, and ammonium chloride is sometimes used in small quantities. Diuretics will wash out potassium and other nutrients with the urine and your depression and fatigue will therefore get worse; taking tranquillizers and anti-depressants runs the risk of side-effects.

Some women find that their symptoms lessen when they go on the Pill, and progesterone is sometimes given to try and right the hormone balance. Bromocriptine, which limits the hormone prolactin, has side effects which include nausea, vomiting, dizziness, a fall in blood pressure and 'there is little benefit to be gained in the Pre-menstrual Syndrome by its use'.[1]

Vitamin B6 supplementation is being given for PMT at St Thomas's Hospital. In 1979 this clinic tested B6, comparing it with the hormone treatment available. The trial took seven months. In those treated with hormones, an improvement with mild side-effects was noted in 73% of the cases. In those given B6, the improvement was 63% overall, with *no side-effects*.

It is now possible to buy B6 supplements over the counter in a chemist or health food shop. Dr M.G. Brush of St Thomas's gives the following instructions for taking it:

'The typical adult case should start with 2 × 20mg tablets at breakfast time and 2 × 20mg tablets with the evening meal, or just before bedtime. If this dose is not sufficiently helpful, the dose should be adjusted to one 50mg tablet at breakfast and one 50mg tablet in the evening.' Dr Brush recommends the B6 to be started three days before the expected onset of PMT symptoms and discontinued when the symptoms would normally disappear, which is usually one to three days after the period has started. If a smaller dose has been used to start with, it can be increased by one tablet a day if the symptoms become more severe just before the time of the period, and this would mean that you would take 3 a day instead of 2. He states that about 75% to 80% of PMT patients are helped by this treatment once the correct dose for the individual is established. Apparently no significant side-effects have been noted apart from some gastric acidity at doses of about 200mg a day. Dr Brush warns that this level should not be exceeded except in the most exceptional circumstances; it has recently been suggested that mega-doses of B6 can cause liver damage. B6 has been found particularly helpful for irritability, pre-menstrual headache, breast tenderness and skin outbreaks.

Calcium tablets during the ten days before menstruation will correct the drop in blood calcium level and may help with headaches and pain during your period. To avoid water retention, cut down on salt for ten days before – too much salt is bad for you at any time.

Current research at St Thomas's Hospital also shows that evening primrose oil is often an effective treatment for the symptoms of PMT, including breast pain (SEE *Evening Primrose Oil* pages 111–14).

The Pre-menstrual Syndrome can often be helped by excellent nutrition – like everything else. So see that you are getting all the B vitamins in wheat germ, brewer's yeast, liver. Avoid fatty foods; it has been shown with laboratory animals that a high fat diet puts up the need for vitamin B6, and this may be the case with humans, too. Alcohol and refined sugar use up the B vitamins as well.

Visit your health food store and find out about the herbal teas such as camomile, raspberry leaf and dandelion, which help water retention and sore breasts, and fennel, winter savory, borage and sage for depression and tension. Don't try to gather your own herbs and make teas without a book of instruction.

There is a specific herbal remedy for PMT – Vitex Agnus Castus – which works by gently stimulating the pituitary to produce the right hormones at the right time (SEE *Additional therapies* at the end of this section). It is effective and absolutely harmless.

For further advice on diet and supplements, please consult a naturopath (SEE appendix page 405) or a nutritionally aware doctor. Please also SEE the appendix if you wish to consult a qualified medical herbalist.

Finally, try to reduce the strain on yourself before your period. Try to get some free time when you can really relax.

Additional therapies

Herbalism: Vitex Agnus Castus is produced by Inter-Medics Limited, 52 Walsworth Road, Hitchin, Hertfordshire, and is obtainable by prescription through a naturopath, medical herbalist or other qualified natural therapeutics practitioner.

Homoeopathy: SEE appendix, page 405.

Deep breathing, Yoga, Relaxation, for tension: SEE appendix page 405.

Stress

'Certain stress diseases are lethal', according to Peter Blythe in his book *Stress*, 'and can kill just as successfully as a well-aimed bullet.' The thirteenth report of the World Health Organization lists, among others, the following illnesses generally accepted as physical manifestations of stress: hypertension (high blood pressure), coronary thrombosis, migraine, hay fever and other allergies, and menstrual disorders.

Stress can often feel exhilarating. The intense concentration and flat-out effort of the athlete, that marvellous feeling when you rise to a challenge and come through with flying colours, the tightening of the throat when you clap the kids in their first school play – all these are stresses, but who would be without them?

But imagine a long queue of cars. You are stuck behind the wheel of one of them, moving an inch at a time while on the pavement old ladies, toddlers and snails flash past. *You are going to miss your train.*

Or you are at a meeting. 'We've got to cut our staff,' says the managing director. You wonder – *could he mean me?*

To understand stress, we need to go back to the time when we were just one animal among others. When early people were threatened with danger, it was a matter of life and death to get away in time. They had to be able to stalk and catch their prey, too, and defend tree or cave against invaders. So they needed resources of speed and stamina which they could call upon immediately.

The body changes built in to help these early people are with us now – and they are called the Fight or Flight response. The body reacts to any kind of stress *in the same way*. Messages from the pituitary gland to the adrenals result in the instant release of stress hormones which cause proteins and fats to be broken down for immediate energy. The blood sugar and blood pressure go up, the first so that energy is available and the second so that nutrients can be pushed quickly into the tissues. Minerals are withdrawn from the bones, breathing and heart rate quicken and blood flow increases to the arms and legs. Digestion and excretion are suspended.

This is the first stage of our reaction to stress, the Alarm Reaction. The second stage, the Stage of Resistance, is when the body repairs itself after exertion or shock, using the raw materials it has to hand. The third stage is when we experience exhaustion.

Stress is not always a life and death matter now. You can always miss that train. Strictly speaking, however, stress is caused by *any* change in environmental conditions which needs an adjustment from us. Our lives, therefore, are full of small reactions to stress – small adaptations to change – mostly hardly perceptible and often pleasant. Like the slight shivers we get in the cold, or the surge of pleasure when we see someone we love. These body changes cope with the minor shifts in our surrounding circumstances which are an inescapable part of living. As Hans Selye, world authority on stress, has said, 'complete freedom from stress is death'.

The Fight or Flight Response was absolutely essential to our primitive ancestors when agility and quick reactions meant the difference between life and death, or food and starvation. But now things are different. Instead of attacking our enemies with a stone axe, we rely on words, or perhaps just a smile through clenched teeth. It's no good, either, throwing the telephone through the window when that order is late. It's sure to fall on somebody underneath. Stuck in that traffic jam you need not brute force, but patience.

One major cause of physical and psychological stress, therefore, is the body's preparation for fast, vigorous action, without any follow-through. Under frequent stresses, when energy is not used, muscle contractions can become a permanent part of the way we hold ourselves and the autonomic (involuntary) nervous system is affected so that breathing becomes constricted and digestion and excretion impaired. This also happens of course if a person is habitually nervous and tense. On top of this is the fact that our bodies are not much good at judging how long we have been tense, so that the muscular contraction will continue long after the cause of it has passed.

The modern world is a shifting place. Our institutions – marriage, religion, law and order – are being severely battered and we have to choose for ourselves what to believe and how to live. Technology is changing our surroundings and moving us around faster and faster, with more and more noise. We are stockpiling weapons which could wipe us out. Our bodies are assaulted daily by the chemicals in the environment and in our food.

Change, too, is a major cause of stress. Make a list of the big changes in your life – were any of them followed by illness? Tests carried out by Dr Richard Rahe with the US navy established that those who had undergone the most changes had suffered the most illnesses. Upheavals in your life, whether pleasant or unpleasant, demand adaptations from you and, as we have seen, adaptation causes stress.

There are many ways we can minimize or avoid unwanted stress. Perhaps the woman holding down a job and looking after a home and family should ask herself if this double life is really necessary. Of course there is always someone next door who does four times as much and thrives on it. But how much stress can *you* stand? The business executive who brings work home would do well to arrange some time in his life when he shuts the door on his responsibilities.

Do you enjoy what you are doing? Selye's recipe for flourishing under stress is to spend your life doing something that really matters to you, and doing it well.

Stress and nutrition
All nutrients are needed in larger amounts during stress. Deficiencies of protein, any of the B vitamins especially pantothenic acid, or vitamins A or E prevent the body from coping well. Vitamin C is essential, to protect the adrenal

glands and help them produce the stress hormones. It also detoxifies any harmful substances present in the body and its protective effects are very marked. Vitamin D and the minerals calcium, zinc, magnesium, iron, potassium, phosphorus and in particular calcium are needed too.

Leaving aside isolated nutrients, there are certain foods which, researchers have established, will guard against the ill-effects of stress. There is, for instance, a very active 'anti-stress' factor in liver, and wheat germ, kidneys, brewer's yeast, green leafy vegetables and soya flour containing its own oil will all give a measure of protection. It has been found that laboratory animals can be protected by these foods in circumstances where individual vitamins or minerals are ineffective. This is an argument for getting nutrients in a natural balance so that they can work as a team. This natural balance can be found in a whole food diet (SEE *Whole Foods* pages 101–6). The way we eat comes first – and any supplements we may need in addition come second.

Always chew your food slowly and thoroughly, particularly when you are tired or tense, and make sure that you enjoy your meal in relaxed surroundings. If you are really upset or exhausted it is better not to try to eat at all. There is absolutely no danger in missing a meal from time to time.

Readers may be interested in the energy drink described in the *Fatigue* section (pages 303–9). If you do not want to go without food entirely then you will enjoy this drink.

Additional therapies
Relaxation is essential to combat stress. This may take the form of a hobby or a reorganization of your life-style. Many people however prefer to learn a deliberate technique: SEE appendix page 405.
The biochemic tissue salt Kali Phos (alone or in combination) will nourish and steady your nerves (please SEE *Biochemic tissue salts* pages 107–8).

Varicose Veins and Piles

Varicose veins are swollen, knotted and sometimes very painful. They usually form in the legs, but you can get them in the veins in the lower trunk and deeper inside the body; in fact anywhere where there are veins.

People with varicose veins will usually feel tired and unable to stand for long periods. Their legs are often uncomfortable and unsightly. Varicose veins are one of the most common Western diseases. A study in a Michigan community showed that 44% of the women aged between 30 and 50 years and 24% of the men in the same age-group had varicose veins. After 50, 64% of the women and 42% of the men had developed the condition.

Only about 5% of rural Africans suffer from these veins, but they are equally common among both blacks and whites living in the West, who both eat a refined diet.

What happens?

Varicosities affect the veins and not the arteries. One of the reasons for this is that the veins, unlike the arteries, lack an elastic coat and are therefore more vulnerable. The arteries carry clean blood on its outward journey from the heart and it is pushed forcefully along by the heartbeat. It is the task of the veins to push the dirty blood back to the heart without the help of the heartbeat, which has largely spent itself by then. They accomplish this partly by small, non-return valves every inch or so along the course of a vein which prevent the blood from flowing downwards and partly by the relaxation and contraction of the muscles surrounding them. The veins just underneath the skin surface are less supported by surrounding tissues and are more likely to become varicose.

As a result of the over-consumption of refined foods the blood becomes thickened, sluggish and acid. This 'colloidal blood' (a term coined by naturopaths) sets up a slight inflammation. Part or all of a valve can break off, which puts a severe strain on the vein and causes it to become twisted and swollen. The health of the veins is further worsened by a deficient diet, which starves the tissues of the vitamins and minerals they need.

Undoubtedly another major cause is constipation.

Nearly a century ago, Dr T.R. Allinson related constipation to a lack of fibre in the diet and it is obvious now that our refined diet, stripped of the fibre we need for a healthy working bowel, is responsible for the modern prevalence of constipation (SEE *Fibre* pages 35–42 and *Constipation* pages 382–6). It is thought that an overloaded bowel obstructs the return of blood through the veins by pressing on them. It is also likely that when a person strains in an effort to defecate the abdominal pressure puts further strain on the veins; even a strenuous exercise like weightlifting raises abdominal pressure less than straining at stool.

Another important factor is the condition of the liver. Part of the liver's job is to help with the return of blood to the heart, and if it is engorged and fatty it will not function properly. Liver function is always taken into account in the naturopathic treatment of varicose veins.

There are several secondary factors which do not cause the condition but which make it worse. These include pregnancy and childbirth, prolonged standing, a severe blow, obesity or even sudden weight loss (which removes support from the abdominal organs, allowing them to sag and press on the veins) and the wearing of tight constricting garments. Even a slight dislocation of knee or pelvis can cause trouble. Lack of exercise leads to poor muscle tone so that standing is tolerated badly by the body and the muscles which help the blood on its return journey are under-used. Emotional upsets and suppressed anger are thought to make matters worse; the leg veins are overloaded with blood ready to kick but since we do not generally go around kicking each other this release is not permitted.

Damage to the venous system is always serious because it will almost certainly spread. Another danger is that a broken piece of valve from the vein wall may be carried round the body in the bloodstream and can lodge in a vital part, causing a heart block or choking an important artery. Varicosity also results in poor circulation of the skin at the affected part. In time the skin may thin and break and an ulcer may form. Thinning of the vein wall itself may mean that even a light abrasion can cause a pin-point wound where the blood comes away in a fine spray but in large quantities. Never, therefore, rub varicose veins, and if you want them massaged, go to a qualified practitioner.

Surgical treatment

Varicose veins can be injected or 'stripped' – which means that
they are removed by a surgeon who cuts the vein at the top and
at the bottom of the leg and then pulls it out. Neither of these
procedures does anything to alleviate the original cause of the
trouble, and simply deprives the affected area of part of its
circulation. More varicosities tend to form within a few years.

The nutritional approach

Once veins have become varicose they cannot be regenerated,
but the condition can be arrested and the pain and tiredness
removed.

Fasting is an ideal way to begin treatment. Please read the
Fasting section (pages 159–63) carefully and set yourself a
pattern of, say, a one-day fast once a week or once a fortnight.
If this is not possible for you, eat nothing but fruit and drink
only fruit juices for 24 hours one day a week. In between your
fasts or fruit days, follow the Food Therapy Plan (pages 396–
401). This diet is designed to purify the blood and supply it at
the same time with all the nutrients essential for health. It will
leave the liver unhampered and able to work well, and will
banish constipation. Please observe the following modifications to the Plan:

1 All flesh foods should be stopped; they put a strain on the
liver.

2 Avoid citrus fruits and very acid foods, i.e. oranges,
lemons, grapefruits, satsumas, rhubarb, plums.

3 Unless your stools are soft and easily expelled and you are
definitely not constipated, add some bran to your breakfast
(SEE *Constipation* for amounts).

If you are tired before meals, rest for 20 minutes or so if you
can. This diet, with your fasts or fruit days, should be
continued until your veins are no longer swollen and painful.

Vitamin E is valuable for alleviating the swelling and
discomfort.

When varicose veins have been injected, additional
networks of veins are called into play to substitute and this
process is helped by vitamin E. The effects of Vitamin E
therapy may not appear until about three or four months after
you start taking it.

A more recent discovery is the value of bioflavonoids, often
called vitamin P. These substances are found in fresh fruits

and vegetables and especially in the pith of oranges, grapefruits and lemons, in the whiteish pulpy part of a green pepper and in tangerine juice. As a supplement, they are obtainable as rutin capsules. Bioflavonoids relieve the pain and swelling and have been shown to improve venous tone and increase capillary wall resistance. [1]

Lastly, a useful remedy for the tiredness and pain of varicose veins is the biochemic tissue salt, Calc. Fluor. Combination obtainable, like the other supplements above, at your health food store, or at a chemist under the brand name of Elasto (SEE *Biochemic tissue salts* page 107–8).

Before you undertake your Food Therapy, it will be necessary for you to understand how and why it works. Please, therefore, read the *Nature Cure* section (pages 391–6) first.

Please note that the dietary treatment is on general lines only and that you may also need additional vitamins and minerals. For individual guidance on both your Food Therapy plan and any necessary supplements, please consult a naturopath (SEE appendix) or a nutritionally aware doctor.

Additional therapies for both varicose veins and piles are listed at the end of the *Piles* section.

Piles

Piles (haemorrhoids) are one of the commonest ailments in the West. Half of all Americans over the age of 50 have them. Piles are much less common in Third World countries and relatively rare among tribal communities. They often form during pregnancy.

In many cases piles stay inside the rectum until they become inflamed when they protrude and cause great pain, especially during defecation.

Piles were previously thought to be varicosities in the anus. Recent research however suggests that the cushions surrounding the upper end of the anal canal which prevent the unwanted escape of faeces can become swollen and forced out of place further down the canal, so that they emerge from the anal opening.

The usual medical treatment is either an injection to form a scar which will obstruct the distended tissue, or surgery to remove it. Suppositories can be effective with small piles. But like varicose veins, piles can re-appear after such treatment because it has not removed the cause of the trouble.

Nutritional treatment

The main cause of piles is constipation. Straining in an attempt to evacuate dry, difficult faeces creates great pressure within the abdominal walls and fills the anal cushions with blood, making them swell. The hard faecal mass pushing past them then forces them downwards.

In his book *Don't Forget Fibre in your Diet* surgeon Denis Burkitt states that most patients with piles will need no further treatment once they have switched to a high-fibre diet which produces soft stools that can be passed without straining. Refined, white flour from which the fibre has been milled is therefore implicated in piles.

The Food Therapy plan in this book is high in natural fibre. If, however, you are constipated and have to strain then please add additional bran to your diet: SEE *Constipation* for detailed instructions.

Another major reason for piles is a disordered liver. In his book *The Nature Cure Treatment for Varicose Veins and Ulcers* naturopath J. Russell Sneddon states that the naturopathic treatment of piles must include the treatment of the liver too. The Food Therapy plan of unadulterated foods with plenty of fresh fruits and vegetables and less animal protein is ideal for the liver.

Bioflavonoids have been used to treat piles.[2] Often called vitamin P, these substances are closely associated with vitamin C and are found mostly in the pith and flesh of green peppers and citrus and other fruits. They are also obtainable as a supplement, rutin.

Piles during pregnancy have been prevented by 10mg of vitamin B6 a day.

The biochemic tissue salt, Calc. Fluor. Combination, helps to strengthen weakened tissues and is therefore useful for piles. It is obtainable at your health food store.

Before you undertake your Food Therapy, it will be useful for you to know how and why it works. Please therefore read the *Nature Cure* section first, pages 391–6.

If you think you have piles, it is best to make sure. 'Cancer of the rectum at an early, curable stage gives similar symptoms,' writes Peter Wingate in the *Penguin Medical Encyclopedia*. You may in any case wish to consult a naturopath (SEE appendix page 405) or nutritionally aware doctor for advice, both on the diet and on any supplements you may need.

Additional therapies for both varicose veins and piles

Acupuncture: SEE appendix page 405.

Deep breathing: venous sufferers are notoriously shallow breathers, SEE appendix page 405.

Exercise, for varicose veins. The best thing is to keep moving. The muscles can then massage the veins and help them send the blood back to the heart. Constricted sitting and standing are bad for varicose veins. SEE appendix page 405.

Herbalism: SEE appendix page 405.

Homoeopathy: SEE appendix page 405.

Osteopathy: SEE appendix page 405.

Yoga: any inverted position is excellent: SEE *Exercise*, appendix page 405.

Water therapy: for varicose veins: a cold hip bath twice a week; stay in for about 30 seconds, resting the feet on the end of the bath out of the water. Spray the legs with cold water for one minute every morning.

For piles: if the piles are external and inflamed, take a hot soapy hip bath for about 15 minutes, resting the feet on the end of the bath out of the water. Gently ease the pile mass back into the rectum when possible. Sometimes it is necessasry to persevere with 2 or 3 hot baths before this can be done.

After the pile mass has gone back into the body, take a 30-second cold hip bath, keeping the feet out of the water. Follow this with a cold spray each morning; one minute on the area between the rectum and the genitals and one minute on the actual rectal area.

Recommended reading for both varicose veins and piles

The Nature Cure Treatment for Varicose Veins and Ulcers by J. Russell Sneddon (Thorsons 1979).

Other books mentioned in this section

Don't Forget Fibre in Your Diet by Denis Burkitt (Martin Dunitz, USA, 1979).

Penguin Medical Encyclopedia ed. Peter Wingate (Penguin 1976).

PART FOUR

Nature Cure
and
Food Therapy

Nature Cure

To the present-day orthodox doctor, illness is an entity – something that sneaks into the body and causes havoc, or a malfunction that gums up the body's works. Largely by the use of drugs, he tries either to destroy this malevolent entity or to suppress the symptoms of malfunction.

But the father of medicine, Hippocrates, insisted that doctors should above all things do no harm to their patients. In view of the side-effects of our drugs, and the fact that over 10% of all illness is estimated to be caused by *prescribed* drugs, is this principle still operating today?

Treatment with drugs concentrates on the symptoms, doing little or nothing about the deep-seated causes of illness. Drugs contain toxins so that, as well as having to cope with the illness, the body's eliminative capacity is called upon to deal with the drug, too. Drugs simply give the body more work to do, and suppress the symptom which is its attempt to heal itself. Recurring symptoms show that the cause of the illness is still there and, particularly with drug treatment, these recurrences can lead to the chronic degenerative diseases which plague us so much now, including heart disease, high blood pressure, kidney disease and cancer. In an article in the *Daily Telegraph* of 28 May 1974, Doctors Murdoch and Gray of Edinburgh City Hospital stated that only about one in seven of the known infections of man can be adequately treated by drugs; and Dr Drysdale of the British College of Naturopathy and Osteopathy told me that about 85% of drugs could be dispensed with, and the remaining 15% used in a more intelligent way.

The naturopath, however, seeks a reason for illness. It is this *cause*, this *reason*, that is important. Why has the germ succeeded in making this particular person ill, when it is unsuccessful with others? Or why is the sick person's body working so badly that he shows the symptoms of high blood pressure, or heart disease, or migraine?

In nature cure the individual, not the illness, is the prime focus of attention. Why is this person ill? What in his life-style – the way he eats, relaxes, exercises, relates to other people – is weakening him and distorting his health?

The naturopath's job is to persuade his patient to see this connection between life-style and health, and to accept the need for changes which he asks his patient to implement – and *continue to implement*.

For in nature cure, results are achieved by the patient. He shares responsibility with his practitioner.

Diet, exercise and relaxation, water treatment, a positive attitude – these are gentle, unspectacular methods. The late Dr Bernard Allinson was once asked if nature cure could perform miracles. 'Instant miracles, no,' he replied, 'but slow miracles, yes.' Nature cure is gradual and undramatic. Natural healing can regenerate diseased bodies, but it always demands one basic condition; *time*. It will not heal overnight, but, in most cases, heal it will. Unless you are going on a long fast (which will be supervised – please SEE *Fasting* section) nature cure will hold no complications for you.

Nature cure teaches that the body is always working towards health and away from illness. Disease is often an attempt on the part of the body to rid itself of accumulated poisons, or to adjust itself back to health again in some other way. It is no good, therefore, attacking the symptoms themselves; these are but signs of the elimination of toxins or of the body's efforts to right itself. It is the *cause* of illness that matters and must be considered. A symptom such as a fever is a sign of the body's attempt to throw off poisons and infections and thereby heal itself. Many other symptoms are evidence of the body's curative reactions.

Yes, you might say, but what about germs? Surely when we catch a germ and get ill, we should take a drug which can wipe out the germ?

There are germs around us all the time. Unless the body is clogged by toxins, or weakened by exhaustion or the wrong food, it throws off these germs effectively and fast. A certain Professor Pettenkoffer swallowed a test tube full of cholera germs in front of his class of students; you could have heard a pin drop. 'Germs are of no account in cholera,' he announced to his more than appreciative audience, 'the important thing is the disposition of the individual.' His students were fascinated to see him turn up for his lecture the next morning. He suffered no ill effects. The father of the germ theory of disease, Pasteur, said to his attendant shortly before he died, 'The germ is nothing. The soil is everything.' In other words the environment in which the germ finds itself – the state of the host body – determines the success or failure of the germ.

The body, therefore, must first and foremost be restored to health; 'Ignore the symptoms and restore normality; ignore the disease and restore health. Do this and the symptoms and the disease will gradually disappear.'[1]

It is no good thinking of the body as a collection of isolated parts which happen to be joined together. It functions as a whole. Disease attacks the whole person, and it is the whole person – that miraculous complexity of intermingled mind and body – which must be healed. If one organ or part is sick, this will affect the rest. Illness is an upset of the healthy balance of the body. Healing is a return to that balance.

Nature cure, therefore, goes against the modern habit of thinking about the body as a collection of separate systems. However, it agrees with the multi-factorial (many causes) theory of illness.

Since it is the whole person who is being treated, his characteristics must be taken into account. Age, strength, mental attitude – all these things influence him and should be considered. This means of course that books like this one are couched in general terms only. We are all different and, although to be healthy we should all go in the same direction, some of us are going to need detailed individual guidance. If you find that this is true of you, then you can take matters further by consulting the appendix.

Nature cure, or naturopathy, is an attitude to healing. It is not a cult. It is not Shangri La or a shield against life. It is an approach to health which calls for intelligent understanding and self-discipline. It is not guaranteed to work and, when necessary, the resources of conventional medicine should be used.

We have seen that the change in living habits called for in nature cure is up to you. Make no mistake – it is much easier to swallow a pill with your coffee. To restrict your diet for the duration of the treatment (and to modify it thereafter, for which you will need no prompting), to exercise, to learn to relax: these changes to your life need motivation and self-discipline.

It is essential to understand why you are taking these steps, and to accept responsibility for persisting in them. 'We cannot cure anything without the co-operation of the patient,' says Dr

I.P. Drysdale, Vice-Dean of the British College of Naturopathy and Osteopathy.

We have seen that illness is likely to be caused by wrong living of some kind, which has weakened or poisoned the sick person. Diet is a part, a very important, vital part, of the living habits which will make or mar our health. Food helps or impedes every process within us and we are, largely, what we eat. It is food, with several other factors of course, that makes us sick or well. By allowing the body to cleanse itself, and by supplying it with the nutrients it needs to function properly, we will help the body to heal itself. Dietary therapy, therefore, forms the major part of nature cure, and is the subject of this book.

Natural healing methods were known and valued by Hippocrates. But they have been crowded out in our times by the avalanche of drugs which doctors are encouraged to prescribe.

The father of modern European nature cure was Vincent Priessnitz (1799–1851), who was followed by several other pioneers. The American movement began with Dr James Caleb Jackson (1811–1896) and other doctors working in this way included Dr Russel T. Trail and Dr H. Lindlahr.

In 1909 the American Bernard MacFadden came to Britain and opened a health sanatorium in Brighton where he achieved many cures of chronic diseases. After the 1914–18 war British nature cure spread under the leadership of naturopath Stanley Lief, the founder of the British College of Naturopathy and Osteopathy.

'Accuse not nature; she hath done her part; do thou but thine.'
MILTON

The principles of nature cure
1   Nature will heal, given the chance. *Only* nature will heal.
2   All disease is one; an expression of striving for health.
3   Health is the natural state of the body.
4   Each disease, however it may express itself, is caused by one or several of the following:
(a)   excess toxins
(b)   deficiencies of vitamins, minerals, enzymes, glandular secretions, etc.
(c)   abnormal blood circulation
(d)   abnormal innervation (nerve supply)

(e)   traumatic injuries
(f)   inherited weaknesses
(g)   psychological stress.

Acute diseases are usually attempts to throw off toxins. Chronic diseases can be due to the continued suppression of these acute diseases by orthodox medical treatments, or long-term poisoning effected by refined, denatured foods and other pollutants.

The practice of nature cure includes:

1   Fasting*, the simplest and most natural of all healing mechanisms.
2   Dieting (SEE *Food Therapy* section).
3   Water treatment or hydrotherapy.
4   Exercise*, breathing*, skin care, sun and air treatments, relaxation*.
5   Psychotherapy.

Used both together with nature cure and on their own by alternative practitioners are osteopathy*, chiropractic, homoeopathy*, acupuncture* and herbal medicine*.

The healing crisis
Progress during treatment will not be uniform and uneventful. The body is getting rid of rubbish which has been clogging it and these toxins are discharged in the form of heavy colds, boils, diarrhoea, skin eruptions, nausea, with sometimes a headache or a temperature. This may depress you, and you may think you have taken one step forward and two steps back. It can be disconcerting, as friends and relatives tell you that you are obviously worse, and on the wrong track; I went through all this myself when I underwent nature cure.

This healing crisis can be unpleasant. But it is an *important step forward in your recovery.* No drugs must be taken during this time – not even the humble aspirin. Fast on fruit and vegetable juices (SEE the *Fasting* section), taken at intervals of two or three hours. If you are feverish, sponge yourself with tepid water. Your temperature should return to normal within two to three days. Break your fast by taking a little sub-acid (not citrus) fruit, and continue with your dietary plan.

* See index.

The first healing crisis is usually the worst and after this you should notice a marked improvement in your condition. Any further crisis will almost certainly be milder and shorter. Not everyone has a healing crisis, but some people have two or three.

In case all this sounds like a depressing and rather pointless endurance test, please remember that the feeling of well-being that you can expect after your body has freed itself of the toxins accumulated over the years has to be experienced to be believed.

Readers may be encouraged to hear about my own experiences with nature cure. (I had a chronic, not disabling, illness.) After a violent healing crisis, which turned out to be the only one, I was so bursting with energy that I danced around for hours to music in a friend's sitting room while she, patient creature, was busy in the kitchen. It was a happy and liberating experience. I could have taken on the world, and never forgot the lesson that this taught me.

Provided you understand the principles behind your treatment and the need for discipline and patience, you will be able to follow it. Only a fool believes that everything is going to be easy. Anyone who has ever achieved anything through persistence and guts will understand this, and will value the feeling of buoyant vitality and health which is the reward.

Food Therapy: The Diet

(For his valuable advice on the whole of this section, I am indebted to Dr Gordon Latto, M.B., Ch.B., President of the Vegetarian Society.)

On rising   Fruit juice or herb tea. (For further information on all foods marked with an asterisk, please SEE Index.)

Breakfast   Whole cereal such as unsugared muesli*, Weetabix, Shredded Wheat; fresh or dried fruit, natural yogurt*, wheat germ*, bran if added fibre is desired, milk, a little honey*, molasses*, or dark brown unrefined sugar*.

OR

soaked dried fruit (unsweetened; it contains plenty of natural sugar); stewed fresh fruit with honey, molasses or dark brown unrefined sugar if desired. Sedentary workers may prefer this breakfast.

OR

Wholemeal bread of toast with a scraping of butter or margarine and a little honey; fresh or dried fruit.

Mid-morning Fruit or vegetable juice, herb tea, grain coffee, Vecon or other caffeine-free drink. Nothing to eat.

Lunch Interchangeable with supper. Always have at least one salad a day. Large raw mixed salad, if possible including sprouting seeds and grains*. You can make a delicious dressing from some of the following ingredients – cider vinegar*, unrefined oil*, a little Biosalt, Ruthmol or other substitute for ordinary salt, lemon juice, herbs. A yogurt dressing can be made from natural yogurt with chopped chives, mint or parsley, with lemon juice. A jacket potato, or potatoes boiled in their skins (skins to be eaten as well as insides) or wholemeal bread with a scraping of butter or margarine, brown rice, wholemeal pasta or other whole cereals (millet, buckwheat, barley, etc).

To follow fresh or dried fruit, with natural yogurt if you like.

Tea As mid-morning break, or you can have some weak unsugared china tea. Nothing to eat.

Supper (interchangeable with lunch, or you can have a second salad). Cooked vegetables, or a jacket potato, or potatoes boiled in their skins, or brown rice. Add one vegetarian protein (cheese, nuts, eggs, yogurt, mushrooms, pulses, lentils). If you feel you really must have some flesh foods, then eat some lamb's liver* or kidneys, or some fish, not more than once a week.

To follow fresh or dried fruit, with natural yogurt if you wish.

Snacks If you are peckish between meals, take some fruit or vegetable juice or a herbal tea (without sugar). If you are really starving, have some fresh raw fruit.

Supplements If you want to add vitamin and mineral supplements to your treatment, please consult a qualified naturopath (SEE appendix) or a nutritionally aware doctor.

Salt* Salt is a culinary habit and, if you cut it down or out, your food will soon taste even better. Biosalt, Ruthmol or sea salt are obtainable from your health food store and are better for you than ordinary salt.

Fats* Use as sparingly as you can. Keep your unrefined oils in the fridge. Unhydrogenated margarines – available from some health food stores – are better for you.

Milk If cow's milk is not advised, you can buy soya milk from your health food store.

Protein* Flesh foods are complex proteins which can tax the digestion. Meat contains a lot of hidden saturated fat and traces of the hormones and antibiotics given to the animal. These foods are not recommended therefore in a therapeutic regime. In general your protein should be vegetarian; low-fat cheese such as cottage cheese, well-cooked pulses and lentils, unsalted nuts without added oils, eggs, natural yogurt. You will see that this diet probably contains less protein than you are used to. This is deliberate and nothing to worry about.

Fruit Grow your own if you can, without artifical chemicals. When buying fruit wash it well, leaving the skin on where possible. Leave some of the pith on citrus fruits and eat apple pips. Keep all fresh fruit in a cool dark place and eat it as soon as possible, to conserve the vitamin C. Some people find citrus fruits (oranges, satsumas, lemons, grapefruits), plums and rhubarb indigestible and should therefore avoid them. Dried fruit should preferably be without sulphur dioxide or mineral oil.

Vegetables Grow your own if you can, without artificial chemicals. When buying vegetables scrub them well and leave the skin on where possible. Do not soak before cooking. Short-cook them with very little salt and use the cooking water afterwards, for example in soups. Keep them in a cool dark place and eat them as soon as possible.

Salads Again, grow your own if you can, without artificial chemicals. Do not soak the ingredients, cut them up just before use, adding any salad dressing at once to conserve the vitamin C. Keep them in a cool dark place and eat them as soon as possible. Mix your own salad from the following list of suggestions.

Salad ingredients (raw except where otherwise stated) Lettuces of all kinds, endive, spinach, cabbages of all kinds, cauliflower, chicory, brussels sprouts, watercress, mustard and cress, sprouting seeds and grains, celeriac, celery, avocado, mushrooms, sweet corn (cooked), small peas and small sliced runner or French beans, onions, garlic, leeks, radishes, cucumber, tomatoes, peppers, beetroot (raw or cooked), swedes, turnips, carrots (not raw potatoes): any cooked beans – red kidney, adzuki, butter, haricot, etc. (kidney beans must be soaked for at least 18 hours and boiled for at least 15 minutes before eating); cooked chick peas; nasturtium leaves, a few dandelion leaves, parsley, chives, mint, basil, rosemary, etc.; sultanas, raisins, currants, dried apricots, etc.; oranges, grapefruits, satsumas, tangerines, apples, pears, pineapple (not starchy bananas).

I am sure that readers can think of a few more salad suggestions.

Drinking

Try not to take any extra liquid with your meal (unless of course it is soup). There is already enough in the salads and fruits.

Chewing

It is vitally important to chew food thoroughly until it is a soft mass before swallowing it. Solid food must be mixed with saliva, otherwise the taste buds cannot react and you will not taste it. Starch and sugar digestion begin in the mouth, so if we do not chew our food properly we do not digest – or assimilate – starches and sugars properly. A copious flow of saliva helps to wash away particles from the teeth and, when it reaches the stomach, it helps the digestion. Many digestive troubles (fatigue after meals, flatulence, discomfort) are due to insufficient chewing and if we bolt our food we tend to eat more as well, thus running the risk of getting fat. If you have never really chewed your food properly you don't know what you are missing – so follow Gladstone, who laid down a rule of chewing everything 32 times!

Proportions

This diet contains a high proportion of alkali-forming foods – all salads, most fresh fruits, all vegetables and milk. (This includes citrus fruits, whose acids leave the body within an hour or so of being eaten, leaving an alkali residue.) It contains a lesser proportion of acid-forming foods – meat, fish, eggs, cheese, nuts, cereals. The more refined a food is, the more acid it is. Too many acid-forming foods can cause acidosis and lower the body's resistance to illness, whereas the alkalis are very valuable to the body. (There is some evidence that if your diet is predominantly alkaline it may be easier for you to stop smoking. Scientists, however, are cautious at present. [1])

Changing
If you are totally unused to this way of eating, then change to it one meal at a time, leaving a gap of about three weeks before changing the next meal, and so on. If a particular food disagrees with you, leave it out and try it again in a week or two.

When you change your diet to Food Therapy, you may experience some fatigue. The body has to adjust to not being stimulated artificially by coffee, tea and white sugar. This feeling will soon pass.

What is left out?
It will be seen that the following foods must be cut out: all fried foods, convenience and junk foods, all foods containing white flour and other refined cereals, white sugar, strong tea and ordinary coffee, all junk drinks such as cokes, squashes, all sweets, alcohol.

In conclusion
A major problem in Food Therapy is that we are so used to having a different pill for each illness that we can't understand how just one way of eating can be used to treat so many different conditions.

Unhappily, a drug will often only suppress the symptoms of disease, doing nothing about the cause. In addition, its toxic side-effects give the body something else to worry about. But *the body itself will throw off disease – given the chance.* The right diet of cleansing, revitalizing foods will help to give it that chance. For a full explanation of the way that food helps the body to cope with illness in the best way, without drugs, please read the *Nature Cure* section.

The importance of diet and its relation to health are increasingly recognized now. But an acceptance of this common-sense principle is one thing. Another thing altogether is the decision to do something about your illness, starting here and now. To make changes in the way you eat, and to stick to those changes until you feel better.

But don't throw up your hands in horror. The naturopath is not asking you to eat pebbles or donkeys' tails. He is simply asking you to give your body the whole, delicious foods it needs in order to do its job properly and defeat illness. You don't need masochism – only guts.

I expect that for many readers this diet may seem depressingly strict, although others may be eating rather like this already. But it won't be long before your improved wellbeing encourages you to continue eating in this way. This positive feeling, coming when you give your body a chance to right itself, has to be felt to be believed and will make all your efforts and self-discipline worthwhile.

And afterwards? When you feel better, do you heave a sigh of relief, and go back to stuffing yourself with doughnuts and coffee, Insto-Chik and chips? These foods may seem pretty seductive to you now. But when you have changed your diet, and your health, for the better, they will seem less so.

You will probably scoff the occasional doughnut. The Insto-Chik will taste awfully salty and the chips will reek of used-again oil. White sliced Angel-loaf will feel and taste like clobbered-up Kleenex. Instead of a tired wisp of lettuce and a slice of senile tomato, you will be tucking in to crisp delicious salads made of everything the garden or the greengrocer can give you which tastes good and goes together. You will enjoy a bar of chocolate or a gooey cake from time to time. But you won't *need* those foods – ever again.

Finally, this diet is an outline only. Everyone is different in his or her nutritional needs. So if you feel you need further advice and individual guidance, please consult a naturopath or a nutritionally aware doctor.

Recommended reading
The Real Food Cookbook by Vivien and Clifford Quick (Thorsons 1981).
Salads the Year Round by Joy Larkcom (Hamlyn Paperbacks 1980).
The Natural Foods Cookbook by Beatrice Trum Hunter (Faber paperbacks 1977),
The Natural Foods Primer by Beatrice Trum Hunter (Unwin paperbacks 1979).

Acknowledgments

I extend my warmest appreciation and thanks to the following, whose generous help and criticism did so much to shape the book and sustain its author.

Special thanks to: Margaret Brady for her help and advice on the weaning plan in the section 'Children and Food'; Doris Grant for help and advice on the section 'Compatible Eating'; Clifford Quick for information for the 'Cystitis' section; Dr Andrew Lockie for help and advice on the 'Low Blood Sugar' section; Harry Clements for help on the 'Migraine' section. Much of the material in the 'Fasting' section is taken from my article in *Prevention* magazine, 23/1.

Individuals
Dr Denis Burkitt; Dr Malcolm Carruthers; Vera Carruthers, psychotherapist and relaxation expert; Naturopath Boris Chaitow; Dr Michael A. Crawford; Ms Sylvia J. Darke, DHSS; Dr Stephen Davies; Dr I.P. Drysdale, Vice-Dean, British College of Naturopathy and Osteopathy; Naturopath Norman Eddie; Stanley C. Evans, ophthalmic nutritionist; Dr Alec Forbes; Martin Freeth of the BBC; Health writer Doris Grant; Maurice Hanssen; Mrs Janet Hicks, consulting medical herbalist; Dr Dennis M. Jones; Miss M. Knowles; Dr Philip Langton-Lockton; Doctors Barbara and Gordon Latto; Dr E.K. Ledermann; Dr Ronald Livingston; Dr Andrew H. Lockie; Dr Alan Long; Beautician Clare Maxwell-Hudson; Dr Jean Monro; Naturopath T.G. Moule; Dr S.J.L. Mount; Naturopath Clifford Quick; Dr Dick Richards; Bates practitioner Michael Ronan; Ms Judy Sadgrove, *The Lancet*; Osteopath Barry Savory; Naturopath Michael A. Van Straten; Mrs Margaret Strauss; Ms Ann Warren Davis, consulting medical herbalist; and Dr Dorothy West.

Organizations
Asthma Research Council; Booker Health Foods plc; The Boots Company plc; British Medical Association; The British Nutrition Foundation; Cantassium Company Limited; The Chest, Heart and Stroke Association; Committee on Safety of Medicines; Cow and Gate Limited; The Dental Estimates

Board; Dietary Specialities Limited; Efamol Limited; Evening Primrose Oil Company Limited; General Dental Council; The Health Education Council; Health Food Manufacturers' Association; Healthilife Limited; H.J. Heinz Company plc; Höfels Pure Foods Limited; Imperial Cancer Research Fund; Inter-medics Limited; W. Jordans & Son Ltd; Keenwell Limited; G.R. Lane Health Products Limited; The Multiple Sclerosis Society; National Anti-Fluoridation Campaign; The National Childbirth Trust; New Era Laboratories Limited; Overseal Foods Limited; Regenics Limited; Robinson's Baby Food; J.I. Rodale & Co. Limited and The Rodale Press; Rowse Honey Limited; The Society for the Promotion of Natural Health; The Soil Association Limited; Sunwheel Foods Limited; Fauser Vitaquellwerk GMBH & Company; and Weightwatchers (UK) Limited.

Finally, I would like to thank John Scarlett, without whose loving encouragement this book would never have been written.

The illustrations in this book are based on material provided by the following:
The General Dental Council (drawing of the tooth); Miss M. Knowles (drawing of the lungs); Ewan Cameron, Linus Pauling and Weidenfeld & Nicholson (chart of vitamin C usage by cancer patients, from their book *Cancer and Vitamin C*); *Prevention* magazine (drawing of the eye).

Appendix

Acupuncture
The Acupuncture Association of 34 Alderney Street, London SW1V 4EV (telephone 01 834 1012) will supply you with a copy of their register of qualified practitioners for £1.25.

The Traditional Acupuncture Society is at Queensway, Royal Leamington Spa, Warwickshire CV32 5EZ (telephone 0926 22121).

Deep breathing
The Knowles System: write to Miss M. Knowles, 46 Fleetwood Close, Chalfont-St-Giles, Buckinghamshire, HP8 4DR.

Exercise
Above all, let your exercise be something you enjoy; otherwise you won't be able to keep it up. Your local library will have details of evening classes and clubs. Here are some other suggestions:

Alexander technique: SEE *Relaxation* below.
Yoga   The Yoga for Health Foundation at Ickwell Bury, near Northills, Biggleswade, Bedfordshire SG18 9EF (telephone 076727 271). They specialize in therapeutic and relaxation activities and give regular weekend and five-day courses, together with individual tuition.

Recommended reading
The Aerobics Way by Kenneth H. Cooper (Corgi 1977).
Fit for Life by Donald Norfolk (Hamlyn 1981).
Write for a free copy of *Looking After Yourself* (send a 9in × 12in stamped and addressed envelope) to The Health Education Council, 78 New Oxford Street, London WC1A 1AH (telephone 01 637 1881).

Herbalism
Contact the National Institute of Medical Herbalists at 148 Forest Road, Tunbridge Wells, Kent TN2 4EY (telephone 0892 30400) for a qualified medical herbalist.

Homoeopathy

Contact the British Homoeopathic Association at 27a Devonshire Street, London W1N 1RH (telephone 01 935 2163) sending a 9in × 6in stamped and addressed envelope for a list of qualified homoeopathic doctors.

The Hahnemann Society, Humane Education Centre, Avenue Lodge, Bounds Green, London N22 4EU (telephone 01 889 1595) supplies information about homoeopathy. Please send them a 9in × 6in stamped and addressed envelope.

Naturopathy

Contact the British Naturopathic and Osteopathic Assocation – SEE Osteopathy below.

Osteopathy

The British Naturopathic and Osteopathic Association at 6 Netherall Gardens, London NW3 5RR (telephone 01 435 8728) will send a list of qualified practitioner members on receipt of a stamped (15½p stamp) and addressed envelope 9in × 6in and £1. This list is also available in some libraries.

The General Council and Register of Osteopaths at 1–4 Suffolk Street, London SW1Y 4HG (telephone 01 839 2060) will send a list of registered qualified osteopaths on receipt of £1.20.

Relaxation

Essential to combat stress. For those wishing to learn a definite technique, the following information will be useful:

Alexander technique   Postural re-education with far-reaching physical and psychological benefits. Contact Alexander Teaching Association, ATA Centre, 188 Old Street, London EC1V 9BP (telephone 01 250 3038).

Autogenic training   A 'self-generated' system of relaxation, influencing mind and body together. I have practised it myself for several years and can recommend it. Write to the Positive Health Centre, 15 Fitzroy Square, London W1, (telephone 01 388 1007). At the time of writing there is a booklet available from the Centre, *Autogenics*, for £2 including postage.

Biofeedback   A system of stress reduction using a biofeedback instrument. Can be learned in a class or alone. For further details about biofeedback, contact The Psycho-

APPENDIX   407

Biology Institute, 26–28 Wendell Road, London W12 (telephone 01 743 1518). For information about biofeedback instruments, contact Andrew Stephens (1947) Company, 41 Dickson Road, Blackpool FY1 2AP (telephone 0253 23755).

Meditation Consult your local library for classes, or contact the School of Meditation, 158 Holland Park Avenue, London W11 4UH (telephone 01 603 6116). They have centres in Sheffield, Basingstoke and Lincolnshire.

Transcendental Meditation, Roydon Hall, East Peckham, near Tonbridge, Kent CNT N12 5NH (telephone 0622 813243).

Additional therapies
Yoga; SEE *Exercise* above.

Recommended reading
Stress and Relaxation by Jane Madders (Martin Dunitz 1979).

References

Introduction

1 Ivan Illich, *Limits to Medicine*, Marion Boyars, 1977.
2 R. Maxwell, *The Growing Dilemma*, 1975.
3 *Pulse*, vol 40, No 34.
4 Peter Parish, *Medicines: a Guide for Everybody*, Penguin, 1980.
5 *General Practitioner*, 22 August 1980.
6 Sir Derrick Dunlop, *Proceedings of the Royal Society of Medicine* 63 (1970: 1279) and G.L. Klerman, *Proceedings of the 1st World Congress on Environmental Medicine and Biology*.
7 *General Practitioner*, 1 August 1980.
8 Robin M. Murray, *British Journal of Hospital Medicine*, May 1974.
9 The Association of British Pharmaceutical Industries.
10 Department of Health and Social Security.

Fats

1 S.D. Splitter et al, *Metabolism* 17: 1129, 1968.
2 *Vegetarian* and *vegan* diets lower blood cholesterol levels. Single foods with the same effect are legumes, pulses, pectin (found in many fruits and vegetables), seaweed or *kelp*, alfalfa (SEE *Sprouting Seeds*), *garlic, yogurt, brewer's yeast*; SEE Index for references to each word in italics.
3 *American Journal of Clinical Nutrition* 12: 358, 1963.
4 The magazine *Prevention*, 24/4.
5 *Journal of Nutrition* 86: 325, 1965. These rats were fed a diet containing 65% butter.
6 The oil was heated to 200°C for 15 minutes. D. Kritchevsky et al, *Journal of the American Oil Chemistry Society* 38: 74, 1961. D. Kritchevsky et al, *Journal of Atherosclerosis Research* 2: 115, 1962. D. Kritchevsky and Tepper, *Journal of Atherosclerosis Research* 7: 647, 1967.
7 *Nutrition Today*, 2:2, 1967. *Present Knowledge in Nutrition*, The Nutrition Foundation, New York, 1967.
8 N. Joliffe, *Metabolism*, 10: 497, 1961. B. Bronte-Stewart, *Lancet* 1: 521, 1956.

Fibre
1 *Medical Aspects of Dietary Fibre:* a Report by the Royal College of Physicians, Pitman Medical, 1980.
2 *British Medical Journal*, 15 December 1979.
3 The American magazine *Bestways*, May 1980.
4 *British Medical Journal*, 15 December 1979, 1541.
5 D.H. Fisher, *Medical World News*, 14 May 1965, 6: 86. G.A. Leveille and H.E. Sauberlich, *Journal of Nutrition*, 1966 88: 209. G.H. Palmer and D.G. Dixon, *American Journal of Clinical Nutrition*, 1966 18: 437.
6 *Ecology of Food and Nutrition*, 1972, vol 1.

The Modern Food Industry
1 *Cancer Control Journal*, 3, 1 and 2.
2 Lady Eve Balfour, *The Living Soil.*
3 James Lambert Mount, *The Food and Health of Western Man*, Precision Press, 1979.
4 *Ecology of Food and Nutrition*, 1972, vol 1.
5 Schroeder et al, *Journal of Chronic Diseases,* 1967, 20: 179.
6 Dr Richard Mackarness, *Chemical Victims*, Pan Books, 1980.
7 Harris and von Loesecke, *Nutritional Evaluation of Food Processing*, Wiley, 1980. J. Schubert and E.B. Sanders, *Nature*, 1971, 233: 199.
8 *Guidelines for Future Parents*, Foresight. Please SEE Pregnancy, Lactation and Food, Information section, for further information on Foresight.
9 B.F. Feingold, *Why Your Child is Hyper-Active*, Random House, 1974.

Protein
1 *Journal of the American Diabetic Association*, 62 (3), March 1973, page 255.

Salt
1 Study by G. Miller reported in *Prevention*, 22/2.

Tea and Coffee
1 *British Nutrition Foundation Bulletin* No 31.
2 E.K. Ledermann, *Good Health through Natural Therapy*, Pan Books, 1978.

Vitamins and Minerals
1 Roger J. Williams, *Nutrition Against Disease*, Bantam, 1978.

Whole Foods
1 Letter to the author, dated 10 June 1980, from the Soil Association.
2 *British Medical Journal*, 22 September 1979.
3 *British Medical Journal*, vol 2, 730, 1926, and *Indian Journal of Medical Research*, vol 14, 649, 1927.

Brewer's Yeast
1 Adelle Davis, *Let's Eat Right to Keep Fit.*

Cider Vinegar
1 Maurice Hanssen, *Hanssen's Complete Cider Vinegar*, Thorsons.

Evening primrose oil
1 *Medical Hypotheses* 6, 689–709, 1980.
2 J.N. McCormick et al, *Lancet* 2: 508, 1977.
3 C.R. Lovell et al, *Lancet* 31 January 1981.
4 D.F. Wilson et al, *Clinical Research* 21: 829, 1973.
5 I. Colquhoun and S. Bunday, *Medical Hypotheses* 7. 631–6, 1981.
6 M.L. Bierenbaum et al, International Prostagla. lin Conference, Washington DC, May 1979.

Honey
1 Dr Kuan Lee, the National College of Food Technology.

Lecithin
1 *Lancet*, 6 December 1975.
2 *Lancet*, 2 December 1978.

Liver
1 *Journal of Nutrition*, August 1974.
2 *Journal of Nutrition*, vol 35, 1948.

Molasses
1 Adelle Davis, *Let's Eat Right to Keep Fit.*

Spirulina
1 International Congress of Food Science and Technology, September 1974.

Yogurt
1 *Journal of the National Cancer Institute*, February 1980.
2 *American Journal of Digestive Diseases*, vol 22, 1955.
3 *American Journal of Clinical Nutrition*, 1979, vol 32: 19.

Children and Food
1 *Pilot Survey of the Nutrition of Young Children*, 1963: Reports on Public Health and Medical Subjects 118, HMSO, 1968.
2 G.C. Arneil, *Scottish Health Service Studies* No 6, 1967.
3 S. Burman, *Archives of Disease in Childhood*, 1972, 47: 261.
4 L.S. Taitz, *British Medical Journal*, 1971, 1: 315.
5 G.W. Lynch, *Medical Officer* (London), 1969, 121: 41.
6 A.E. Bender et al, *British Medical Journal*, 1972, 2: 383.
7 D.P. Richard and M. Lawson, *British Medical Journal*, 1972, 2: 593.
8 R.J.L. Allen et al, *British Journal of Nutrition*, 1968, 22: 555.
9 D. Grant, 'Vitamin Deficiencies, Mind Pollution and Anti-Social Behaviour', *Health Quarterly*, vol 3, No 3.

Compatible Eating
1 Notably Dr William Howard Hay, *A New Health Era*, Harrap, 1935.

The Eyes and Food
1 Stanley C. Evans, *Nutrition in Eye Health and Disease*, Roberts Publications, 1978.
2 *British Journal of Nutrition*, January 1979.
3 *British Journal of Ophthalmology*, vol 63 No 3, 1979.
4 *Lancet*, 7 January 1978.
5 *British Journal of Nutrition*, January 1979.
6 William Luftig, *How to Cure Eye Disease Without Operation*.
7 Harry Benjamin, *Better Sight Without Glasses,* Thorsons, 1974.

Fasting
1 H.M. Shelton, *Fasting Can Save Your Life*, Natural Hygiene Press, 1964.
2 E. Heun, *Hippokrates Heft*, 15, Stuttgart, 1960.

Hair and Food
1 Irwin I. Lubowe, *The Modern Guide to Skin Care and Beauty*, E.P. Dutton.

Macrobiotics
1 *British Medical Journal*, 3 February 1979.

The Menopause
1 Barbara Evans, *Life Change*, Pan Books, 1979.
2 Baird et al, *Recent Progress in Hormone Research*, 25, 611. Grodin et al, *Journal of Clinical Endocrinology and Metabolism*, 36, 207. Frost et al, *Journal of Investigative Dermatology*, 46, 584.

Older People and Food
1 Interview for the American magazine *Bestways*, August 1980.
2 E.G. Toomey and P.D. White, *American Heart Journal*, 1964, 68: 841.
3 Alen Moyle, *Natural Health for the Elderly*, Thorsons. Now unhappily out of print, but your library may have a copy.
4 *Clinical Endocrinology*, December 1977.
5 James Lambert Mount, *The Food and Health of Western Man*, Precision Press, 1979.

The Pill
1 *Vegetarian Bulletin*, No 24.

Pregnancy, Lactation and Food
1 Jane B. Morgan of the Department of Nutrition, University of Southampton, *British Nutrition Foundation Bulletin*, No 30.
2 Office of Population Censuses and Surveys, DH3/81/1.
3 *Journal of Human Nutrition*, 33, 1979.
4 F. Hale, *Journal of Heredity*, 24: 105, 1933.
5 B. Mackler et al, *Pediatrics*, June 1969.
6 D.J. Naismith and D.C. Ritchie, *Proceedings of the Nutrition Society*, 34, 1975.

REFERENCES 413

7   B.S. Burke et al, *Journal of Nutrition*, 26: 569, 1943. B.S. Burke et al, *American Journal of Obstetrics and Gynaecology*, 46: 38, 1943.
8   R. Luikhart, *American Journal of Obstetrics and Gynaecology*, 52: 428, 1946.
9   David Potterton, writing in the American magazine *Bestways*, January 1981.
10 R.F. Harrell et al, *Metabolism*, 5: 555, 1956.
11 A. Nisenson, *Pedriatrics*, December 1969.
12 *Nutrition Reports International*, November 1974.
13 Dr P.M. Newberne, *Technology Review*, December 1974.
14 *Anatomical Record*, 121: 775, 1955. *Science*, 92: 383, 1940.
15 L. Wertalik et al, *Journal of the American Medical Association*, 27 September 1972.
16 *Journal of Clinical Nutrition*, September–October 1953. *Science*, 16 December 1949.
17 *Executive Health*, January 1976.
18 Dr Alton Ochsner, *Executive Health*, vol XI, No 3, 1974.
19 J. Ritchie et al, *New England Journal of Medicine*, 28 November 1968.
20 *Nutrition Reviews*, 1976.
21 Oberleas et al, 1972.
22 J.A. Halstead and J.C. Smith, *Lancet*, 1970, 1: 322.
22 *Environmental Factors and Foetal Health*, Foresight.
24 *Science*, 97: 312, 1943.
25 Adelle Davis, *Let's Have Healthy Children*, Unwin, 1975.
26 Ibid.
27 William Thomson, *Herbs that Heal*, Scribner, 1977.

Pre-menstrual Tension
1   *Current Medical Research and Opinion*, vol 6, supp 5, 1979.

Skin and Food
1   Roger J. Williams, *Nutrition in a Nutshell*, Dolphin, 1962.
2   *Obstetrical and Gynaecological News*, 1 May 1974.
3   *Medical Tribune*, 3 October 1968.

Teeth and Food
1   England and Wales.
2   General Dental Council.

3   James Lambert Mount, *The Food and Health of Western Man*, Precision Press, 1979.

4   S.L. Slack and W.J. Martin, *British Dental Journal*, 1958, 105, 366.

5   E.J. Cheraskin, *Oral Medicine*, 1966, 21: 173.

6   A paper presented by Dr Dean Burk, founder and former head of the Cytochemistry Department of the National Cancer Institute, at the 4th International Symposium on the Prevention and Detection of Cancer, 29 July 1980.

7   A separate factor has been identified in wholemeal flour that prevents caries (T.H. Grenby, *Archives of Oral Biology*, 1967, 12: 513, and G.N. Jenkins et al, *British Dental Journal*, 1959, 106: 195).

8   Roger J. Williams, *Nutrition Against Disease*, Bantam, 1978.

9   New Mexico Agricultural Experiment Station.

Vegetarian and Vegan Eating

1   R.W. Parker, Assistant Editor, *The Meat Hygienist*.

2   Research done by the National Water Quality Laboratory, Duluth, Minnesota.

3   West and Hayes, *American Journal of Clinical Nutrition*, 1968, 21: 853, etc.

4   Phillips, *Cancer Research*, 35: 3513, November 1975.

5   Surgeon Denis Burkitt, interviewed in the American magazine *Bestways*, May 1980.

6   Robertson et al, *Clinical Science*, 1979, 57, 285.

7   *Vitaminologia*, 1959, 5: 88, and 1958, 4: 81.

8   Letter to the *Lancet*, 1 (7970); 1190, 29 May 1976: F.R. Ellis and T. Sanders.

9   Ellis, Path and Ellis, *The Vegan*, Spring 1972.

Allergies to Food

1   Article in *Here's Health*, September 1979.

2   L.W. Smith et al, *Antibiotic Medicine and Clinical Therapy*, 4: 515, 1957.

3   Roger J. Williams, *Nutrition in a Nutshell*, Dolphin 1962.

Arthritis and Rheumatism

1   Described in the *Proceedings of the Royal Society of Medicine*, vol XXX.

2   N. Zvaifler, *Journal of the American Medical Association*.

3 E.C. Barton-Wright, Arthritis Kochlight Laboratories and the Cantassium Co, 1975.
4 Roger J. Williams, *Nutrition Against Disease*, Bantam, 1978.
5 Adelle Davis, *Let's Get Well*, Unwin, 1975.

Asthma and Hay Fever
1 Asthma Research Council.
2 Health Education Council.
3 F. Bicknell and F. Prescott, *The Vitamins in Medicine*, Lee Foundation for Nutritional Research, 1953.
4 A Houhuys et al, *Journal of Allergy and Clinical Immunology*, April 1973.
5 F. Valic and E. Zuskin, *British Journal of Industrial Medicine*, 30: 1973.
6 I. Szorady, *Acta Paediatrica*, IV, 1, 1963.
7 Dr W.G. Crook, *Can Your Child Read? Is He Hyperactive?*, Pedicenter Press, 1975.
8 Interview in the American magazine *Bestways*, May 1980.

Bronchitis and Emphysema
1 *Studies on Medical and Population Subjects, No 14, vol 1, HMSO, 1958.*
2 James Lambert Mount, *The Food and Health of Western Man*, Precision Press, 1979.
3 *Royal Society of Health Journal*, 1967, 87: 298.
4 Public Health Service, USA, Public. 600, 1963.
5 Clifford Quick, *Nature Cure for Bronchitis and Emphysema*, Thorsons, 1979.
6 H.M. Nitowsky et al, *Bulletin of the Johns Hopkins Hospital*, 98, 361, 1956.
7 Adelle Davis, *Let's Get Well*, Unwin, 1975.

Cancer
1 Office of Population Censuses and Surveys.
2 James Lambert Mount, *The Food and Health of Western Man*, Precision Press, 1979.
3 Folkman, *Annals of Surgery*, 175 (3), 409–16, 1972.
4 Dr R. Livingstone, University of Texas, Report to House Select Committee, 1979.
5 Leon Chaitow, *An End to Cancer?*, Thorsons, 1978.
6 Ewan Cameron and Linus Pauling, *Cancer and Vitamin C*, Weidenfeld and Nicolson, 1979.

7   R. Hoover and J.F. Frameni, 'The Risk of Cancer in Renal Recipients', *Lancet*, 2: 55, 1973.
8   Article in *New Age*, February 1980.
9   *New Scientist*, 13 July 1978.
10 Dr Dean Burk, founder and former head of the Cytochemistry Department of the National Cancer Institute: a paper presented by Dr Burk at the 4th International Symposium on the Prevention and Detection of Cancer, 29 July 1980.
11 Thomas H. Maugh, *Science*, 27 December 1974.
12 *Journal of the National Cancer Institute*, June 1979.
13 Richard A. Passwater, *Cancer and Its Nutritional Therapies*, Pivot, 1978.
14 *British Nutrition Foundation Bulletin*, No 22.
15 *Experimental Cell Biology*, vol 47, 1979.
16 *Cancer Research*, April 1980.
17 *British Nutrition Foundation Bulletin*, No 22.
18 *Medical World News*, 21 June 1968.
19 *Clinical Bulletin*, vol 9, 1979.
20 *Journal of the National Cancer Institute*, February 1980.
21 *The Complete Book of Vitamins*, Rodale Press, 1977.
22 *New Ecologist*, No 6, November–December 1978.
23 R.F. Phillips, *Cancer Research*, No 35.
24 Kenneth R. Pelletier, *Mind as Healer, Mind as Slayer*, - Allen and Unwin, 1977.
25 Simonton, Mathews-Simonton and Creighton, *Getting Well Again*, J.P. Tarcher Inc, 1978.
26 *Lancet*, 1979, 2, 785.
27 *Lancet*, 1979, 1, 706.
28 Kochi et al, *Cancer Treatment Reports*, vol 64, No 1, January 1980.
29 McNaughton Foundation Data submitted to the Food and Drugs Administration, 1970.
30 Max Gerson, *A Cancer Therapy: results of 50 cases*, Totality Books, 1977.

Constipation

1   *Let's Get Well* by Adelle Davis, published by Unwin, 1975.

Diabetes

1   W.J. Butterfield, *Proceedings of the Royal Society of Medicine*, 1964, 57: 195.

2 'Facts Behind the Headlines', *British Nutrition Foundation Bulletin*, No 18.
3 American Diabetic Association, the University Group Diabetes Programme; from *Diabetes*, vol 19, supp 2, 1970.
4 Adelle Davis, *Let's Get Well*, Unwin, 1975.
5 Dr Arnold Bloom, *Diabetes Explained*, Medical and Technical Press, 1971.
6 A.M. Cohen, *Metabolism,* 1961, 10: 50. Cohen and Bavly et al, *Lancet*, 1961, 2: 1399.
7 J.M. Perley and D.M. Kipnis, *Journal of Clinical Investigation*, 1967, 46.
8 During a talk to the Vermont Natural Food and Farming Association Inc, 1971.
9 A.E. Sobel and A. Rosenberg, Polytechnic Institute of Brooklyn: I. Jennings in *Endocrine Metabolism.*
10 *Australian and New Zealand Journal of Medicine*, December 1977.
11 Issue for November 1971.
12 T.L. Kopjas, Journal of the American Geriatrics Society, November 1966.
13 *Netherlands Journal of Medicine*, vol 23, 4, 1980.
14 *Acta Haematlogiea*, vol 62, 1979.
15 *Medical Aspects of Dietary Fibre:* a Report by the Royal College of Physicians, Pitman Medical, 1980.
16 Adelle Davis, *Let's Get Well*, Unwin, 1975.
17 E. Diengott et al, *Endocrinology*, 65, 602, 1959.
18 J.W. Anderson et al, *American Journal of Clinical Nutrition*, 1976, 29. *Diabetes Care*, 1978, 1.
19 *Medical Aspects of Dietary Fibre:* a Report by the Royal College of Physicians, Pitman Medical, 1980.
20 *The Prevention of Coronary Heart Disease*, a Report of the Working Party of the Royal College of Physicians of London and the British Cardiac Society, 1976.

Fatigue
1 Harry Clements, *Stopping Fatigue*, Thorsons, 1978.

Heart and Artery Disease
1 *Lancet*, 22 November 1969, 1088.
2 Dr Julian M. Whitaker, California Heart Treatment Center.
3 Committee on Safety of Medicines.

418   REFERENCES

4 J.J. Barboriak et al, *Natural Nutrition*, 64: 241, 1958.
5 S. Naimi et al, *Natural Nutrition*, 86: 325, 1965.
6 *Journal of Athersclerosis Research*, 4: 289, 1964.
7 *Nutrition Against Disease*, Bantam, 1978. Also T. Nishida et al, *Circulation Research*, 6: 194, 1958, etc.
8 G.J. Christakis et al, *American Journal of Public Health*, 1966, 56: 299.
9 S.D. Talbott et al, *International Medicine*, 54, 257, 1961.
10 E.T. Gale et al, *Geriatrics*, 8, 80, 1953.
11 O. Paul, *Food Nutrition News*, 351, 1, 1964.
12 James Lambert Mount, *The Food and Health of Western Man*, Precision Press, 1979.
13 L.M. Morrison, *Geriatrics*, 13: 12, 1958.
14 Steiner et al, *Circulation*, 5, 605, 1952.
15 B. Sokoloff et al, *Journal of the American Geriatrics Society*, 1966, 14: 1239.
16 *British Heart Journal*, 1972, 34: 238.
17 Gvozdova et al, *Vorprosy Pitanyia*, 25: 40, 1966.
18 A White et al, *Principles of Biochemistry*.
19 L. Kopjas Tibor, *Journal of the American Geriatrics Society*, November 1966.
20 *Nutrition Reviews*, October 1955.
21 I. Bersohn and P.J. Oelofse, *Lancet*, 1: 1020, 1957.
22 T. Crawford and M.D. Crawford, *Lancet*, 1: 229, 1967, etc.
23 D.H. Fisher, *Medical World News*, 14 May 1965, 6: 86.
24 E.G. Toomey and P.D. White, *American Heart Journal*, 1964, 68: 841.
25 Hodges et al, *American Journal of Clinical Nutrition*, 1967, 20: 198, etc.
26 F. Grange et al, *Natural Nutrition*, 86: 313, 1965.
27 Phillips, *Cancer Research*, 35: 3513, November 1975.
28 *Nutrition Against Disease* and Horlick, 1956; Aldersberg, 1943, etc.

High Blood Pressure
1 Health Education Council.
2 From an interview in the American magazine *Bestways*, October 1979.
3 *Journal of the American Medical Association*, 28, 1977, and *American Journal of Epidemiology*, November 1974.
4 *Here's Health*, October 1979.

5 R.A. Womersley et al, *Journal of Clinical Investigation*, 34, 456, 1953. C.D. Darrow et al, *Journal of Clinical Investigation*, 27, 198, 1948.
6 Adelle Davis, *Let's Get Well*, Unwin, 1975.
7 *Lancet*, 10 January 1981.
8 Y. Nichizawa et al, *Journal of Vitaminology*, 3, 106, 1957.
9 *New England Journal of Medicine*, 8 January 1976.
10 *Lancet*, 23 February 1974. *Lancet*, 21 January 1976.

Hyper-active Children

1 J.W.T. Dickerson and Felicity Pepler, *Journal of Human Nutrition*, 1980, 34.
2 Dr Ben F. Feingold, *Why Your Child is Hyper-active*, Random House, 1975.
3 Department of Psychiatry and Pediatrics, State of New York; Downstate Medical Center, Brooklyn; Southbeach Psychiatric Center, New York; and *Modern Medicine,* 30 September 1979.
4 *Modern Medicine*, August 1975.
5 J.M. Swanson et al, *Science*, vol 207, 28 March 1980, p.1485.
6 B. Weiss et al, *Science*, vol 207, 28 March 1980, p.1487.

Low Blood Sugar

1 Hawkins and Pauling (ed.), *Orthomolecular Psychiatry*, W.H. Freeman, 1973.

Migraine

1 Adelle Davis, *Let's Get Well*, Unwin, 1975.
2 R.E,. Hodges et al, *Journal of Clinical Investigation*, 38, 1421, 1959; and R.E. Hodges et al, *American Journal of Clinical Nutrition*, 11, 181, 187, 1962.
3 In *The Women's Holistic Headache Relief Book*, St Martin, 1979.
4 *Archives of Orolaryngology*, vol 75, 1962.
5 F. Clifford Rose and M. Gawel, *Migraine: The Facts*, Oxford University Press, 1981.

Multiple Sclerosis

1 The Multiple Sclerosis Society.
2 Consumer Bulletin, May 1962.

3 Dr E.K. Ledermann, *Good Health Through Natural Therapy*, Pan Books, 1978.
4 *Cancer Control Journal*, vol 2, No 3.
5 *Proceedings of the Nutrition Society*, 1979, 38, 373.
6 *Neurology, Minnesota*, 2: 369–460, September–October 1952.
7 B13 is obtainable from the Cantassium Company, 225 Putney Bridge Road, London SW15 2PY (tel 01-870 0971).
8 *Journal of the American Medical Association*, 5 August 1950.
9 *Journal of the American Medical Association*, 12 September 1958.

Obesity
1 Health Education Council.
2 Roger J. Williams, *Nutrition Against Disease*, Bantam, 1978.
3 Ronald Gatty, The Body Clock Diet, Gollancz, 1980.

Pre-menstrual Tension
1 *Current Medical Research and Opinion*, Vol 6, supp. 5, 1979.

Varicose Veins and Piles
1 *Family Practice News*, 15 March 1974.
2 B.A.D. Wissmer, *Current Therapeutic Research*, August 1963.

Nature Cure
1 Boris Chaitow, *My Healing Secrets*, Health Science Press, 1980.

Food Therapy
1 S. Schachter, *Journal of Experimental Psychology*, January 1977, and *Annals of Internal Medicine*, January 1978.

Index

ACTH (corticotrophin) 232, 355
ARMS (Action for Research into Multiple Sclerosis) 361
acebutalol 327
acetohexamide 294
acupuncture 405
Adaptogens 117
addiction 222
Africa 170, 321, 382
ageing 29, 31, 170, 176–83
air pollution 251
alcohol 21, 27, 64, 189, 190
Aldomet 328
Alibert, Dr J.L. 263
Alimentation, Foundation pour le Progrès de l' 16
allergies 153, 219–29, 241, 360
    Dr Coco's pulse test 223
    to food 219–29, 348–9
    testing 222–4
    total allergy syndrome 222
    treatment 224–5
Allinson, Dr Bernard 392
Allinson, Dr T.R. 383
almonds 84
alternative medicine 15
American Medical Association 340
Ames test (Dr Bruce Ames) 267
amino acids, essential SEE EAAs
amphetamines 334
amyl nitrite 313
anaemia, pernicious 76, 124
Anshutz, Dr E.P. 107
anti-depressants 347
    tricyclic 12
anti-histamines 224, 241
anti-metabolites 260
antibiotics 10, 11, 12, 44, 252–3
appendicitis 36
appendix, inflammation of 22
Apresoline 328
apricots 71, 73, 80
Aquapura water 148
arachidonic acid 25
artery disorders 31, 32
    SEE ALSO heart and artery disease

arthritis 9, 230–8, 343
    rheumatoid 113
Arthritis and Rheumatism Council 230
Asia 321
asparagus 84
aspirin 12, 13, 225, 232, 335
asthma 113, 219, 238–47, 343
Asthma Research Council 246
atenolol 327
Athenaeus 160
atherosclerosis 31, 64
Atkinson, Dr Miles 350
Atromid-S 313
Auriquin 312
Australia 212
avocados 75

BUPA Medical Centre 264
babies, weaning 148–50
    SEE ALSO breast-feeding and pregnancy
baby foods 150
bacteria, intestinal 12, 23
bananas 75
barbiturates 12
Barton-Wright, E.C. (biochemist) 234
Bayer, Dr R. 195
beans 24, 25, 33, 42
Beatson, Sir George (surgeon) 261
beef 72
Behan, Dr 346
Bellerga 347
Best, Sir Charles 64
beta-blockers 313, 327, 347
Beta-cardone 327
Betaloc 327
bethanidine 328
Biermann, June 350
biguanides 295
Bingham, Sheila 48
biochemic tissue salts 107
bioflavonoids SEE vitamin P
Biosalt 87, 92
biotin 79
Bircher-Benner Clinic 230

Bircher-Benner, Dr 125–6
Birth Defects Foundation,
  March of Dimes 190
biscuits 21
blood fat 114, 122
blood pressure 66, 92
  high 324–33
blood sugar 25, 37, 64
  low 22, 229, 240–5, 360
Blythe, Peter 378
bottle-feeding 142
bran 21, 35, 38, 39, 72, 73, 74,
  75, 77, 79, 80, 87, 88, 90, 91,
  96, 97, 98
  analysis table 40
bread 21, 40, 44–7, 87
  wholemeal 39, 42
breast-feeding 141–5, 197–8
breathing 405
Brekhman, Professor (Institute
  of Biologically Active
  Substances, Vladivostok)
  116–7
Brighton 394
Brillat-Savarin 16
British Cardiac Society 33
British Dental Association 205
British Nutrition Foundation
  168, 193, 196, 215, 295
broccoli 71, 84
bronchitis 247–56
Brookhaven National
  Laboratory 61
Brush, Dr M.G. (St Thomas's
  Hospital, London) 376
Bryant, Dr Isaac 263, 271
Bryce-Smith, Professor Derek
  190
Budd, Martin (naturopath) 343
Buddhists 209
Bulgaria 136
Burkitt, Denis (surgeon) 35, 38,
  46, 282, 297, 301, 386
Burn, J.H. 199
Burr, Dr George (University of
  Minnesota) 201
butazolidin 232
butter 24, 26, 32, 71, 83

cabbage 71, 84, 85
cadmium 46
  poisoning 190

Cafergot 347
cake 21
calcium 31, 40, 46, 86
Cameron, Allan 48, 82, 260, 262,
  272–5
Canadian Medical Association
  59
cancer 9, 30, 31, 32, 33, 38, 50,
  55, 59, 66, 80–1, 82, 100, 112,
  172, 256–81
  environmental factors 263
  Gerson therapy 277–81
  and laetrile 275–7
  and the mind 269–70
  orthodox treatments 257–63
  and vitamin C 272–5
Cancer, Eppley Institute of
  Research in 268
Cancer, International Union
  against 30
cantaloupe 85
carbohydrates 21–23
Carli, Audrey (medical
  journalist) 332
carotenoids 31
carrots 70, 71, 84, 85
Catapres 328
cauliflower 85
cereals 35
  breakfast 21, 42
  whole 80, 91, 97, 98, 99
  wholegrain 88
Chad 132
Chaitow, Leon (naturopath) 219,
  226, 261, 276, 329–30, 355
cheese 26, 73, 87, 96, 97
cherries 71
Chest, Heart and Stroke
  Association 255, 327
Chichester, Sir Francis 162
chick peas 96
children 145–51
China 108, 116, 309
chlorophyll 31
chlorothiazide 296
Choledyl 240
cholesterol 22, 25–9, 31, 32, 38,
  39, 50, 66, 109, 115
  and age 178
  and EFAs 28
  effect on blood vessels 26
  and vitamin B 27

choline 27, 78
chromium 96, 109
cider vinegar 110
cislinoleic acid 33
citrus fruits 78
Clements, Harry (naturopath) 304–5, 351
climate and arthritis 233
clofibrate 12, 313
clonidine 328, 347
cobalt 97
coconut oil 24
cod ovaries 74
Codesol 240
coffee 65–7
    grain 67
Coleman, Dr Vernon 189
Columbia University 193
Comfort, Alex 170
compatible eating 151–5, 227
constipation 22, 36, 282–6
copper 31, 97
corn 71, 84
corticosteroids 12, 224, 240, 355
cortisone 232, 296
Cott, Dr Allan (psychiatric consultant, Institute of Child Development, New York) 337
Cox, Dr Hugh J.E. 338
cramps, leg 29
Crawford, Dr Michael (Nuffield Laboratory of Comparative Medicine) 24, 25, 50, 102, 358–9
cream 24, 26
Cromolyn 225
Cuba 208
custard 28
cystitis 286–91
cytotoxic therapy 260

DGLA (dihomogammalinolenic acid) 111
DHA (docosahexaenoic acid) 25
DHSS (Department of Health and Social Security) 143
dairy foods 52, 57
    SEE ALSO INDIVIDUAL NAMES
Dalldorf, Dr Gilbert 320
Davies, Dr Stephen 338
Davis, Adelle (nutritionist) 27, 108, 125, 189, 197–8, 201,

227, 234, 245, 295, 322, 349
Denmark 9
Dental Estimates Board 204
Department of Health and Social Security SEE DHSS
Deseril 346
Devil's claw 237
Dexamed 334
dexamphetamine 334
Dexedrine 334
DiCyab, Dr E. 194
diabetes 9, 10, 22, 36, 37, 64, 108, 112, 115, 118, 291–302, 342
Diabetic Association, British 293, 302
Dibotin 295
digitalis 312
digitoxin 312
digoxin 312
dihomogammalinolenic acid SEE DGLA
Dimelor 294
Dinshah, Jay (founder, American Vegetarian Society) 209
diphtheria 9
Disease Control, US National Center for 294
disodium cromoglycate 225
Dixarit 328, 347
doctors 13–15
Doisy, Richard 108
Dong diet 235
Dong, Dr Colin 235
Dopamet 328
Downs, Dr Robert (Southwest Center of the Healing Arts, Albuquerque) 177, 245, 275, 328–9, 336, 344
Draper, Dr Peter (Director, Unit for the Study of Health Policy, Guy's Hospital, London) 311
drugs 9, 10–13, 172, 178, 224–5, 232, 239–41, 252–3, 259–61, 285, 288, 294–6, 304, 312–13, 327–9, 334–5, 342, 346–8, 355, 376, 391, 394
    advertising 13
    cure symptoms, not illness 11
    painkillers 13
    side-effects 11, 12
    SEE ALSO INDIVIDUAL DRUGS

Drysdale, Dr I.P. (Vice-Dean, British College of Naturopathy 11, 230, 391, 394

EAAs 52, 56
EEC (European Economic Community) 119, 210
EFAs 24–25, 26, 28, 33, 85
EPA (eicosapentaenoic acid) 25
Eagle, Robert 225
Ecuador 322
eczema 25, 113, 135
Eddy, Dr Walter H. 320
Efamol 113
Effergot 347
eggs 24, 26, 52, 53, 57, 70, 71, 72, 73, 74, 75, 76, 77, 78, 79, 83, 84, 89, 96
   powdered 28
Egypt 114
eleutherococcus 117
Elliott, Dr W.A. 234
Ellis, Dr John M. 193, 235
Ellis, F.R. 322
emphysema 247–56
energy drink 308
England and Wales 9, 145, 250, 325
ephedrine 239
ergotamine 347
Ershoff, Dr Benjamin 124
Esbatal 328
Eskimos 29
essential fatty acids SEE EFAs
Europe 309, 394
Evans, Dr Barbara 171, 184
Evans, Stanley C. (Bates Association of Eyesight Training) 159
evening primrose oil 111–14
Evers, Dr Joseph 356, 357, 361
Evers diet 357
Evian water 148
exercise 27, 104, 405
   table 366
eyes 155–9
   disorders 29

FAS SEE foetal alcohol syndrome
fasting 159–63, 373, 384
fat, body 21, 23, 24
fatigue 303–9

fats 21, 22, 23–35, 38
   animal 26
   and free-range animals 24
   hydrogenated 33
   polyunsaturated 28, 30, 32
   summary 34
   triglycerides 22
   vegetable 26
   SEE ALSO fatty acids
fatty acids
   essential SEE EFAs
   monounsaturated 24
   polyunsaturated 24, 122
   saturated 24, 32
   trans- 33
Feingold, Dr Ben (chief allergist, Kaiser Permanent Medical Center, San Francisco) 49, 335–6, 338
Femergin 347
fertilizers, artificial 43–4
fibre
   dietary 21, 22, 27, 32–3, 35–42
   and disease 37–9
   in foods, percentage table 41
fish 24, 52, 71, 73, 75, 76, 78, 79, 83, 87, 88, 96, 97
   smoked 28
flour 21, 35
   extraction rates 45
   nutrient losses table 45
   white 21
   wholemeal 21
   wholewheat 42
fluoridation 206–7
foetal alcohol syndrome (FAS) 190
folic acid 12, 76
food
   canned 48
   convenience 48–51
   fast 33
   fried 26, 33, 50
   frozen 48–9
   preserved 50
   snack 33
   whole 42, 92, 101–6
food additives 46–51, 137, 146, 267–8, 335, 349
   and allergies 221
food industry, modern 15, 42–51
food processing 25, 63

food therapy 396–401
Food and Drug Administration
    (USA) 67, 190, 337
Food, Nutrition and Health,
    White House Conference on
    (1969) 189
Forbes, Dr Alec 7, 16, 300
Foresight (charity) 199
France 132
free radicals 32
free-range animals 24
fructose 118
fruits 21, 35, 38, 74, 82, 85, 92,
    98, 99
    citrus 77
    dried 42, 88

GLA SEE linolenic acid, gamma
gall bladder, inflammation of 22
gallstones 38
Gant, Dr Norman F.
    (Southwestern Medical School,
    Dallas) 197
garlic 99, 114–15
Gatty, Ronald (researcher) 372
Geneva University 115
German, Dr Donald (Clinical
    Professor of Radiology,
    University of Missouri School
    of Medicine) 269
Germany 47, 123, 313
Gerson, Dr Max 59, 277–80, 359
Gerson therapy 277–81
Gibson, Dr R.G. 237
ginseng 116–17
Gladstone, W.E. 399
Glucophage 295
glucose 118
    tolerance test 343
glyceryl trinitrite 313
glycosides 117
Gobley, Maurice 121
gold injections 232
Goodall, Dr Jane 211
Gothenburg University, Sweden
    208
gout 64, 233
grains 57
    whole 33, 72
    SEE ALSO sprouting seeds and
    grains
Grant, Doris 147

Grant, Dr Ellen (Charing Cross
    Hospital, London) 331, 347,
    350
Gray, Dr (Edinburgh City
    Hospital) 391
Greece 114, 160
green leaves 24, 25, 33
guanethidine 328
Guillebaud, Dr John 185, 186
gum disease 204

HDLs (high-density lipoproteins)
    25, 27, 122
HRT (hormone replacement
    therapy) 171–2
haemorrhoids SEE piles
hair 163–6
    disorders 25
ham 72
Hardwick, Professor H.L. 204
Hare, Dr D.C. (Royal Free
    Hospital, London) 230
Harefield Hospital 312
Harvard School of Public Health
    192
hay fever 219, 238–47, 343
Health Education Council 13
Health and Diet Food Company
    127
Health, Education and Welfare,
    US Department of 340
health, public 10
hearing disorders 29
heart and artery disease 22, 115,
    309–24
    heart disease 9, 29, 32, 36, 37,
    64, 114, 292–3
heart transplants 311–12
herbal medicine 405
Herbert, Professor Martin
    (director, Child Treatment
    Research Unit, University of
    Leicester) 338
hereditary factors 27
Herman, Dr Robert 344
hiatus hernia 38
Hindus 209
Hippocrates 391, 394
Hippocratic oath 10
Hitler, Adolf 209
Hodge, Dr Gordon K.

(University of New Mexico) 337
homoeopathy 107, 406
honey 21, 91, 92, 117–20
    table of contents 118
hormone 22, 26
    replacement therapy SEE HRT
    synthetic 44
    therapy 261–2
    treatment 347
Horrobin, David F. (Clinical
    Research Institute, Montreal)
    33, 111–14
Huggins, Charles 261
Hunger and Malnutrition, US
    Citizen Board of Inquiry into
    147
Hunzas 103–4, 179, 269, 322
hydralazine 328
hyper-active children 333–9
Hyper-active Children's Support
    Group 338–9
hyperventilation 222
hypoglycaemia SEE blood sugar,
    low
Hypovase 328
Hytten, F.E. 190

iatrogenic illness 12
immune system 25
immunization 9, 10
immunotherapy 262
Inderal 327
India 103, 108, 127, 170, 269,
    309, 322
indocid (indomethacin) 232
inositol 27, 78
insulin 10, 22, 293–4
Intal 225, 240, 241
Inter-Medics Ltd 174
intestinal disorders 47, 115
iodine 87
Iran 40
iron 31, 46, 88
Ismelin 328
isoprenaline 239
Israel 297

Jackson, Dr James Caleb 394
Jamaica 233
Japan 9, 59, 120, 132, 166
Jarvis, Dr D.C. 110
Jones, Hardin B. (Professor of

Medical Physics and
    Physiology, University of
    California) 259, 261
Judaism, orthodox 375
juices, fruit and vegetable 21,
    129–31
    table of properties and effects
    130

kale 71
Kanimura, Dr M. 245
Kaufman, Dr William 234
Keen, Professor Harry (Guy's
    Hospital, London) 293
kelp 87, 120–1
Kennedy, Ian 14, 313
kidneys, inflammation of 22
Klenner, Dr Fred R. (Fellow,
    American Association for the
    Advancement of Science) 194,
    333, 355, 359
Klosterneuburg Hospital 128
Knight, Dr Granville F. 245
Knowles breath training method
    246, 255
Krebs, Dr Ernst 275

LDLs (low-density lipoproteins)
    27
La Leche League of Great
    Britain 145
labetolol 327
lactation 188–99
    SEE ALSO breast-feeding
Langford, Dr Herbert
    (University of Mississippi) 59
Latto, Conrad 38
Latto, Dr Gordon (President,
    Vegetarian Society) 396
lauric acid 32
laxatives 285
lead 44
    poisoning 190
lecithin 28, 30, 31, 78, 121–3
    and cholesterol 27
Ledermann, Dr E.K. 16, 67, 356
legumes 21, 89
    SEE ALSO INDIVIDUAL NAMES
lentils 42, 91, 96
lettuce 71
Levine, Dr R. 299
Librium 189

Lief, Stanley (founder, British College of Naturopathy and Osteopathy) 394
lima beans 77, 96
Lingraine 347
Linn, Dr Richard T. (University of New Mexico) 337
linoleic acid 24, 25
linolenic acid 25, 30
gamma (GLA) 111
lipoproteins
high-density SEE HDLs
low-density SEE LDLs
liver 71, 80, 82, 91, 123–4
Lockie, Dr Andrew 343
Lomusol 240
London Hospital Medical College 331
Lopresor 327
Los Viejos 179, 322
Lubowe, Dr Irwin I. (dermatologist) 165, 201
lumbago 231
Lynch, Dr G. Roche (Home Office pathologist) 50

MacDougall diet 357
MacFadden, Bernard 394
Mackarness, Dr Richard 42, 47, 67, 221, 364
Mackie, Alastair (Director-General, Health Education Council) 311
macrobiotics 166–8
magnesium, 28, 31, 90
Mahler, Dr Halfdan (Director-General, World Health Organization) 15
Malvern water 148
manganese 97
Mann, Dr George V. 299
Manner, Dr Harold (University of Chicago) 275
Maoris 127
margarine 33, 83
Marie Curie Foundation 347
Masai 315
McCance and Widdowson 47
McCarrison, Robert 102, 103, 179, 269
McMichael, Sir John 32
measles 9, 10

meat 9, 21, 24, 26, 52, 73, 75, 76, 77, 78, 79, 84, 85, 88, 96, 97, 98
organ 70, 72, 74
smoked 28
Medical Research Council 47, 316
Medicines Act (1971) 11
Medihaler Iso 239
Medihaler-Ergotamine 347
megavitamins 100
menopause 168–74
mental illness 100
mercury 44
metaprolol 327
metformin 295
methyldopa 328
methylphenidate 334
methysergide 346
Mexico 132, 318
Miami University School of Medicine 201
migraine 67, 342, 345–53
and food 348–9
and vitamin therapy 349
Migril 347
milk 21, 24, 26, 70, 71, 73, 74, 76, 79, 82, 83, 87, 90, 92, 97, 99
UHT (ultra heat-treated) 102
breast 25, 99
differences between human and cow's 141
goat's 102
raw 102
skimmed 72
soya 102
whole powdered 28
minerals 21, 22, 30, 43, 48–9, 68–70, 86–99
trace 96–9
table of content in foods 94–5
SEE ALSO INDIVIDUAL NAMES
Ministry of Health 145
Minnesota, University of 55
Mogadon 189
molasses 63, 72, 75, 77, 78, 79, 87, 89, 90, 124–5
molybdenum 98
Moolenburgh, Dr H. (physician) 276
Morgan, Jane E. (nutritionist) 190

rtality, perinatal 188
oule, Terry (naturopath) 242
Mount, Dr James Lambert
(nutritionist) 145, 198, 206,
297, 322
Moyle, Alan (naturopath) 180,
284
muesli 125–7, 230
Muller, Dr T. (Hospices Civils,
Strasbourg) 195
multiple sclerosis 113, 353–63
Multiple Sclerosis Society 361
Multiple Sclerosis, Action for
Research into SEE ARMS
Munro, Dr Daniel 227
Murdoch, Dr (Edinburgh City
Hospital) 391
mushrooms 96
myristic acid 32

NHS SEE National Health
Service
nails 175
Nalcrom 225
National Childbirth Trust 144
National Health Service 13
National Institute of Research
and Dairying, Reading 102
naturopathy 33, 108, 160, 351,
391–6, 406
Net Protein Utilization SEE
protein, NPU
Netherlands 9, 299
New Zealand 127
New Zealand green lipped mussel
extract 237
Newberry, Dr P.D. 154
niacin SEE vitamin B3
Nicholls, Dr A.B. (University of
Montreal) 180
nickel 99
Nieper, Dr Hans 275
night cramps 12
nitrates 50
nitrites 50
nitroglycerin 313
Nixon, Dr Peter (Charing Cross
Hospital, London) 222
Norbrium 189
Norway 9, 313
Nuelin 240
nutrients, Recommended Daily
Allowances 59
nutrition 16–19, 226–9, 233–7,
243–6, 253–5, 264–9, 288–90,
296–302, 305–8, 313–21,
330–2, 343–4, 351–2, 356–61,
369–73, 377, 380–1, 384–7
Nutrition Society 214
Nutrition and Human Needs, US
Senate Select Committee on
(1977) 23
nuts 24, 25, 35, 42, 52, 72, 73,
75, 77, 79, 87, 89, 90, 91, 96,
97, 98, 99

O'Shea, Dr James 337
obesity 9, 21, 36, 37, 363–74
Odens, Dr Max 254
Ohsawa, George 166
oil, sesame 31
oils 24, 29–32
commercial 'polyunsaturated'
vegetable 31
fish 25, 71
fish liver 70, 83
fruit and vegetable 25
mineral 30
refined 29–31
salted refined 33
unrefined 30–1, 84, 98, 99
SEE ALSO INDIVIDUAL NAMES
Opren 232
Orbach, Susie 367
organic farming 43–4, 102
orotic acid SEE vitamin B13
orthomolecular therapy 100
Osler, Sir William 13
Osteopaths, General Council and
Register of 231
osteopathy 406
Oster, Dr (cardiologist) 323
Oxford University–Vegetarian
Society research project 213
oxprenolol 327

PABA (para-aminobenzoic acid)
77
PGs SEE prostaglandins
PMT SEE pre-menstrual tension
pacifarins 133
pain-killers 355
Painter, Neil (surgeon, Manor
House Hospital, London) 283

palm oil 24
palmitic acid 32
pancake mixes 28
pangamic acid SEE vitamin B15
pantothenic acid SEE vitamin B5
papaya 85
Papworth Hospital 312
para-aminobenzoic acid SEE
  PABA
paracetamol 13
Paris, University of 117
Parish, Peter 10, 240, 241, 312
parsley 84
Passwater, Dr Richard 26, 82,
  267, 318
pasta, wholegrain 42
Pasteur, Louis 392
pastry 21, 26
Pauling, Linus 82, 100, 147, 260,
  262, 272–5
Pawan, Dr Gaston 17, 179
peaches 71, 74, 75, 78
peas 42, 73, 79, 85
  split 72
pectin 38
penicillin 12
Pennsylvania, Medical College
  of 120
peppers, green 85
pesticides 44, 102
Petkov, Professor (Institute of
  Advanced Medical Training,
  Sofia) 116
Pfeiffer, Dr Carl 254
phenacetin 13
phenformin 295
phenylbutazone 232
phospholipids 31
phosphorus 91
phytate 39–42
phytic acid 46
Pickard, Dr Barbara 198
piles 22, 37, 385–7
Pill, the (contraceptive) 28,
  183–8, 189, 287, 296, 311,
  350, 376
  side-effects 184–6
pindolol 327
pizotifen 347
polio 10
pollen 118, 127–8
Pollitabs 127

Pope, Alexander 209
Porter, Dr Seymour 337
Poskanzer, Dr David C.
  (Departments of Preventive
  Medicine and Neurology,
  Harvard Medical School) 355
potassium 91, 110
  table of content in foods 60
potatoes 21, 73, 77, 85
Prazosin 328
pre-menstrual tension (PMT)
  374–8
prednisolone 240
Prednosol 240
Predsol 240
pregnancy 188–99
preserves 21
Price, Weston A. 191
Priessnitz, Vincent 394
Pritikin, Nathan (Longevity
  Center, Los Angeles) 322–3
propolis 128
propranolol 327, 347
prostaglandins (PGs) 25, 111–14
protein 24, 28, 51–7
  NPU 53
  needs 54–5
  sources 52–3
  table of content in foods 53
proteins, complementary 56–7
prunes 75
pulses 21, 52, 72, 75
  SEE ALSO INDIVIDUAL NAMES
pyridoxine SEE vitamin B6

Quick, Clifford 235, 290
Quincardine 312
quinidine 312
quinine 12

radiotherapy 258
Rahe, Dr Richard 380
raisins 75
Randolph, Dr Ted 364
Rastinon 294
Reid, Dr 346
Reinhold, Dr John (Pennsylvania
  Nutrition Research Project) 39
relaxation 406
reserpine 12, 328
rheumatism 9, 230–8
riboflavin SEE vitamin B2

ce, brown 21, 42
Ritalin 334
Rowe, Dr 320
Royal College of Physicians 33, 36–9, 300
royal jelly 74, 131
Rubin, Dr Philip 259
Ruthmol 92
Rynacrom 225, 240

Safety of Medicines, Committee on 12
Sakai, Dr 132
salbutamol 239–40
salt 57–61
    deficiency 58
    and potassium 59–61
    refined 61
Samburus 29
Sanders, Dr Tom (Queen Elizabeth College, London) 25, 215, 322
Sanomigran 347
sardines 87
sausages, smoked 28
Saventrine 239
scarlet fever 9
schizophrenia 343
Schizophrenia Association 113
schoolchildren 145, 150
Schuessler, Dr W.H. 107
Scotland 145
seaweed 87
    dried 121
Sebrell, Dr W.H. 193
Sectral 327
sedatives 347
seeds 24, 25, 33, 52, 57, 78, 80, 84, 87, 89, 90, 91, 96, 97
    SEE ALSO INDIVIDUAL NAMES AND sprouting seeds and grains
selenium 31, 98, 109
Selye, Dr Hans 173, 235, 379, 380
Serpasil 328
sesame seeds 74
Seventh Day Adventists 212, 215, 322
Shaw, George Bernard 163, 209
Sheiham, Dr (London Hospital Medical College Dental School) 207
Shute, Dr Evan (Director, Shute Foundation for Medical Research) 298, 299
Shute, Dr Wilfred E. 195, 299, 318
silicon 99
Simonton, Carl (radiation oncologist) 269–70
skin 200–2
    disorders 25, 67, 219
sleep, drug-induced 13
Smithells, Professor R.W. (Leeds University) 192
smoking 27, 185, 189
Sneddon, J. Russell (naturopath) 386
sodium 92
    table of content in foods 60
sodium cromoglycate 240, 241
soil 42–3, 102
Soil Association 106
Somalis 29
Sotacor 327
sotalol 327
soya 52
soybeans 72, 74, 75, 77, 78, 85, 87, 90, 91, 96
spina bifida 185
spinach 71, 84, 85
spirulina 52, 76, 132–3
sprouting seeds and grains 52, 72, 73, 74, 75, 79, 84, 87, 89, 96, 133–5
St Thomas's Hospital, London 113, 375–7
Stanway, Dr Andrew 33
starch 21, 24, 36
stomach disorders 67, 219
stress 117, 378–81
sucrose 22
sugar 21, 24, 36, 61–5
    addiction 65
    white 21, 22
    SEE ALSO blood sugar, low
Sugiara, Dr Kanematsu (Sloan-Kettering Institute) 276
sulpha drugs 12
sulphonylureas 294–5
sunflower seeds 38, 72, 73, 74, 75, 83
surgery 259, 384

Sussman, Vic 212
Sustac 313
Sweden 9, 129, 170, 299
Switzerland 9
Symonds, Sr Charles (National
    Hospital for Nervous
    Diseases) 356

Tannenbaum, Dr Albert 268
Tanzania 315
tea 65–7
    herbal 67
teeth 38, 62–3, 118, 202–9
    Anglo-Saxon 204
Ternormin 327
theophylline 240
thiamine SEE vitamin B1
Third World 9, 29, 36, 283
    SEE ALSO INDIVIDUAL NAMES
thrombosis 38
tin 99
Tipton, Dr Isabel H. 319
tolbutamide 294, 295
tomatoes 73, 85
Toohey, Barbara 350
Towell, Dr Hugh 60
Trandate 327
tranquillizers 13, 44, 355
Trasicor 327
trinitrin 313
Trowell, Dr Hugh 235
Tufts University School of
    Medicine 315
turnips 77

UK 9, 33, 115, 123, 146, 172,
    176, 188, 190, 210, 238, 247,
    256, 282, 292, 309, 313, 333,
    338, 345, 353
    SEE ALSO England and Wales
USA 9, 59, 147, 115, 128, 172,
    190, 208, 301, 309, 318, 321,
    333, 382, 394
USSR 115, 116, 254, 307
Ultracortenol 240

Vaddadi, Dr Kenneth
    (psychiatrist) 113
Valium 189
vanadium 99
varicose veins 22, 382–7
vasodilators 32

Vegan Society 216
vegan diet 54, 209–16
vegetables 21, 35, 38, 73, 74, 77,
    78, 79, 82, 92, 97, 98, 99
    green 70, 87, 89, 90, 96, 97
    raw 104
vegetarian diet 56, 209–16
Vegetarian Society 216
vegetarians 38
venereal disease 12
Ventolin 239
Vessey, Professor Martin 311
Visek, Dr W.J. (Cornell
    University) 55
Visken 327
vitamins 21, 22, 48–9, 68–85
    A 23, 70
    B 12, 23
    B1 (thiamine) 71
    B2 (riboflavin) 72
    B3 (niacin) 73
    B5 (pantothenic acid) 74
    B6 (pyridoxine) 27, 28, 74
    B12 75
    B13 (orotic acid) 79
    B15 (pangamic acid) 80
    B17 80
        SEE ALSO laetrile
    C (ascorbic acid) 12, 31, 81
    D 23, 26, 82
    E 23, 30, 31, 83
    F SEE EFAs
    H SEE biotin
    K 12, 23, 85
    P (bioflavonoids) 85
    fat-soluble 26
    table of content in foods 94–5
Vitex Agnus Castus 173, 377–8
Vogel, Dr (dentist) 208

WHO (World Health
    Organization) 313, 378
Waerland, Dr Are 358
Wales SEE England and Wales
Walnuts 84
Washburn, S.L. (physical
    anthropologist) 211
water 148
watercress 71
watermelon 71
weight, body 27
    table 368

West, the 9, 35–6, 47, 104, 145, 170, 179, 191, 210, 283, 292, 293, 297, 309, 382
    diseases of 21
West, Dr Dorothy 228
wheat germ 52, 72, 73, 74, 75, 77, 78, 79, 80, 84, 87, 88, 90, 91, 96, 97, 98, 99, 135–6
whey 79
wholefood 216
wholegrains 52, 73, 74, 75, 77, 78, 79, 84, 90, 96
whooping cough 9, 10
Wilkinson, Dr Marcia (Princess Margaret Migraine Clinic, London) 347
Williams, Roger J. (biochemist) 29, 31, 102, 146, 148, 182, 191, 194, 200, 228, 234, 314, 316, 319, 322, 363
Wingate, Peter 386

Woollam, Dr David (Emmanuel College, Cambridge) 190
World Health Organization SEE WHO

yeast, brewer's 52, 72, 73, 74, 75, 77, 78, 79, 80, 89, 90, 91, 92, 96, 97, 108–10
Yemenites 297
Yin-Yang 166
yoga 405
yogurt 73, 87, 136–8
    pasteurized 137
Yudkin, John 15, 58, 64, 158, 233, 297, 316, 370

zinc 12, 39, 46, 93
Zorn, Professor (Physical and Chemical Institute, University of Jena) 237